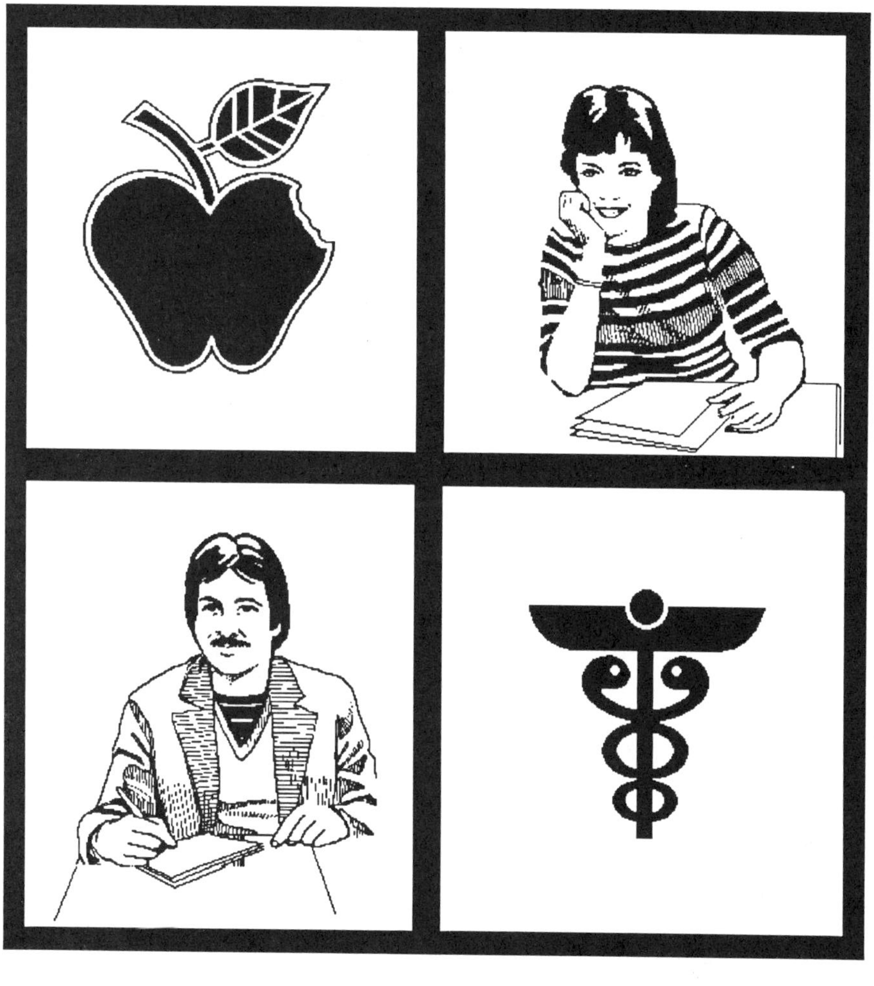

ACKNOWLEDGEMENTS

With this final step in a long and rewarding journey the author takes the opportunity to acknowledge the many who have extended assistance along the way. First I wish to give thanks to my mentor, Dr. Ray Watters, who served for many years as the chairman of the Department of Health Sciences at Brigham Young University. The course for which this book was originally written, School Health For Secondary Teachers, was one of his primary interests. Little did I know when I enrolled in his class that one day I would write a text for that course. He counseled me well when I was his student and remained an inspiration long after he hired me as a new faculty member and assigned me to teach that course. Although now retired, Ray and his wife Madge remain as cherished friends.

I wish also to thank McKay Rollins, my current department chairman, and all my colleagues in the Department of Health Scienceds at Brigham Young University. They are great people to work with and their examples have provided encouragement at each step in this journey. I particularly appreciate the help extended by Robert Burgener, Steve Heiner, and Richard Hurley who also teach the School Health for Secondary Teachers. A parallel course for elementary teachers is taught by Keith Karren, Ronald Rhodes, McKay Rollins, and Richard Salazar. All students who certify as school teachers at Brigham Young University must take a health course from one of these superb teachers. Paul Coon, Brent Hafen, and Altone Thygerson provide instruction and leadership for the students with Health Majors in Secondary Education.

The major contributors to this book are the students in my School Health classes over the past 20 years. Collectively they have seen this product grow from random in-class handouts to a commercially published text. This text was originally published by BYU Continuing Education under the title *School Health for Secondary Teachers.* It was published as the text for students enrolled in the independent study course, but was also made available for on-campus students. The efforts of Ralph A. Rowley, Ronald F. Malan, and Ralph V. Larson and their textbook production staff at BYU Independent Study must be recognized. Student needs have always been the motivation behind this writing project, whether in the form of handouts, packet, or textbook. Many of the ideas originated as handouts prepared by individual students and student committees. One must acknowledge the role of student questions and class discussions in the development of this project.

Finally and most importantly, I thank my wife, Norene, and my loving family. Without Norene's patience, encouragement, ideas, and typing skills; this book would have never been completed. She stood by patiently while I spent time writing that should have been spent on family activities and responsibilities. She typed, edited, and re-typed many of the handouts that preceded this text long before computers and word processors were used for manuscript production. For this and for her constant love I give humble thanks.

HEALTH ISSUES

FOR

SECONDARY TEACHERS

Ray A. Petersen

Brigham Young University

KENDALL/HUNT PUBLISHING COMPANY

2460 Kerper Boulevard P.O. Box 539 Dubuque, Iowa 52004-0539

Health Issues for Secondary Teachers

This text was originally published in 1990 with the title *School Health For Secondary Teachers* by the Department of Independent Study, Division of Continuing Education, Brigham Young University, Provo, Utah.

This edition has been printed directly from camera-ready copy.

ISBN 0-8403-6867-4

Printed in the United States of America.
10 9 8 7 6 5 4 3 2

TABLE OF CONTENTS

PREFACE

PURPOSE

The primary purpose of this book is to help prepare prospective secondary teachers to assume health-related responsibilities of the teaching profession. This book also serves as a personal health text for teachers. It is a **School Health** text and a **Personal Health** text.

OBJECTIVES

One of the principle objectives of modern education is to help maintain and promote the health of the pupils and other members of lthe school community. The school's have three major health-related responsibilities. The first is to protect the students and staff from any harm that may occur while they are at school or involved in school activities. The school must be safe. The second stems from the fact that health contributes to effective learning and poor health hinders learning. The students must be healthy. The third is to promote the health knowledge, attitudes, and practices of students today so they will become healthy contributing adults tomorrow. The students must be prepared for life.

DUTY

As a teacher, you will be partially responsible for the health and welfare of your students while they are in your classroom or under your supervision. You will also help prepare them for the future by helping to promote good health today. To do this you must be an example of a healthy lifestyle. Furthermore, you will be more effective as a teacher if you healthy. You will be more alert and better able to maintain the interest of your. You will also be more aware of the students interests and needs. Teaching is a stressful profession, but that stress minimized by good personal health practices.

DEDICATION

With your decision to become a school teacher you have joined a dedicated profession. Do not become a teacher unless you are motivated by principles that are altruistic in nature. Even though society may not fully recognize your worth, there are personal rewards for those who commit their life to teaching the youth. Congratulate on your decision, hopefully this book will contribute to your professional career and your personal life.

CERTIFICATION

This text is designed for use in those states which have a health education requirement for teacher certification on the secondary level. In some states that requirement is met any personal health class, but in other states that course must include information in specific content areas. This text was written originally as the textbook for the course, *School Health For Secondary Teachers*, which is taught on campus and through independent Study at Brigham Young University. That course meets the health education requirement for secondary teacher certification in those states which have the most definitive requirements such as Utah and California. It includes information pertaining to adolescent health, teacher health, and the school health program. It also deals thoroughly with such issues as teenage suicide, substance abuse, sex education, child abuse, learning disorders, nutrition, and school safety.

Some states have a teacher certification requirement in health education for elementary school teachers, but unfortunately no such requirement for secondary teachers. Where no requirement exists, this book would be a valuable addition to the school library or the teachers personal library.

ATTITUDES

Because this book provides a comprehensive coverage of many common health topics, the reader may be familiar with much of the material. However, a review may be beneficial. Other topics will be new and unique. Since many of the details covered are too specific to commit to memory, parts of this book may best serve as a resource for future reference. This book deals not only with facts, but also with attitudes. If you have the personality to become a teacher you will have already incorporated many of the attitudes discussed in this book into your life and this book may provide effective reinforcement.

ISSUES

The title of this book deserves mention. The words *health* and *secondary teachers* were obvious choices, but *issues* is the key word. Nouns such as concerns, considerations, problems, questions, topic, and duties were all considered, but issue is also a verb which originally meant to go forth, to emanate, to emerge, or to dispense. It stresses the beginning of

UNIT 1

THE SCHOOL HEALTH PROGRAM

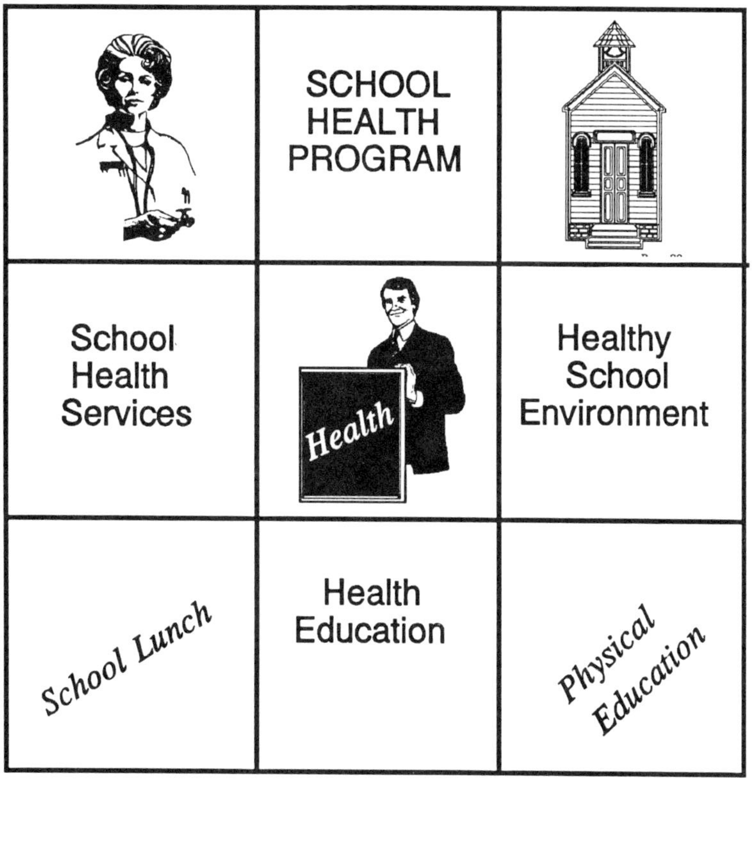

"The prepared course of action taken by the school in the interest of the health of the child and school personnel."

C. L. Anderson

SCHOOL HEALTH PROGRAM

The definition of health used by C.L. Anderson suggests that the school health program may differ from school to school. Each state passes its own laws pertaining to the school health programs. Each school district establishes its own school health policies. Yet, today in this country most school health programs have common components.

The school is recognized as an agency for promoting health. Certain facets of a school's health program are based on legal requirements and others are inherent in the school's resolve to do its job well. Many people in the school setting contribute to school health, but none more than the classroom teacher.

The **Joint Committee on Health Problems in Education of the National Education Association** and the **American Medical Association** has published a booklet, *Suggested School Health Policies,* which provides a basic framework for a school health program. Its suggestions can be adapted to meet the needs of a particular school. The lessons in this unit deal with this basic plan.

The school health program in your school is, in a practical sense, whatever your school does to meet its health related responsibilities. Usually there are three phases of a school health program: school health services, school health education, and a healthy school environment. Your effectiveness as a teacher will be partially determined by how well you contribute to school health.

Your concept of health can influence your role as a teacher.

This unit should help you understand the various aspects of school health today. You will look at the various organizations that have an interest in the health programs within the schools. But first, you should try to understand how your concept of health can influence your role as a teacher.

To put this into perspective, you will look briefly at the history of the school health movement and the laws relating to school health. You will look at the health needs and interests of adolescents. And finally, you will see how you can respond to the potential health problems frequently encountered by students and teachers in the secondary schools.

This unit serves as an introduction to the other three units in the course. The school health program provides a framework for preventing and dealing with the health problems that will be explored later in more detail.

At the conclusion of this unit the student should be able to meet the objectives on the following page. They may be used as a study guide for this unit.

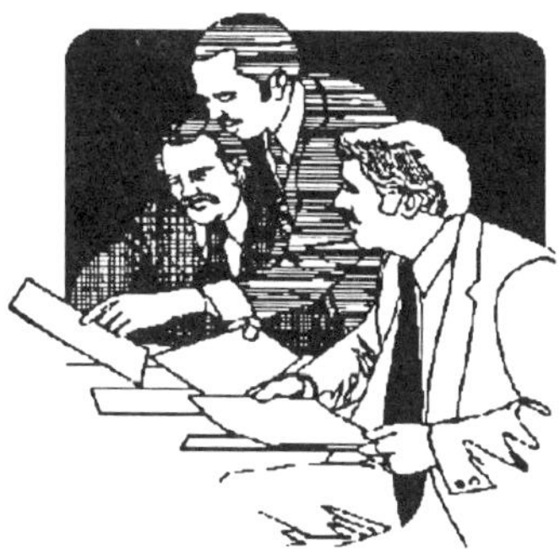

OBJECTIVES

1. A CONCEPT OF HEALTH

DISCUSS THE MODERN CONCEPT OF HEALTH AS IT APPLIES TO THE SCHOOLS.

- Contrast the modern concept of health with earlier definitions.
- State the World Health Organization's definition of health.
- List and describe the significant points of health.
- List the five dimensions of health and give examples of reciprocal relationships.
- Describe how the subjects you will teach can be used to foster health knowledge, attitudes, and practices among your students.

2. THE SCHOOL HEALTH MOVEMENT

DISCUSS HOW HISTORICAL EVENTS AND MOVEMENTS HAVE CONTRIBUTED TO THE PRESENT SCHOOL AND COMMUNITY HEALTH PROGRAMS.

- Give examples of how past health beliefs have influenced health practices today.
- Compare the phases in public health and the periods in the school health.
- Summarize the health related goals stated in the prominent objectives of education.

3. THE LAW AND SCHOOL HEALTH

EXPLAIN THE ROLE OF LAWS AND GOVERNMENT AS IT RELATES TO YOUR RESPONSIBILITIES IN THE SCHOOL HEALTH PROGRAM.

- Outline the role of government in relationship to the school health program.
- Describe the types of laws affecting the school health program.

4. ENVIRONMENT

OUTLINE THE ROLE OF A CLASSROOM TEACHER IN PROMOTING A HEALTHY SCHOOL ENVIRONMENT.

- Explain the teacher's role in promoting a healthy physical environment.
- Explain theteachers's role in promoting a healthy psychological environment.

- Give examples of student practices not conducive to a healthy school environment.

5. SERVICES

SHOW HOW AN EFFECTIVE SCHOOL HEALTH SERVICE CAN HELP TEACHERS ACHIEVE THE GOALS OF EDUCATION.

- List reasons why schools are involved in health services.
- Compare the role of the school health service to the role of the parents.
- Describe the areas of the school health service in which a teacher is most likely to be involved.

6. EDUCATION

DISCUSS THE CHARACTERISTICS OF A CREDITABLE SCHOOL HEALTH EDUCATION PROGRAM.

- Explain why comprehensive health education is a vital part of the curriculum.
- Compare the various curriculum approaches for providing health education.
- List the basic characteristics of effective health education.
- Identify opportunities within your teaching area to provide health instruction.

7. POLICIES

DESCRIBE THE ORGANIZATION OF THE SCHOOL HEALTH PROGRAM AS IT RELATES TO POLICIES AND PERSONNEL.

- Define school health policies and indicate areas where health policies are needed.
- Describe the role relationships of school health within the local school organization.

8. RECOGNIZING HEALTH PROBLEMS

IDENTIFY THE MOST FREQUENT AND SIGNIFICANT HEALTH PROBLEMS AMONG SECONDARY STUDENTS.

- Describe the health status of teenagers as compared to the general populace.
- Explain how a school health program can alleviate common health problems.

True Education

Character is the aim of true education, and science, history, and literature are but means to accomplish this desired end. . . . True education seeks to make men and women not only good mathematicians, proficient linguists, profound scientists, and brilliant literary lights, but also honest men with virtue, temperance, and brotherly love. It seeks to make men and women who prize truth, justice, wisdom, benevolence, and self-control as the choicest acquisitions of a successful life.

Gaining knowledge is one thing, and applying it is another. Wisdom is the right application of knowledge. . . . A man may possess a profound knowledge . . . . pertaining to general and natural sciences, but if he has not, with his knowledge, that nobility of soul which promotes him to deal justly with his fellow men, to practice virtue and honesty in personal life, he is not a truly educated man.

What, then, is true education? It is the awakening of a love for truth, a just sense of duty, opening the eyes of the soul to the great purposes and end of life. It is not teaching the individual to love the good for personal sake; it is to teach him to love the good for the sake of the good itself; to be virtuous in action because he is so in heart; to love and serve God supremely, not from fear, but from delight in His perfect character.

Upon the teacher rests much of the responsibility of lifting society to this higher level. . . . Teachers, yours is the responsibility to teach not only by precept, but by example! Ralph Waldo Emerson, reputedly the wisest American, said, "Character is higher than intellect. A great soul will be fit to live as well as to think." *Instructor,* August 1961

--David O. McKay

Chapter 1

A CONCEPT OF HEALTH

WHAT DO YOU MEAN BY HEALTH?

The definition of health has undergone a significant change over the past century. Let's look back a few years to see the change that has taken place in the concept of health. Dr. C.E. Turner, a prominent author of health education textbooks, provides us with two contrasting definitions of health. Both reflect the prevailing definitions of the time.

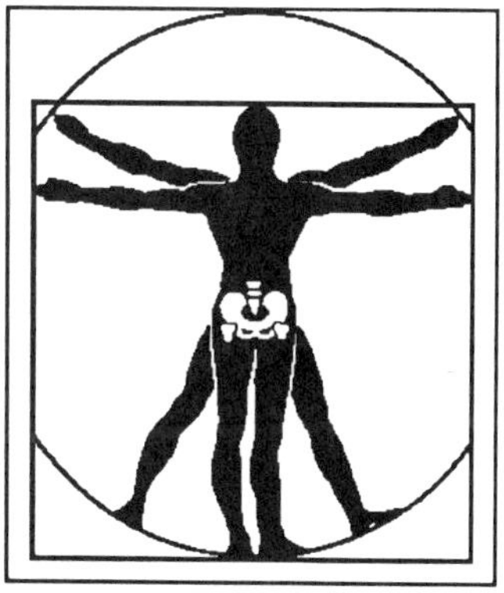

The first was a common definition of health in 1924:

> ***Health is the normal functioning of all parts of the body, complete physical fitness.***

The second was a the way authorities defined health in 1947:

> ***Health is that complete fitness of the body, soundness of mind, and wholesomeness of emotions, which makes possible the highest quality of effective living and of service.***

The first presents a singular dimension of health--the physical. By 1947, a three-dimensional model of health was being accepted. The definition of health adopted by the World Health Organization in 1947 is still widely used.

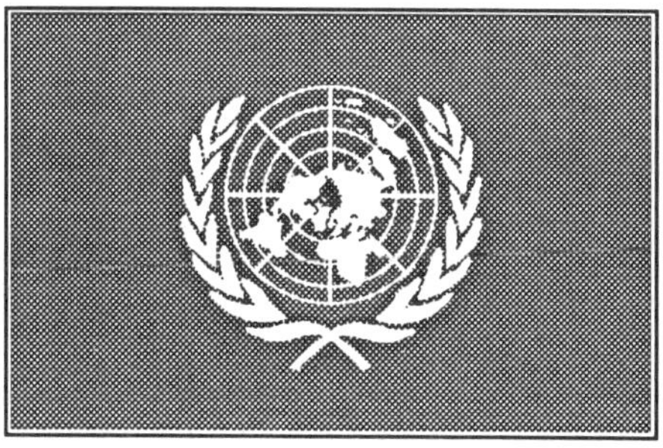

> ***Health is a state of complete physical, mental, and social well-being, and not merely the absence of disease or infirmity.***

The School Health Study, conducted in the mid-1960s, was one of the most comprehensive curriculum studies ever conducted in this country. It used the following definition of health:

> ***Health is a quality of life involving dynamic interaction and interdependence among the individual's physical well-being, his mental and emotional reactions, and the social complex in which he exists.***

The definitions of health used by several contemporary authors suggest that health can be defined most simply as "*the quality of life.*"

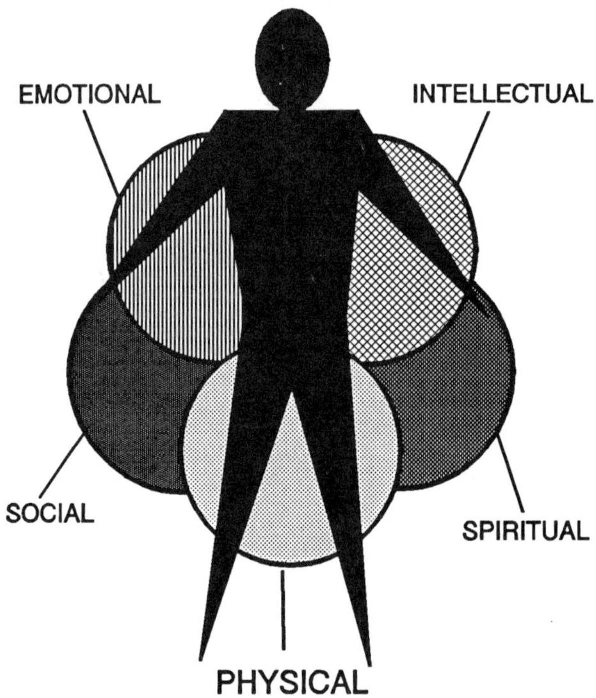

Since the mid-1960s, most definitions of health include the multidimensional view of health. Since the early 1900s the definition of health has changed from a single dimension, to a three-dimension, to a five-dimension model. The modern definition of health recognizes the spiritual dimension and differentiates between the emotional and intellectual components of mental health.

THE MULTIDIMENSIONAL VIEW OF HEALTH

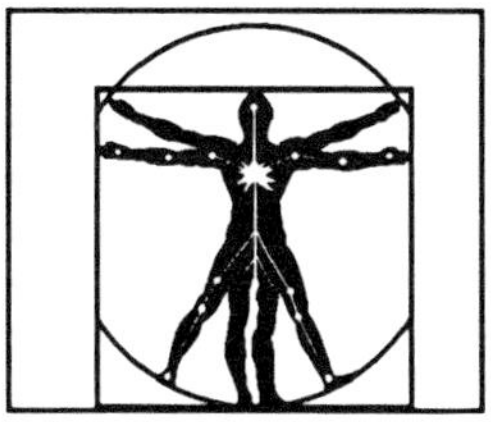

Physical. We know more about the physical dimension than the other four dimensions. The tangible body is easiest to study, and we have been studying it longest. The physical deals with cells, tissues, organs, and systems and their functions.

Social. Man is a social creature and the quality of our life is very much dependent upon the quality of our interpersonal relationships. The things we do and the way we feel physically is influenced a great deal by social influences. Just as strong muscles are important to physical health, social skills such as effective communication skills are important to social health.

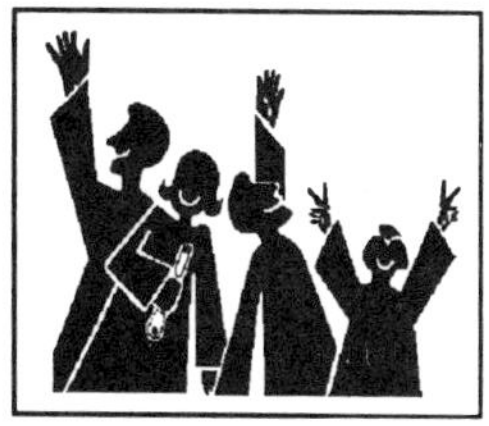

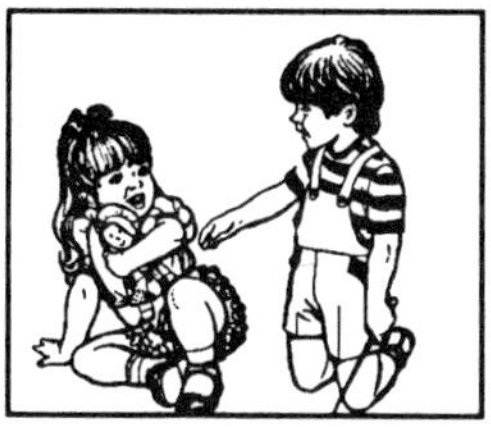

Emotional. The term "mental health" may include both the emotional and intellectual dimensions, yet each are significantly different. Emotions are intense feelings accompanied by physical reactions. Much of our behavior is motivated by our emotions. Poor emotional health may interfere with an individual's ability to concentrate and solve intellectual pursuits.

Intellectual. Our ability to reason and to recall pertinent information is associated with our intellectual health. It may be measured by I.Q. tests and demonstrated by GPAs and ACT scores. It is objective and analytical. Good intellectual health enables an individual to solve problems that might otherwise cause emotional or social disturbances.

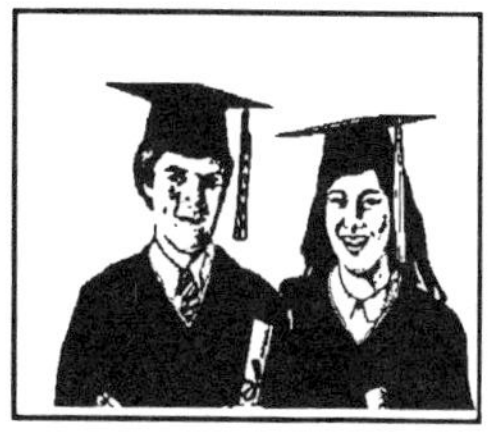

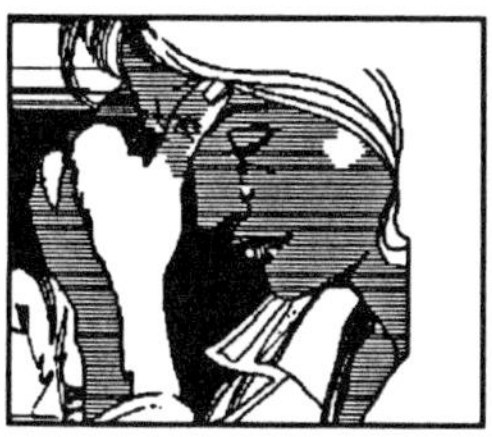

Spiritual. The spiritual or moral dimension distinguishes between right and wrong. It provides the basis for determining values and ethical conduct.

Mankind will change...
The spiritual gives direction to change.
Without it change will be chaotic.
With it change will be progressive.

SPIRITUAL HEALTH

A religious background may prepare some people to understand the spiritual dimension. They may believe in the separate entity of the spirit, that birth represents the uniting of the body and the spirit to form the soul, that death is the temporary separation of the body and the spirit, and those who are spiritually in tune may receive inspired communication from the divine spirit.

People without this religious background, however, are not without a spiritual dimension. Even atheists have a spiritual or moral dimension. It is based on the concept that man and his culture is constantly changing, and it is the spiritual dimension that gives purpose and direction to this evolution. Without the spiritual dimension these changes may be chaotic and regressive, but with the spiritual dimension these changes may be progressive and concerned with the well-being of mankind.

People constantly face the task of making difficult but important decisions about complex health issues. This task is much easier when all decisions about health are tied to a central purpose or philosophy. When each question about health behavior is viewed independently, the decisions are more difficult and the results are less consistent. The spiritual dimension integrates the various components of life into a complete and meaningful whole.

An event that affects one dimension may also affect other dimensions. Growth does not always occur evenly; one dimension may experience a growth spurt and another may rest on a plateau or regress. People who have not experienced growth in a certain dimension may deny the importance of that dimension, but a person striving to reach his or her potential will develop in all five dimensions.

DIMENSIONS OF HEALTH

The acceptance of a modern definition of health tends to increase the health-related responsibilities of secondary school teachers. Today, health is viewed as the quality of life involving the reciprocal relationships among the physical, intellectual, emotional, social, and moral dimensions of man. A teacher is responsible for the growth and development of the whole student. An effective teacher is familiar with the needs and characteristics of each of the dimensions of health. Just as the physical dimension requires food and exercise, the other dimensions also require nutrition and challenge in order to grow, develop, and remain healthy. We are much more familiar with the physical muscles and the types of nutrients and activities necessary to develop them than we are with the other four dimensions. But what are the muscles in the other dimensions? What are the foods and exercises in the other dimensions?

> Just as the physical body requires food and exercise to grow, the other dimensions also demand appropriate nourishment and exertion to mature.

We know most about the physical dimension. That is why, a few years ago, health was thought of as having to do with the physical body. Physical health is essential to the other dimensions. Physical health is also affected by other dimensions. The intellectual dimension involves the use of the nervous system in sensual perception, memory, reasoning, logic, and other cognitive skills.

Emotions are intense feelings accompanied by body reactions; the more intense the emotion, the greater the body reaction. The endocrine system, the nervous system, and the vital functions of the body are affected. The student's emotional state can have a profound effect upon his or her intellectual ability, and a person's ability to perceive and reason has an effect upon his or her feelings.

The intellectual and emotional dimensions are often referred to, either separately or collectively, as mental health.

How one feels physically and emotionally has a direct relationship to one's social health--how he or she relates to other people.

Moral health also relates to social health. Moral health deals with standards of "right and wrong" and governs relationships with others. It gives meaning and purpose; it gives direction to man's existence. Darwin said, "Man has evolved." That was significant, but he also said, "Man is evolving." That was even more significant. Our culture is changing and the moral dimension gives direction to that change. It governs one's relationship to himself, his relationships with others, and his relationship to Deity.

A DESCRIPTION OF HEALTH

As we analyze and compare the definitions and descriptions of health, we see that a modern concept of health includes the following points.

UNITY	Health is the quality of the total functioning of the whole individual. A teacher should be concerned with the whole, not just a part of the student. For example, do you teach math, or do you teach Johnny math?
DIMENSIONS	Health is the result of the interactions between the physical, intellectual, emotional, social, and moral dimensions of man. If you, the teacher, are concerned about the total growth and development of your students, you will help them grow in all five dimensions.
FACTORS	Health is influenced by hereditary, environmental, and personal factors. By knowing the factors that influence the interrelationships among the various dimensions of health, the teacher is in a position not only to assist his students with health problems, but also to help prevent health problems.
DYNAMIC	Health is constantly changing on a continuum ranging from mortality on one end to various levels of illness (morbidity) to optimal health on the other end. Teachers have the responsibility of observing the dynamics of student health in the various dimensions, so that the student who is ill can be referred to proper assistance.
KEY	Health is a key that enables one to live effectively, to reach goals and potentials, and to achieve a personally satisfying and socially useful life. Health should not be thought of as an end in itself, but as an enjoyable means to an end. A teacher should value his students' health, because the quality of their health will determine how well they will be able to learn the information related to the academic course of study.

WELLNESS

During the first half of this century, a list of the leading causes of death was dominated by communicable diseases such as pneumonia, influenza, tuberculosis, diarrhea, enteritis, and diphtheria. There were also frequent epidemics of smallpox, poliomyelitis, and pertussis as well as measles, mumps, rubella and strep infections. Two words, sanitation and immunization, are primarily responsible for reducing the major killers of the early 1900s.

The communicable diseases have been replaced by chronic diseases. Today's top killers include heart disease, cancer, stroke, diabetes, atherosclerosis, cirrhosis of the liver, and emphysema. Among those between the ages of one and thirty-eight, accidents are the leading cause of death. In the high school and college age group, accidents, suicide, and homicide are the top three killers. A new approach is needed to combat these killers. New lines must be drawn. The battlefield is no longer traditional public health, the arena is personal health.
The new target is personal lifestyles. The new approach has been called the "Wellness Movement."

A recent study identifying the leading causes of death among western nations found that human biological factors (hereditary defects) accounted for 27 percent of the deaths. Environmental factors (pollution, etc.) accounted for 19 percent. Health service organizations were accountable for 11 percent of the deaths (including iatrogenic or doctor-induced conditions), but lifestyle factors led the list by being responsible for 43 percent of the deaths. Lifestyle consists of the health-related behavior patterns over which individuals have personal decision-making control. When self-imposed risks result in illness or death, the victim's lifestyle is said to be the cause. Since lifestyle is the number one cause of death and disease, efforts to change lifestyle is the new direction.

To understand the wellness movement, one must first make a distinction between the word *health* and the word *wellness*. When health is defined as a *state of being* or the "freedom from disease," the goal is a standard of mediocrity. When wellness is defined as *a process* of striving for a "quality of life," the goal is a standard of inspiration. When our goal is to overcome or avoid disease by treatment or prevention, we rely to a large extent on professionals. When our goal is to reach our *potential* by following a quality lifestyle, we rely on our own personal commitment.

The wellness movement is dedicated to improving people's lifestyles. It embraces the multidimensional concept of man, and endeavors to help people change their behavior. It realizes that behavior modification is based on the tripod of health education: knowledge, attitudes, and practices. The effective school health programs are those that have caught the spirit and vision of the wellness movement.

Dr. Jonas Salk, one of the great heroes of our times, is primarily responsible for the development of the polio vaccine. He stated the following ideas in a talk given at an annual convention of the American School Health Association. *Journal of School Health,*

Regardless of background, all children have in common the fact that they are active in the process of growth and development. In a sense, they are in a stage of plasticity; they are capable of being shaped by the conditions in which they grow and develop.

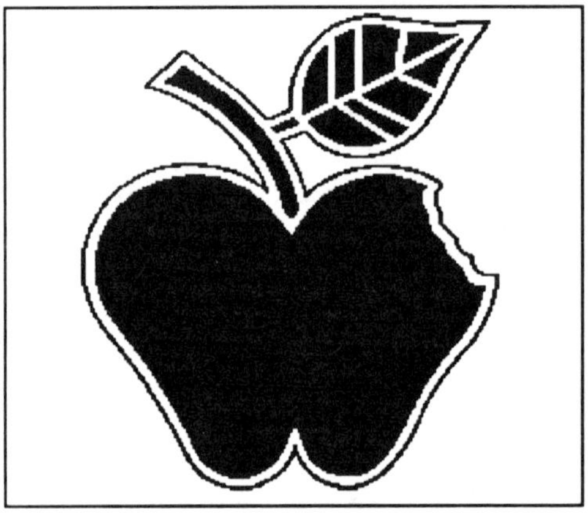

The objective of this stage of life is to develop interdependent relationships with other people and things in their environment. Many complex considerations pertaining to the body, the mind, the emotions, the child's relationships with others, and the diversity of opinion as to what is "right or wrong," enter into the achievement of this goal.

Health is not merely a passive state of freedom from disease; rather it is an active condition of growth, development, and evolution. Health is not an abstraction, but something specific and concrete; not the absence of a negative condition or disease, but a positive state of health.

What we need most is an attitude that values health and well-being.

A study of living systems reveals that health in man is an interdependent phenomenon in which the well-being of each of us is dependent upon the well-being of others. Healthy groups, whether it be cells or man, cannot exist unless predominantly composed of healthy members.

To the extent that disease exists in a community, the community will expend resources, time, and attention to fighting the disease. The time has come when we must think not in terms of ourselves alone or others as being separate from ourselves, but, for our own health, we must think of others.

Because of our present knowledge for reducing the probability of disease and premature death, there is now far greater opportunity than ever before for devoting attention to the enhancement of health. For example, just as certain diseases are contagious and are transmitted from person to person, let us think of health as being similarly transmissible. Think of health as if it were "contagious" in the sense that it could spread within a group.

> Health education can be a form of immunization...

This means a state in which the potential of the individual is developing in a balanced way so that he may cope with the vicissitudes of life and function fully in the service of life.

The "herd-effect" in contagious diseases operates to spread immunity. A similar phenomenon may also operate in the spread of health. In the case of vaccination for the control of epidemics, it is not necessary to vaccinate 100 percent of the people to prevent an outbreak. With polio it was found that if 85 percent of the children in a neighborhood were immunized, the community as a whole was protected. This is attributed to the reduced number of disseminators of the virus. As the number of susceptibles is reduced, the number of disseminators is reduced and the spread of the disease is arrested.

Health education can be a form of immunization also. More needs to be learned and more needs to be done to prevent the waste of disease. We have a long way to go, but the schools are a good place to start.

The "plastic" child can begin to develop habits of thinking as well as habits of behaving that will favor maintaining a state of health. A great deal of pathology later develops as a result of unhealthy experiences in the early years. More needs to be done to prevent poor health not only in children, but also in adults. What we need most is an attitude that values health and well-being.

Dr. Salk's ideas suggest a modern concept of health as it applies to the role of secondary school teachers.

> The"herd-effect" in contagious diseases operates to spread immunity. A similar phenomenon may also operate in the spread of health.

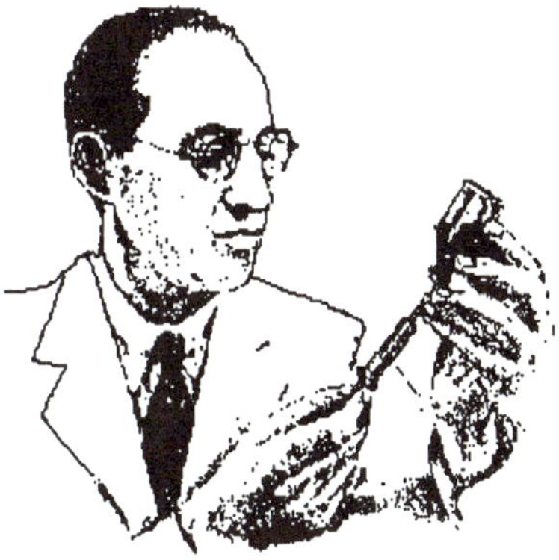

STUDY HELPS

These significant terms may be of assistance to you as you study.

attitudes
character
dimensions
dynamic
emotional
factors
intellectual
key
knowledge

lifestyle
potential
physical
practices
social
spiritual
unity
wellness

"contagious"
"herd-effect"
"true education"
single-dimensional
three-dimensional
multidimensional

David McKay
Jonas Salk

---

1. How would you define health?

2. How does health differ from wellness?

3. Is the modern definition of health really new, or did the modern concept of health also exist in earlier civilizations?

4. How does the acceptance of a modern definition of health alter the role of a school teacher.

Chapter 2

THE SCHOOL HEALTH MOVEMENT

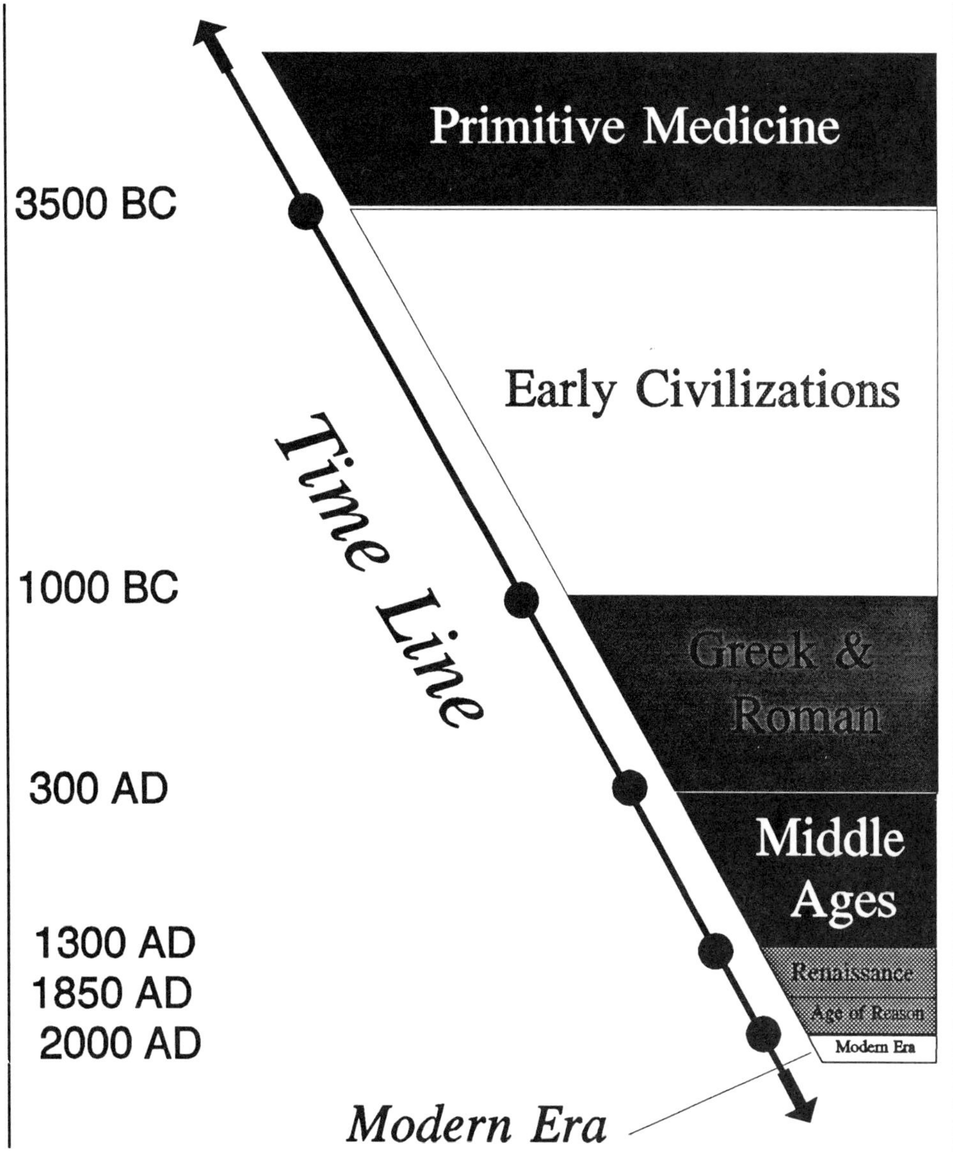

A HISTORICAL PERSPECTIVE

This chapter is a summary of the history of health and medicine form primitive times to today. It deals with people's attitudes about themselves and about the problem of disease. It provides a perspective that we might better understand humanities struggle to conquer disease and acquire the benefits of health and wellness.

THE PRIMITIVE MEDICINE MAN (4000 BC)

If you were living more than 6000 years ago when you became ill, you would probably visit the village shaman. The shaman or medicine man was a combination priest and physician. He would tell you what made you ill and perform some religious rituals to heal you. He would explain that your illness was due to evil spirits or angry gods. He would use rituals to cast out the demons or to compensate for broken taboos.

Historians rely on legendary accounts to tell us of primitive medical practices. In some ways, there are similarities between the primitive medicine of 6000 years ago and native tribal medicine in some corners of the world today. Even in the most modern countries, people still hold to beliefs about health that date back to primitive man. To better understand medicine in the past is to better understand medicine today.

Shaman

Even before the dawn of civilization, health and religion were intertwined in the beliefs and rituals of the primitive villagers. As people of that day observed sickness and death, they turned to the medicine man not only for help but for an explanation. In his dual role as priest and physician, the shaman's explanation involved demons, evil spirits, taboos, superstitions, and angry gods. The people also believed the medicine man had power to cast out evil spirits, to compensate for broken taboos, to overcome evil spells, and to please the gods. Sometimes it was thought that the disease was caused by magic or witchcraft coming from the sick person's enemies. So the medicine man practiced a form of counter magic to ward off the enemies' magic.

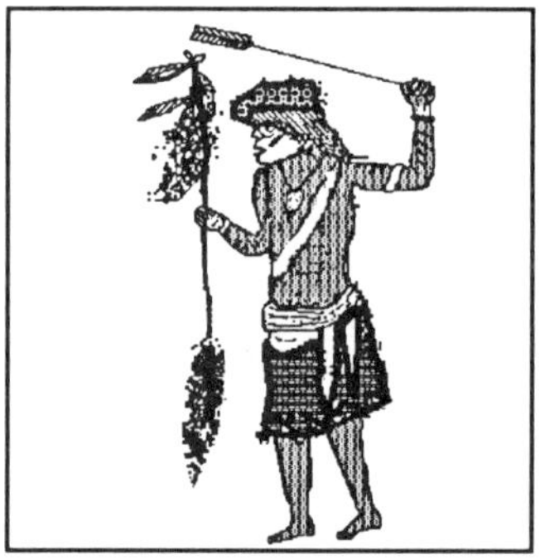

Early logic suggested that people become sick when there was something in the body that did not belong there or because something necessary for health was removed from the body. Treatment was to remove or restore the foreign or missing part. With injuries,

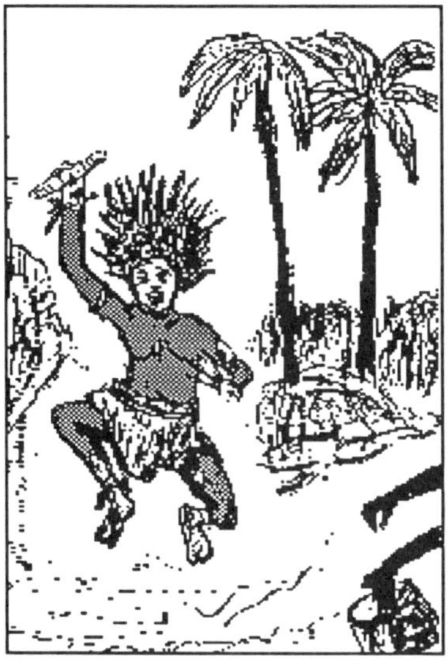

people could understood the cause of the illness and self-care was sufficient. But when they could not observe the cause of their illness, they attributed it to the magic of their enemies or to evil spirits. Their enemies, they believed, were using supernatural powers that could not be detected by ordinary senses to put something into or take something out of their bodies to cause the illness. They would then go to the shaman, medicine man, or witch doctor who had the powers and understanding to perform the healing.

The medicine man exploited people's superstitions, manipulated their imaginations, and created a trance state that would respond to the powers of suggestion. The rituals involved dancing, singing, painting, and a variety of charms, fetishes, effigies, and spells. The medicine man might also put himself into a trance state in order to "divine" the cause of the illness. No doubt his reputation and success were enhanced when he treated the wide variety of illnesses, including psychic disorders, which are more responsive to the power of suggestion. In such cases, the patient might be more apt to benefit from the treatment if he had confidence in the medicine man who performed it.

When the ancient priest-physician tried to heal a person, he first tried to determine if the patient had broken any taboos or if the sickness had been caused by a demon. Then he would try to treat the patient with spells, incantations, and rituals including dancing, singing, rattling bones, drawing pictures, and scattering dust and ashes. With time baths, massages, poultices, and herbal infusions were combined with the religious rituals. Eventually, mixtures made from seeds, bark, roots, and inorganic matter that actually had therapeutic properties were used.

The observant medicine men noticed that some potions used in the rituals were more effective than others. The therapeutic value of certain substances was gradually recognized. But to protect his role, the priest-physician maintained the people's faith in his magic rituals rather than in the natural healing properties of the medication.

Generally the treatments used by the medicine men were more successful in dealing with problems of the mind and the spirit than the body. But as they gradually recognized the therapeutic value of certain mixtures, the medicine men became more effective in treating physical problems. They began to abandon some approaches and look for new approaches. This haphazard method eventually led to the discovery of some effective treatments that are still in use by physicians in one form or another.

Progress was slow because circumstances made observations confusing. It was difficult to determine whether recovery occurred because of a treatment or because of some other factor. The medicine man and his successors have sometimes been given credit falsely. Many conditions give a treatment the appearance of success. For example:

- Many diseases are self-limiting and given a little rest and time the body will heal itself. With such diseases almost any treatment would appear to work.

- A spontaneous remission occurs when a chronic disease appears to go away for a while only to reappear again perhaps months later. In the meantime, people may give false credit to a treatment for the apparent recovery.

- People who have a disease of a psychological origin may respond well to a little special attention. The tender love and care (TLC) that accompanies any treatment might satisfy the patient's emotional needs. The symptoms disappear and the treatment falsely gets the credit.

- The power of suggestion or *placebo effect* was employed by the primitive medicine man as well as his many successors. The act of taking a pill sometimes triggers a physiological response that cures the ailment, even when the pill contained no therapeutic ingredient. This effect occurs frequently enough for people to give the treatment undue credit.

- When there are multiple factors involved, it is difficult to give credit to the right factor. The credit that should be given to one factor may be given falsely to another. The herbs used in the ritual may have produced the cure, but the medicine man's magic may get the credit.

Even when the treatment is worthless, there may be conditions present that give it the appearance of success. In the primitive villages those conditions were present enough of the time to maintain peoples confidence in their medicine man's healing power. To further protect his image, the medicine man had something else going for him. If the patient did not recover, the outcome was accepted as the will of the gods and was not associated with ineffective treatment.

This fatalistic approach and the inability to distinguish between coincidental relationship and the cause and effect relationship inhibited the progress of medicine for centuries.

During those thousands of years before the evolution of civilizations, each medicine man worked independently. The succession to the role of shaman succeeded along family lines. The son received apprenticeship training from his father or grandfather. Besides that, there was little sharing of information. Treatments were selected at random or by hunch. Successful treatments occurred more by coincidence than by wise planning.

In time, physicians learned to share their discoveries and ideas with each other. Physicians in the more advanced cultures realized the value of observation and reasoning. Some uniformity in theories and practices occurred. Therapeutic approaches were accepted or rejected depending on the presence or absence of evidence that they worked. There were, however, differences of opinion and disagreements as to what constituted evidence or proof. Each culture seemed to excel along certain lines, and different systems of healing developed in various parts of the world.

If the ancient medicine man enjoyed any advantage over his more rational successors, it was in his relationship to the transcendental. While most modern physicians in practice reject the idea of supernatural healing, others find the idea of extrasensory communication to be at least an interesting hypothesis. The tales of healing by native medicine men in Africa, Australia, and America today and by religious leaders throughout history are well known. Perhaps there is still more we can learn from the shaman.

MEDICINE AMONG EARLY CIVILIZATIONS (4000 - 750 BC)

As recorded history transcends the generalities of the primitive era, distinctive healing systems emerge. However, the popularity of the various systems of healing throughout history resembles the coming and going of the tide. Recorded medical history started in the cradles of civilization.

Mesopotamia and Babylonia

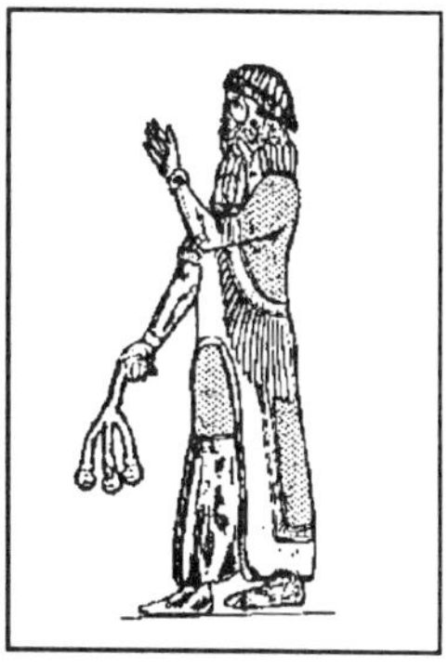

In early Mesopotamia a system of healing was practiced which embraced both the natural and the supernatural. Religion and magic were reflected on one end of the spectrum, and science and learning were reflected on the other. Health and disease were considered cosmic phenomena related to the universe. A sick person would first go to a diviner who would determine whether the sick person should see an exorcist to drive out demons or a physician to treat the ailment with medicine or surgery.

The Babylonians also approached healing from both ends of the spectrum, but it was much more organized and subject to the influence of the community leaders. The physicians organized into a profession and were subject to a code of conduct. King Hammurabi established the Code of Hammurabi which included a code of ethics governing physicians. The code regarded the rights of the citizens more than the prosperity of the physician. The code set maximum fees for services and prescribed penalties for unsuccessful treatments. The penalties varied according to the status of the patient. If a bondsman died while under the care of a surgeon, the surgeon would have to replace the bondsman. If a freeman died, the surgeon would have his hands cut off so he could not repeat the mistake. Strict public health regulations were also enforced.

Egypt

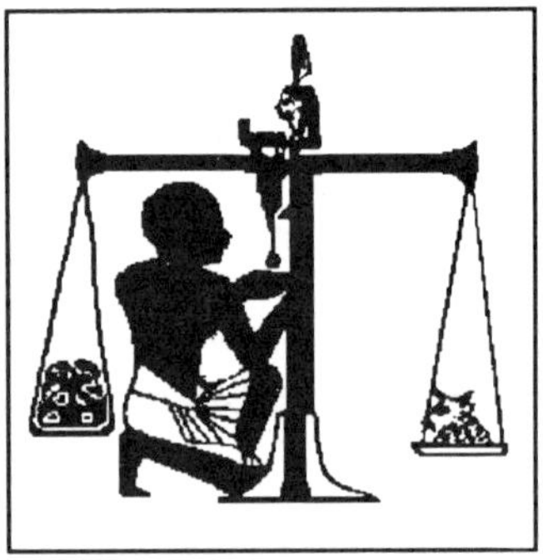

Early Egyptians had an extensive knowledge of anatomy, physiology, and drugs. They used herbs extensively in the form of pills, beverages, and suppositories. Their knowledge of pharmacology was demonstrated by their advanced techniques for preserving the body after death. They knew the value of hygiene, and a code of sanitation was enforced. Early Egyptian medical techniques were basically rational with little reliance on magic, but later medicine in Egypt split into factions. One faction abandoned the rational therapies in favor of the irrational, superstition, sorcery, magical, and religious rituals, while the other continued the rational tradition.

There was much competition between the natural physicians on one side and the priests on the other. The two groups contended to protect both their pocketbooks and their prestige and sought to discredit the other. The rational physicians based their claims on natural law and could promise only what they could deliver. The priests, not limited by what they knew or what could be proven, could promise anything. Given their influence as spokesmen for deity, the priests seemed to win out. People were attracted by the color, flair, and excitement of the priests and magicians. People are often more apt to follow something they do not understand than something they understand. The truth may be simple, modest, and common, but the unknown is only limited by the bounds of one's imagination.

In Egypt as in other cultures, the practice of medicine progressed as the whole civilization developed. But as the morals of the society depreciated, political corruption occurred and economic conditions degenerated, the practice of medicine also became perverted.

India and China

Near the same time farther to the east in the land now known as Pakistan and India, the Hindu civilization was developing. It followed a form of medicine that was quite advanced and closely linked with their religion. Health practices were a part of their lifestyle.

Acupuncture, practiced in China today, is part of a system of healing that dates back 5000 years. It is a theory of health and disease that deals with a balance between two opposite natural forces, the Yin and the Yang. If a person maintains a balance or harmony between the Yin and the Yang, he or she will be healthy. If the Yin or Yang gets out of balance, illness appears. Acupuncture needles are inserted into certain areas of the body to restore the balance between the two forces.

The Chinese are also credited with a unique method of paying for medical services. People pay the physicians to keep them healthy. Then when a person gets sick, they stop payment until they are restored to health again. This encourages a form of medicine that emphasizes promoting health rather than curing disease.

Peru

The ancient Peruvians also had some advanced health practices. Their physicians practiced a form of medicine that included drilling a hole through the skull and capping the hole with a metal plate. The purpose of the surgery is uncertain, perhaps to let evil spirits out, perhaps to deal with the trauma of an accident, or perhaps to perform actual brain surgery. But skeletal remains showing bone growth around the metal plate is evidence that the person lived for many years after the surgery.

Hebrews

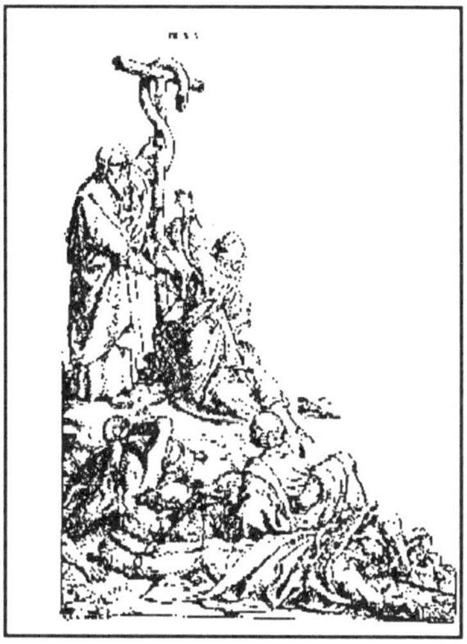

Another example of advanced health practices in ancient times is the Hebrews. Under Moses, the Hebrews followed a health code that was far ahead of its time. They credited its source as the God of Israel in direct revelation to Moses in the form of commandments. The Law of Moses, recorded in the book of Leviticus, pertained to food selection and standards of sanitation. For example, they were to isolate patients with ceratin diseases, wash their hands, eat beef but not pork. They were to burn the clothing and bedding of those who died. They were even commanded to rest their bodies one day a week. The God of Israel expected his people to preserve their health and thus practice preventive medicine. They understood what they should do, but not why. They operated on faith. The why was not understood until the advent of the germ theory thousands of years later. Medical history notes that the Hebrew contribution was in the area of preventive medicine and health maintenance rather than in a system of healing. The modern symbol of the medical profession, the *caduceus* or rod with entwined serpents, comes at least in part from the Hebrews under Moses. (Art in Babylon, Egypt, Mexico, and Greece also portrays a snake in connection with healing.) The account (Numbers 21:6-9) indicates that many people were dying from the bites of snakes. The people went to Moses for help, and he inquired of the Lord.

> ***And the Lord said unto Moses, make thee a fiery serpent and set it upon a pole: and it shall come to pass, that everyone that is bitten, when he looketh upon it, shall live. And Moses made a serpent of brass, and put it upon a pole, and it came to pass, that if a serpent had bitten any man, when he beheld the serpent, he lived.***

Numbers 21:6-9

GREEK AND ROMAN CIVILIZATIONS (750 BC -- 300 AD)

In Greece as in some of the earlier civilizations, there were two types of healers. One group was the physicians who followed the natural approach using medications and other physical therapies. The other group was the priests who used supernatural approaches including purification, appeals to the gods, and temple worship.

GRECIAN MYTHOLOGY

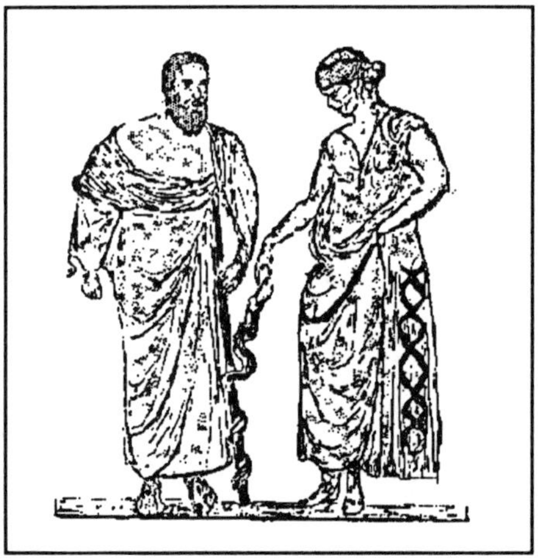

In the Louvre in Paris, France there stands a reproduction of an ancient Grecian sculpture representing the mythical god Aesculapius (es kyoo lay pee us) and the mythical goddess Hygeia. This sculpture represents the polarity between two basic approaches to health care, prevention, and treatment.

In ancient times people explained natural events with myths about gods, goddesses, and heroes. Myths differed from stories, tales, and legends in that people considered the myths sacred and true. Religious leaders, in order to explain certain occurrences and to encourage certain values, had much to do with the origin and perpetuation of the myths. The myths tell us much about the values of cultures. For hundreds of years the Greeks and Romans shared a rather complex system of myths of which some have influenced the history of health and medicine.

At first, Aesculapius was a very successful and popular mortal physician. In life he was regarded as a hero (the son of Apollo), and after his death, he became the first god of healing. The physicians of Greece prayed to Aesculapius for the power to heal. In art Aesculapius was usually portrayed holding a serpent-entwined staff. The serpent was an ancient symbol of health because it could shed its skin and appear young and healthy again. Because of the popularity of Aesculapius, the leaders of the religious cults were able to fuse the religious and natural cures for a time. Healing temples were built and adorned with statues of Aesculapius. People would come to the temples, participate in purification rights, sleep, see visions, and be healed. It was believed that if they saw visions of Aesculapius, his children or snakes, they would be healed. To make sure people would see visions, the temple priests would enter the rooms dressed as a god and let snakes loose in the room. They felt if the cure worked, the deception was justified. No doubt the cure worked well when the sickness was the type that would respond well to suggestion. Some of these healing centers flourished throughout the Roman era.

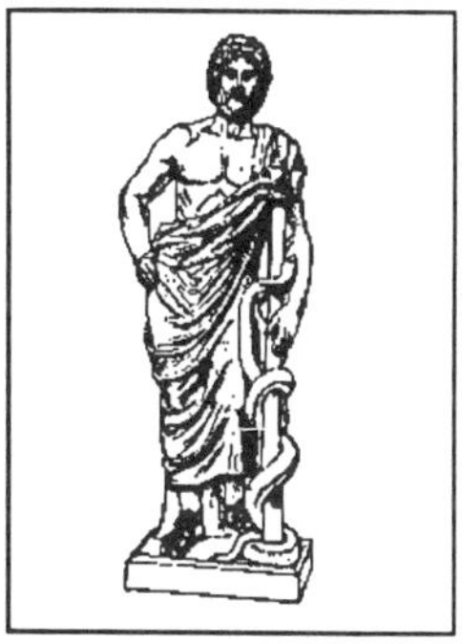

Hygeia, the Athenian goddess of health, was considered to be the wife of Aesculapius at times and at other times to be his daughter. She symbolized what results from living according to natural laws. Hygeia appealed to man to apply reason to his living. To her was attributed the philosophy that people can live well and healthy, if they live according to wisdom.

Hygeia represents a positive or preventive approach. People can gain and retain health if they apply their intelligence and wisdom. Aesculapius, on the other hand, represents a negative or creative approach. People turn to the physician for a cure after they have become ill because they have failed to live wisely. Throughout history the curative approach has prevailed, people usually go to a physician for treatment, not for prevention.

GREEK MEDICINE

Hippocrates

The Grecian civilization contributed much more than mythology to the history of medicine. The physician Hippocrates had such an influence on the principles of medicine that he is known as the *Father of Medicine.* The Oath of Hippocrates is still taken by graduating medical students today. He is given credit for establishing the treatment of disease as a science and establishing it as a profession.

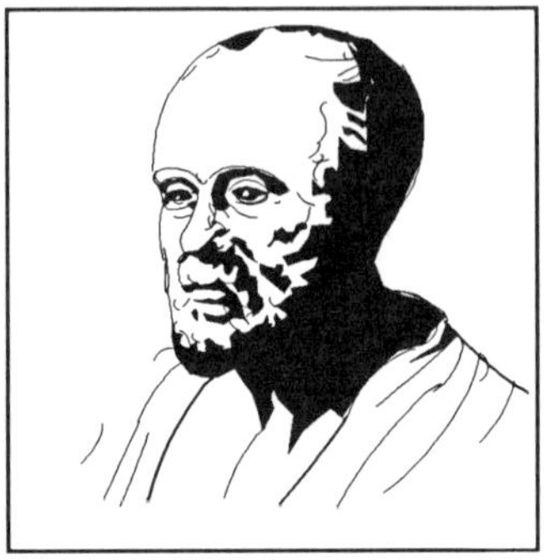

Had Hippocrates lived in another time and place, his ideas would have been ignored. But in Greece during the fifth century BC, the climate was right. The counsel of Socrates to "know thyself" had motivated an emphasis on personal health. Medical schools were established and accepted as the most effective means of training new physicians. Prior to this time, most physicians had been trained through apprenticeships, but the hospital-based medical schools brought many patients together in a setting where they could be thoroughly observed and compared. It also brought leading medical theorists together so they could reason and conduct research. Various treatments could be studied and compared. As some theories were accepted, others were rejected, and the curriculum in the medical schools started to become standardized.

The body of medical knowledge that emerged in Greece was more complete than in any previous civilization, and it was to remain intact for another fifteen hundred years. That is not to say that there was complete agreement among physicians, far from it. Nor is it to say that the body of knowledge was accurate, not by today's standards.

Diagnosis was based on finding an imbalance in the four body humors (blood, phlegm, yellow bile, and black bile), the four elements (water, air, fire, and earth), the four seasons (winter, spring, summer, and autumn), and the four conditions (hot, cold, wet, and dry). If all were in balance the person was healthy. Disease was due to an excess or deficiency in one of the above. Medications were used to restore the balance, but there was a conflict between the use of allopathic and homeopathic medicines. Homeopathic medications would produce results in the body similar to the patient's symptoms. Allopathic medications would produce results in the body that were opposite to the patient's symptoms.

Hippocrates was a great teacher of physicians. His greatest contributions to medicine were in the area of clinical diagnosis and prognosis. He urged the physicians not to have preconceived notions about the cause of or treatment for a disease. Instead, he taught the physicians to observe their patients carefully and to record and study their findings. He emphasized the quality of the physician-patient relationship. He recognized the physician's limited role in assisting the patient's natural life forces. He emphasized the use of diet, rest, massages, and baths and turned to medications and surgery only as a last resort. He taught his students to treat the patient with respect and dignity, to benefit the patient or at least do no harm, to be willing to lose a fee rather than trouble a sick person about it, and to neglect no opportunity to serve the poor and the stranger. Hippocrates' teachings were recorded and passed down for generations. Perhaps there is still much that physicians of today can learn from Hippocrates.

Galen

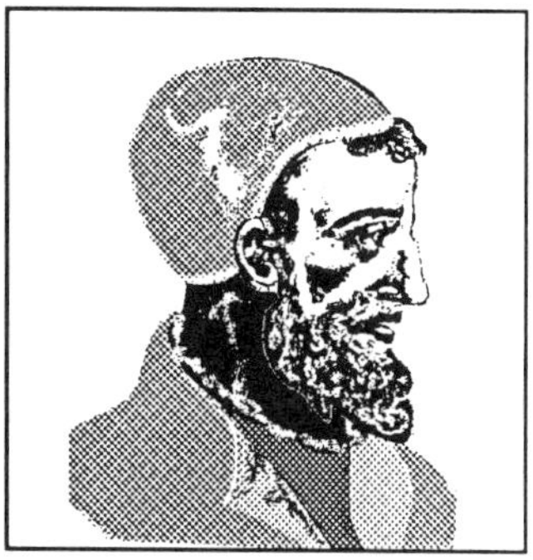

When Rome replaced Greece as the ruler of the Mediterranean world, the emphasis changed from personal health to community health. This change was marked by aqueducts, sewers, and army hospitals. Greek physicians were welcome in Rome, but the most famous was Galen. He ranks second only to Hippocrates in the history of medicine. He continued the principles and pursuits of Hippocrates and made additional contributions in the area of human anatomy and physiology. Human dissection was illegal, so he made extrapolations from his studies of animals. He served as a surgeon for gladiators, and as a healer he was very successful. His fame spread, and he became physician to the emperor. This sealed his reputation, and as he became more famous, he also became more arrogant and dogmatic. He proclaimed his theories as though they were fact. Though he made many discoveries, he also promoted many false ideas, and this had a detrimental influence on the history of medicine. He was a prolific writer and lecturer, and his teaching remained unquestioned for over a century.

From the time of Hippocrates (400 BC), medicine moved forward along a rational basis, but shortly after Galen's death (200 AD), medical progress stopped. New political and religious alignments contributed to the change. First, Christianity became the official religion of the Roman Empire, and then the empire split into the eastern empire with its capital in Constantinople and the western empire with its capital in Rome.

In the eastern empire, the Eastern Orthodox Church encouraged missionary activities among their Arabian neighbors. The Arabians did not accept Christianity, but they did accept their medical practices. So the medicine of Greece continued in Arabia for hundreds of years.

HEALTH IN THE MIDDLE AGES (300-1300 AD)

The Middle Ages refers to the period of time in western Europe between the fall of Rome in about A.D. 400 to the 1500s. It is also sometimes called the medieval period or the Dark Ages. Dark aptly describes the health conditions in Europe during the Middle Ages. The practice of medicine as a profession ceased, and health conditions deteriorated. The personal and community health practices emphasized in the Greek and Roman periods were abandoned. Sanitation was terrible, disease was rampant, and there were no physicians to care for the sick. Health conditions became deplorable.

"The Christian Influence"

To many it is surprising that historians credited this change to "Christian influence." Why are people surprised by these allegations? First, Christianity grew out of the Hebrew culture, and no group in history paid more attention to health than the Hebrews. Second, Christ was not only known as the greatest healer of all time, but His teachings also emphasized health. Through the parable of the *Good Samaritan*, He taught His followers to care for the health needs of even the unfortunate stranger. The writings of Paul to the Corinthians further emphasized the importance of health in the doctrine of Christ.

> ***Know ye not that ye are the temple of God, and that the spirit of God dwelleth in you? If any man defile the temple of God, him shall God destroy; for the temple of God is holy, which temple ye are... Know ye not that your body is the temple of the Holy Ghost which is in you?***

Three hundred years later the church reversed its emphasis on health. It was improper to be concerned about health or the body, that would have been carnal or worldly. They were to be concerned about the spirit and the next life. Disease had almost become a state of grace. Through suffering one could share the agony of Jesus on the cross. By suffering in this life, one could earn greater rewards in the hereafter. Sickness was a means of redemption; a way of being purged of sin.

Christians did not pay attention to health practices such as food and water sources, diet, or amount of rest. They did not clean their bodies, their clothing or their homes. They did not bathe. Their underclothing was sewn on and there it remained until it partially decomposed. Then a new garment was sewn over the top of the old. Homes were not kept much better. Food from the table fell to the floor where it mixed with other debris such as human or animal excrement and was eventually covered with a new layer of grass clippings or sawdust. This made an excellent place for the yet undiscovered microorganisms to grow. Europe experienced plagues and epidemics like it has not known before or since. One report stated that within a year and a half, half of the population of Europe died in a devastating epidemic.

When people became sick, they did not go to physicians. There were no physicians. Anyone who tried to practice medicine became an outcast. If a person died, they died unto Christ. For a thousand years, there was no organized efforts to give relief to those who were suffering. Finally, toward the end of the Middle Ages, attitudes started to change. Faced with an overwhelming need, sisters and monks began to provide nursing type custodial care to those who were sick. Eventually, monastery hospitals were established, but they provided nursing, not healing. In time, however, the monks and nuns began to introduce herbs grown in the monastery gardens to their nursing practices. Gradually, lay helpers were allowed to assist in the monastery hospitals. They developed some skill in administering simple herbal remedies and in performing menial surgical tasks. In the meantime the people's faith in the church as the sole source of healing began to dwindle. They sought help outside the church. Those who had learned the skills in the monastery hospitals began to help people in the community. Again the role of healer in the community was established.

The lay healers sought information from any source. During the Middle Ages, the monks had faithfully recopied the manuscripts containing the teachings of Hippocrates and Galen. Once again the ideas of these Greek heroes became the standard for medical practice. The four humor system was the basic approach. Galen's theory of polymedication, the more ingredients the better, was followed. When a drug did not appear to work, bleeding became the standard treatment. Eventually, medical schools were established and medical doctors from Arabia were imported as teachers.

MEDICINE DURING THE RENAISSANCE (1300-1600 AD)

Since the fall of the Roman empire, Europe had been divided into small feudal states. Yet the Catholic church maintained a powerful control through all Europe. The Renaissance was an age of adventure, curiosity, and challenge. It spread throughout Europe during the fourteenth, fifteenth, and sixteenth centuries. It set aside the customs in art, religion, politics, and medicine that had been there for over 1000 years. This was the period of Michelangelo, da Vinci, Columbus, Luther, and the printing press. In this period, three physicians risked being ostracized by the medical profession and challenged the teachings of Galen.

Paracelsus

A physician by the name of Philippus Paracelsus, born in Zurich in 1493, was impressed by the purity of the teachings of Hippocrates in contrast to the complicated writings of Galen. He did not believe in using drugs except in emergencies, and then he sought to find the best drug for a specific situation. He did not believe in polymedication. He became zealous in his work and was at first generally regarded as a heretic, but gradually he gained a following. Today, medicine recognizes the contributions of Paracelsus in starting to move medicine out of the Dark Ages. Medical historians have referred to Paracelsus as the Martin Luther of medicine.

Vesalius

A greater challenge to the works of Galen came from Andraes Vesalius. Born in Brussels in 1514, he became famous for his contributions to the study of anatomy. As a youth, he was involved in dissecting small animals, and as a medical student he stole the buried bodies of criminals. At an early age, he became a professor of surgery and anatomy.

At first, he was not a revolutionary--he sought to show his students that Galen had been right--but his observations showed that in many ways Galen was far from the truth. Galen had done well in attempting to describe something he had not seen, but Vesalius thought it important to correct the errors. Although he verified his findings, the older anatomists and physicians had difficulty accepting his work. Galen's anatomy continued to be taught in the universities until the 1600s.

<u>Pare</u>

Prior to the days of Ambrose Pare, surgery was the lowest order in the medical field. Even during earlier civilizations, physicians rarely performed surgery. Often a slave or servant performed the surgery under a physician's direction. At this time, the local barber usually served as the local surgeon. The red and white on the barber pole repres-ented the blood and bandages. They pulled teeth, lanced boils, cauterized wounds, set broken bones, and performed amputations. Sometimes the blacksmith was called on to perform the surgical tasks that physicians felt were beneath their dignity. Pare, the son of a barber, made a notable contribution to the art and science of medicine. As a surgeon in the French army, Pare had a lot of experience surgically treating gunshot wounds. He discovered many new surgical procedures, and this launched him into a new career discovering and teaching surgical techniques. In 1552 he became surgeon to the king. His work elevated surgery to a respected level as a medical specialty.

The contributions of Paracelsus, Vesalius, and Pare were recognized more in later years than in their own time. In most ways, medicine and health made little progress during the Renaissance.

MEDICINE IN THE AGE OF REASON (1600-1850 AD)

The seventeenth century began a time in world history called the Age of Reason. It began as an intellectual revolution. Ideas, new and old, had to stand the test of reason. People tried to find better ways of doing things. This led to political revolution. New freedoms found expression in the inventions of the tools and methods that gave birth to the Industrial Revolution. The most important outcome of the Age of Reason was, however, the dawn of experimental science.

The word *science* can mean either a system of inquiry or a body of knowledge. Scientists observe the relationships between events. For example, If event B precedes event A, scientists try to determine whether event A caused event B, or if their occurrence in sequence was merely a coincidence. Science uses various methods to test relationships. Clinical observation was the method advocated by Hippocrates. Observation is a valuable method. It did much to further medical science, but it has serious limitations in the pursuit of truth. The Age of Reason made three major contributions to science. It produced instruments of measurement that greatly increased the power of observation; it produced a model for controlled experiments; and it developed a system to mathematically analyze data.

Galileo and Newton

Galileo and Newton were not medical scientists, but they indirectly contributed much to the advancement of medical science. They developed the experimental model that was used much later by medical science. Galileo is regarded as the father of modern experimental science. The first step in his method was to establish a theory or hypothesis and then utilize a variety of procedures to test the theory. The procedures controlled the variables and provided reliability and validity. Newton helped by developing a system of mathematics for statistical analysis that would not only explain occurrence but would also accurately predict events.

Harvey

William Harvey was the English physician who discovered how blood circulates. His discovery was another contradiction of what was being taught in the medical schools. Harvey was afraid that publishing his findings might jeopardize his career. He waited years to establish his reputation before publishing his discoveries in 1628, and even then he was criticized by his colleagues and his medical practice diminished. Yet the climate for accepting good research was changing, and Harvey lived to see his discoveries applauded.

van Leeuwenhoek

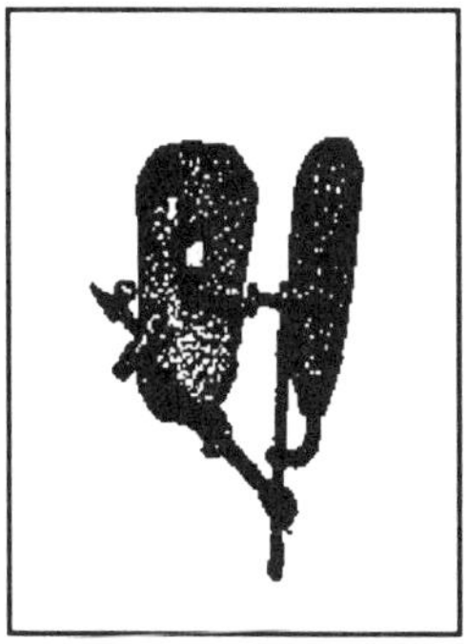

Although medical science made few advances during the Renaissance, other scientific achievements of that period prepared the way for future medical discoveries. For example, a Dutch amateur scientist named Antonie van Leeuwenhoek improvised a microscope that made it possible to see things too small to be observed by the unaided eye. His writings about the "little animals" were accepted by the Royal Society for the Advancement of Science in 1665. Another important instrument for medical observation or measurement was the clinical thermometer developed by Socrates in 1714. René Laennec made the first stethoscope from a hollow wooden tube in 1816.

Jenner

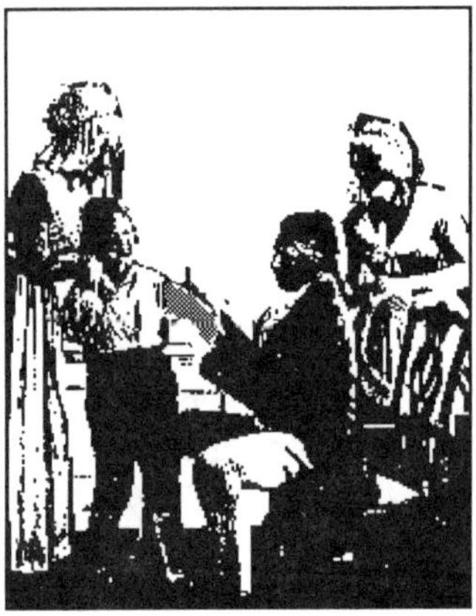

Edward Jenner made a significant early contribution to preventive medicine in 1796. At that time, it was estimated that one in five people in Europe died of smallpox. Half of the survivors bore pox marks for the rest of their lives. Jenner, an English country doctor, ob-served that the farm girls who milked the cows did not get the dread disease because they had been exposed to cowpox. He performed an experiment that was to place him among the heroes of medicine. He transferred pus from a cowpox lesion into the flesh of two young boys. A few days later he injected the boys with smallpox germs. When the disease did not develop, he had successfully introduced the smallpox vaccination. He later was recognized as the father of immunizations.

Lind

Another preventive measure involved the importance of maintaining a balanced diet. In 1757 James Lind, a physician in the British Navy, discovered that the disease scurvy could be prevented if the sailors were given a ration of limes or other citrus fruit. The authorities had difficulty accepting Lind's discovery, because the remedy was so simple. Eventually because of this discovery, the British sailors were called "limes," and Lind was recognized for making one of the first contributions to the science of nutrition.

MEDICAL GUILDS AND QUACKERY

Although there were isolated examples of medical breakthroughs during the Age of Reason, medicine as a whole progressed rather slowly. The smallpox immunizations introduced by Jenner in 1796, for example, were still not available to everyone until midway through the twentieth century when the disease was finally eradicated. Eventually, the scientific method would be used to distinguish between reliable and unreliable medical procedures, but not yet. In the meantime, the practice of medicine had few constraints. The discoveries by Paracelsus, Vesalius, Pare and others discredited the traditional restrictions, and the new restrictions based on scientific evidence were not yet in place. Approaches to healing proliferated and the Age of Reason was also the golden age for quackery.

To help deal with the problem, ethical physicians established guilds. A guild was an association of people with common interests such as craftsman or merchants. They were organized to protect the mutual interests of the members. The guilds also served to protect the public from unethical and incompetent providers. Guilds tried to keep nonmembers from practicing the craft. They also limited membership so members would be assured of work. To eliminate competition among members, they standardized fees, established rules, and instituted training requirements. A university education was a prerequisite to membership in the physicians' guilds and the mark of distinction between orthodox physicians and quacks.

MEDICINE IN AMERICA

At the time of the Revolutionary War, medical care in the United States was provided by a few immigrant doctors trained in European universities, a few native sons who had traveled to Europe for university training, a few physicians who had learned medicine through apprenticeships, and a few self-taught practitioners.

Rush

The first medical school in the United States was established at the University of Philadelphia in 1765 by Doctor Benjamin Rush, a signer of the Declaration of Independence. That school, like the universities in Europe, taught the philosophies of Hippocrates and Galen, maintaining that the four humors were the key to medical success. The standard treatments were blood letting, vomiting, and purging. The chief medication was calomel, a mercury chloride mixture, which was used to purge the body of poisons.

Thomson

Among the self-taught practitioners was a man named Samuel Thomson. He formulated his own healing system using herbs as medications and developed a large practice. He received a patent for his system in 1809 and published several books. For twenty dollars, a person could buy his book and the patent rights to become a Thomsonian Practitioner. In Ohio in 1835, half of the population were advocates of Thomsonian medicine.

Because of men such as Thomson, opposition to orthodox medicine was mounting. Men like Post, Kellogg, and Graham, the founders of the cereal industry, were strong critics of orthodox medicine and advocated proper diet as the alternative. Thomson was opposed to the establishment of schools to teach medicine. He wanted a system of lay practitioners. He felt the herbal approach was safer and more effective than the methods taught in the medical schools. He was not alone in his opposition to orthodox medicine. Several schools of homeopathic medicine were established in the United States in the early 1800s, and homeopathic physicians were opposed to traditional medicine. The discontent among the people, however, was reflected in a statement made by Thomas Jefferson. After paying close attention to the practice of medicine in the United States and in Europe, Jefferson said, "Not only a reformation in medicine is necessary, but a revolution."

It was the advent of the scientific method for the purpose of distinguishing fact from fallacy that brought about the revolution. The American Medical Association was founded in 1847. Its role was not only to protect the profession but also to protect the public from unscrupulous practitioners. It established the position that for a new theory to be accepted there must be verifiable evidence that it worked. The burden of proof was on the promoter of the new idea. Although medical science could not accurately say that an unproven theory was false, it took the position that the theory remained questionable until it was proven true.

The American Medical Association

During the next half century, the AMA did much to revolutionize medicine. It tackled the problem of unproven methods on several fronts. It encouraged states to require doctors to be licensed and to accept graduation from an accredited medical school as the basis for licensure. It worked to improve the curriculum in medical schools. Schools that did not teach scientifically based concepts were not to be accredited.

It was not easy to protect the public from unscientific procedures, particularly when they had been a part of orthodox medicine for centuries. For example, orthodox physicians clung tenaciously to their old panacea calomel. During the Civil War, an army doctor conducted research that showed calomel to be not only ineffective but also dangerous. With this information, the U.S. Surgeon General ordered the removal of the supply of calomel. Orthodox medicine was offended and succeeded in getting the Surgeon General fired. It was another fifteen years before the use of calomel by orthodox physicians was completely halted.

Morton

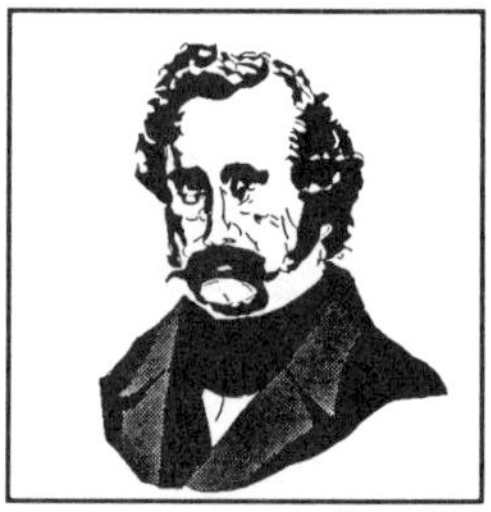

The first major contribution to medicine to come from America was anesthesia. Prior to anesthesia, pain during an operation was the major difficulty of surgery, so anesthesia was a major breakthrough. During the 1840s, several individuals claimed credit for introducing anesthesia, but a dentist, William Morton, is generally given the credit. He assembled a board of eminent surgeons at the Boston Medical Center in 1846 to observe his experiment. It worked, and the use of anesthesia spread rapidly both in the United States and in Europe. This opened the way for tremendous advances in surgery.

THE MEDICAL REVOLUTION

Near the beginning of the Middle Ages, medicine experienced a period when many of the previously-known principles were abandoned. Then early in the Modern Era medicine experienced a period when many of the previously-known principles were rediscovered. Since then modern scientific medicine has produced new information at a rate that is staggering to the imagination.

MODERN MEDICINE
(1850 -->)

The period of modern medicine started near the middle of the nineteenth century. Its beginning was marked by the acceptance of the scientific method in medicine. It meant that medical theories must stand the test of science and that unsubstantiated old theories were to be rejected. It opened the way for new breakthroughs to occur in medicine. With modern medical science, more medical discoveries have taken place in the last hundred years than during all of the rest of history combined. In fact, the medicine of the 1850s had more similarities to the medicine of Greece (more than two thousand years earlier) than to today's medicine (less than one hundred and fifty years later).

Pasteur

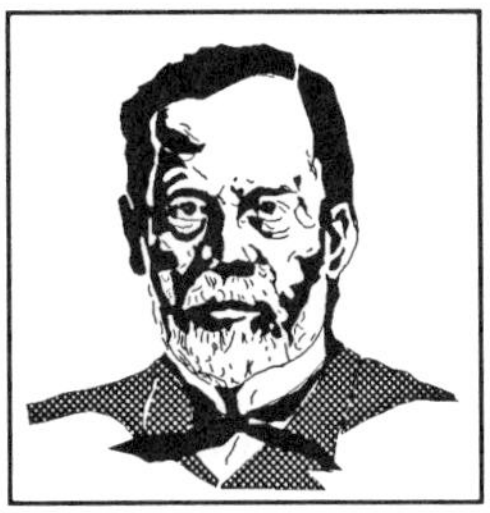

Probably no name in medical history stands out as much as Louis Pasteur of France. He was not a physician, but a great scientist. Between 1850 and 1890, Pasteur made many great contributions to chemistry, industry, and medicine, but perhaps his greatest contribution was in the example he set as a scientific researcher. Others before him had presented ideas about microorganisms causing disease, but Pasteur came at the right time and place and possessed the right aptitude for research to do something about the problem. His meticulous research transformed disconnected ideas into a complex and well-structured theory that revolutionized medicine.

Others as early as the Romans had theorized that invisible organisms or agents too small to be seen were the reason for the epidemics, but lacking the tools of research they could not support their theories. The invention and perfection of the microscope made it possible to see the "tiny animals" as Pasteur called them. Pasteur was a chemist with an interest in probing the mysteries of bacteriology. He was the first to disprove the theory of

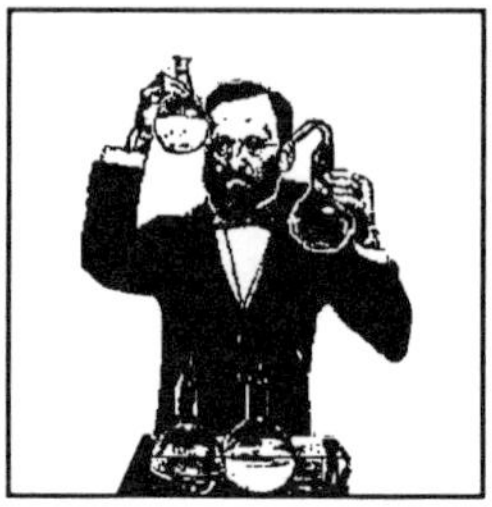

spontaneous generation and prove that living things come only from living things. He showed that bacteria live almost everywhere, but their spread can be controlled. The application of his theories saved the silk industry when he showed how to eliminate germs from the silk nurseries. He saved the sheep industry when he developed a vaccine for the disease anthrax. He also developed vaccinations for chicken cholera and rabies. But perhaps he is best known for developing pasteurization. The idea of using heat to kill bacteria was first used in the wine industry, but now it is the basis for the modern dairy industry.

Pasteur's many scientific accomplishments can be summarized in his major contribution to medicine, the germ theory of disease. This theory was not easily accepted by traditionalists, but eventually medical science was to accept his theory as fact. Certain diseases are caused by microscopic organisms called pathogens. Pasteur is an example of a scientist who became famous in his own lifetime.

Lister

Joseph Lister, a surgeon who also had an interest in bacteriology, read of Pasteur's works with interest, and in the 1860s developed antiseptic techniques that revolutionized surgery. At that time, surgeons paid little attention to cleanliness. Patients were operated on without any attempts to remove the dirt and grime that may have been on their bodies. Surgeons did not wash their hands or clean their instruments and their aprons and operating tables were covered with splashes of blood and pus from countless operations. The most trivial operation was likely to introduce infection with a death rate as high as fifty percent.

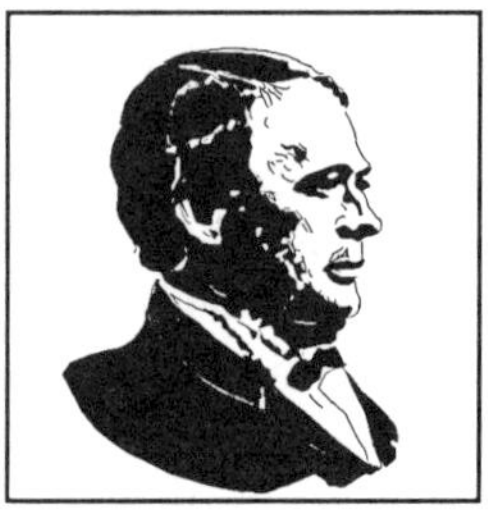

Lister's idea was to spray the air in the operating room with carbolic acid to kill the germs and advocated that surgeons should wash their hands, instruments, and the patients with this solution. At first, his fellow surgeons viewed his ideas with contempt, but when the mortality rate from his operations dropped to four percent his ideas were accepted. Antiseptics so revolutionized surgery that the history of surgery is divided into pre-Lister and post-Lister periods. As the first physician to be honored by England with the title of knight, Sir Joseph Lister became the father of antiseptic surgery.

Simmelweis

While Lister's story is one of success, many physicians who introduced new ideas were not as fortunate. Ignes Phillip Simmelweis was a Hungarian physician who specialized in obstetrics. Although he was a contemporary of Pasteur and Lister, there is no evidence that

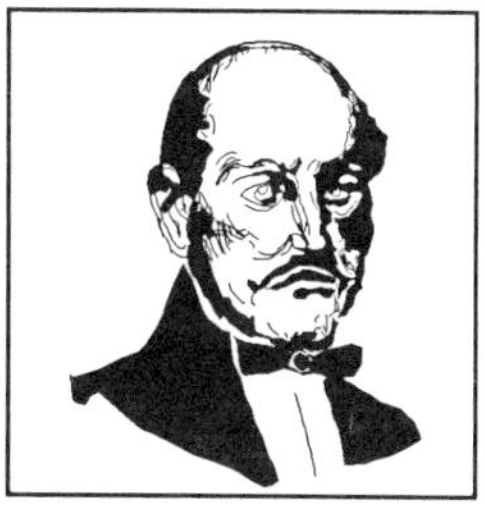

he knew of their works. He was concerned about the number of mothers who contracted "childbirth fever" while staying in a hospital to deliver a baby and soon died of the dread disease. Simmelweis observed that the disease rate was high in the wards attended by physicians but was rare in the wards attended by midwives and almost nonexistent in rural home deliveries. He also noted that a physician friend died from a fever associated with a wound accidentally encountered while performing a postmortem. His friend exhibited the same signs and symptoms as the mothers who died with childbirth fever. He realized that the physicians would go directly from doing postmortem to the maternity ward and conduct pelvic examinations, thus spreading disease to the expectant mothers.

Simmelweis tested his theory by having the physicians wash their hands thoroughly before and after each examination. Immediately, the incidence of childbirth fever dropped dramatically. But when he tried to convince other physicians that they should do likewise, his ideas were rejected. He maintained his stand and published his works in 1860, but opponents to his ideas attacked him fiercely. He had a reasonable hypothesis and he backed it with evidence, but he was too blunt in his criticism of his colleagues. He called them murderers. They retaliated and fought his ideas bitterly. His ideas were eventually recognized as being right, but not before he died in a hospital for the mentally ill. His insanity was due to the guilt he felt when so many women suffered and died, because he was unable to convince his colleagues to follow a few simple procedures.

Koch

Robert Koch is recognized as the founder of bacteriology as a separate science. This German physician developed new techniques for incubating and staining bacteria in a laboratory. He developed a technique known as Koch's postulates for isolating and identifying the microorganism causing a specific disease. This technique involved extracting the microorganisms from the person or animal that was diseased, growing the organisms in the laboratory, then introducing the organisms into a second healthy animal. If the second animal developed the same disease symptoms as the first, the organism had been identified. Knowing the identity of the responsible organism is necessary before appropriate treatment can be started.

Reed

Walter Reed was a medical officer in the United States Army. In 1898 he headed a commission to study typhoid fever. Scientific experiments found that flies were the most important carrier of the infection. In 1900 he headed a commission to investigate an epidemic of yellow fever among American troops in Cuba. Reed supervised a series of daring experiments in which volunteers were infected by yellow fever germs. The experiments showed that yellow fever was spread by mosquito bites. The experiments also demonstrated a successful way of controlling the disease.

Roentgen

In 1901 a German professor of physics named Wilhelm Roentgen won the first Nobel Prize in physics for his discovery of X-rays. Within a year after this scientific breakthrough, X-ray equipment was being employed as a diagnostic tool by physicians around the world.

Goldberg

When Dr. Joseph Goldberg, a surgeon in the United States Public Health Service, discovered that the disease pellagra was due to protein deficiency, he pointed other researchers toward the discovery of the essential nutrients.

Banting and Best

In 1921 two Canadian researchers, Doctors Frederick Banting and Charles Best, found that insulin controlled sugar diabetes. When their experiments produced a method to mass-produce insulin, their discoveries gave life to millions of diabetics.

Flemming

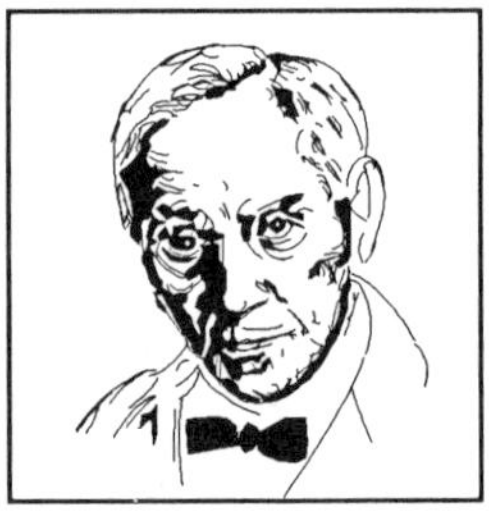

Dr. Alexander Flemming, a British bacteriologist, made some observations in 1928 that led to the discovery of penicillin in 1940. One day some mold accidentally started growing in a petri dish full of bacteria cultures. Flemming noticed a clear substance around the mold that was destroying the bacteria. The substance produced by the mold was later called penicillin. He started to do research on the subject, but funding was not available so he set the research aside. A few years later during World War II, it became obvious that the army with the best treatment for infection in wounds would have a decided advantage. Suddenly there was great interest in Flemming's discovery, so research was renewed in 1940. When it was concluded that wartorn England was not the best place for the research, the project was transferred to the United States. By 1943, there was enough penicillin to meet the military needs for all of the Allies as well as for urgent civilian cases. Since then, the development of antibiotics has been spectacular. It has brought great changes to the practice of medicine.

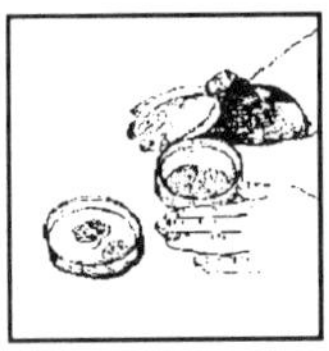

Salk

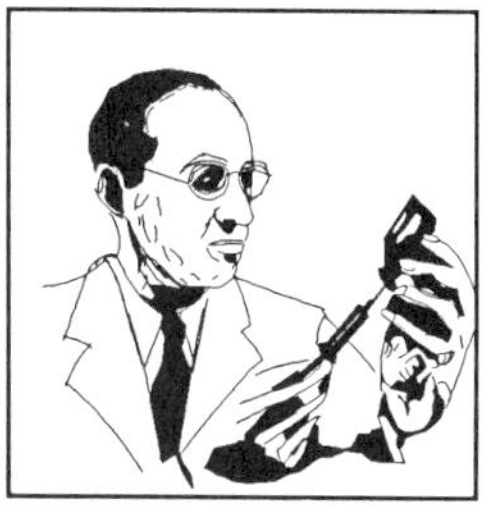

The human race has known polio since the beginning of civilization, but during the 1940s terrifying epidemics swept the U.S. killing and crippling thousands each year. This gigantic problem led to something new in medical research, the team approach. Dr. Jonas Salk led the team. The team was divided into groups, each attacking the problem from different angles. The research was financed by the National Foundation (March of Dimes). Dr. Salk had a vaccine ready for mass testing in 1954. Dr. Salk is still conducting important team research at his research center near San Diego, California.

Cooper

Future books on medical history will probably list the name of Kenneth Cooper among the heros of medicine. In 1968, Kenneth Cooper, a physician in the United States Air Force, wrote a book with the title *Aerobics.* In his book, Cooper cited research that showed the value of cardiovascular fitness in preventing heart disease. This book did much to encourage the physical fitness movement in this country. The effect was remarkable. People started jogging and engaging in other aerobic exercises. Cooper is a key contributor to the new disease prevention approach in medicine, an approach that emphasizes personal lifestyle management.

SPACE AGE MEDICINE

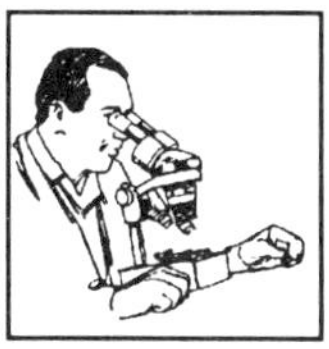

For over a hundred years now, the scientific method of investigation in medicine has been well accepted. It has been adding new information to the body of medical knowledge at a astonishing rate. So many scientific breakthroughs have occurred recently that it is difficult to isolate the most significant. It is also difficult to give credit to single individuals, because most medical achievements today are the result of a team effort. For example, to whom will future historians give credit for the first permanent replacement artificial heart: Dr. Kolff who assembled the team, Dr. Jarvis who designed the heart, Dr. de Vries who headed the surgical team, Dr. Barney Clark who was the first recipient, the University of Utah's Division of Artificial Organs who sponsored the research, or some other individual or group on down the road who may perfect the procedure?

Much of today's medicine is referred to as space age medicine. It includes artificial organs, test tube babies, biofeedback, laser surgery, insulin pumps, and CT scans (computerized tomography) to name just a few. Inter-esting discoveries are being made about the effect of personality and social relationships on physical health and longevity. But space age medicine is not without its special problems. One is the gap between what medical technology has discovered and what physicians do in their daily practice. Some procedures are technologically achievable but financially prohibitive. Space age medicine also faces many new problems such as new environment pollutants, AIDS and other new diseases, and changing consumer practices.

As historians look back at the medicine of today, it will be judged by its ability to encourage patients to follow a lifestyle that is conducive to health and wellness. This includes efforts to improve people's health knowledge, attitudes, and practices. Health education in the schools, at the worksites, in clinics and hospitals, and throughout the communities is a key to many of medicine's space age challenges.

HEALTH EDUCATION

This historical perspective started with a glance back to a point when history began to fade into speculation. It looks at a time when independent families merged into small communities and people began to examine the forces that influenced life. They wondered about the forces related to death and disease. They wondered what enabled some people to live long and remain healthy. Those behaviors that contributed to a longer and healthier life became part of the taboos of the culture. The village shaman's role was to define and encourage compliance with those taboos. In his combined role as a priest and physician, he also served as a teacher. In a practical sense the shaman was the first health educator.

In time, others assumed the role of religious leader and health educator, and the physician's role was confined to healing. In some ways, this restricted role was less effective in dealing with the whole person who is a combination of mind, body, and spirit. But in other ways, it helped because it enabled physicians to concentrate on that which was discernible through the senses and not have to deal with that which was intuitive, required speculation, or was perceived through extrasensory perception. Nevertheless, throughout history, the most successful practicing physicians maintained a balance between the art and the science of medicine.

Eventually, taboos evolved into civil laws and religious doctrine. Throughout the generations, those who interpreted and enforced the laws and taught the religious doctrine also served as informal health educators.

Influential philosophers of the eighteenth century promoted the worth of each human life and the importance of the individual for the well-being of society. The reason *why* we should concerned about health was established. Next came the *how*. The discoveries of medical science in the nineteenth century established principles of personal and community health. The problem was finding a *way* to get the people to put those principles into practice.

The novel *Oliver Twist*, written by Charles Dickens in 1839, helped society recognize its health problems. It showed the plight of the many orphans whose parents had died at an early age due to the unsafe and unsanitary conditions of the day. A few years earlier, 1832, Edwin Chadwick was commissioned to prepare a report of the sanitary conditions in London. The report documented the problem and suggested that instruction in hygiene and safety in the schools was a means of dealing with the problem. In 1850 the *Report of the Sanitary Commission of Massachusetts* by Lemuel Shattock of Boston called for mandatory instruction in hygiene in the public schools in the Commonwealth of Massachusetts. Horace Mann, America's great school reformer, had recognized health education as a part of the solution to the problem. Several of his reports between 1837 and 1843 had urged mandatory programs in hygiene education.

Although the early calls for health education did not take effect immediately, gradually the quantity and quality of health education in the schools improved. Over the years, many nationally recognized groups have met to determine the goals of education. Such groups as the National Education Association, the National Association of Secondary School Principals, the American Council on Education and others have each listed health outcomes among the highest objectives of education.

Physicians, nurses, and others involved in medicine have nearly always supplemented their primary objective with some informal health education, and they will continue to do so. But as a result of the emphasis on health education, a new and distinct role in the health field was established. People were hired, assigned, and trained to be health educators. Today professional health educators work in school, community, worksite, and clinical settings. There are school health educators, community health educators, health promotion specialists, and patient health educators. Health education is an applied science. It extracts facts from the medical and behavioral sciences and applies them to the needs of the learner. All professional health educators should have a common generic academic background plus some specialty course work.

The **phases** in the history of public health and the **periods** in the history of school health have paralleled each other since the beginning of the modern era of medicine in approximately 1850.

PHASES OF PUBLIC HEALTH

MIASMA (1850 - 1880)

Miasma means bad air. At this time, it was believed that disease was caused by night air and noxious odors. This was partially true for mosquitos came out at night and spread disease. Also, decaying garbage produced bad odors as well as disease-producing microorganisms.

BACTERIOLOGICAL (1880 - 1920)

By this time the theories of disease presented by Pasteur, Lister, Koch, and others had been accepted.

POSITIVE HEALTH (1920 - 1960)

The positive health phase started with the application of many preventive measures. Immunization and sanitation did much to extend life expectancy.

SOCIAL ENGINEERING (1960 --->)

The social engineering phase started when it was realized that lifestyle changes would be needed to improve personal and community health. Polio can be prevented with comparatively less effort than preventing heart disease. Social engineering is changing people's lifestyles and that involves health education.

PERIODS OF SCHOOL HEALTH

RECOGNITION (1850 - 1880)

At this time, it became recognized that schools could and should play an important role in promoting health. Health education emphasized sanitation and safety.

EXPLORATION (1880 - 1920)

The role of school health was still being explored. The child study movement was underway. Health education emphasized physical education and drug education.

EXPANSION (1920 - 1935)

The role of school health expanded into a multiphased program. More organizations became involved. More studies were conducted.

INTEGRATION (1935 --->)

The multiphased program became integrated into the current three-phased school health program: services, education, and environ-ment. Advancements were made in the professional preparation for health educators. The status of the health class in the curriculum improved.

SIGNIFICANT EVENTS IN THE HISTORY OF SCHOOL HEALTH

1850

- **Lemuel Shattock Report**, *Report of the Sanitary Commission of Massachusetts*, was issued in 1850. It recommended the teaching of health in the public schools.

1871

- Massachusetts became the **first state to pass a law requiring classes in physiology and hygiene** in all public schools.

1872

- The American Public Health Association (**APHA**) was established in 1872. Although it showed concern for the health of the school child, it was primarily a public health organization. In 1942, a school health section was established.

1918

- The **Child Health Organization** founded in 1918 brought a new look to school health. In 1918, it replaced the term *hygiene* with *health education.*

1919

- The National Education Association (**NEA**) established the Department of Child Study (the name was later changed to the **Department of Child Hygiene**).

1921

- The **NEA-AMA Joint Committee on Health Problems in Education** was established. The Joint committee of the National Education and the American Medical Association published several books setting minimal standards for a school health programs.

1937

- In 1895 the NEA established the Department of Physical Education (at that time physical education and health education were almost synonymous). In 1937, the Department of Physical Education became the American Association for Health, Physical Education, and Recreation (**AAHPER**). The Health Education Division published a professional journal called *Health Education.* Years later AAHPER became the American Alliance for Health, Physical Education, Recreation, and Dance (**AAHPERD**). The Health Education Division became the Association for the Advancement of Health Education (**AAHE**).

1938 ■ The American Association of School Physicians (organized in 1927) expanded to become the American School Health Association (**ASHA**). It serves school physicians, school nurses, and school health educators and publishes the *Journal of School Health.*

1950 ■ The Society of Public Health Educators (**SOPHE**) was organized. Although its primary interest is public health education, it has a secondary interest in school health.

1961 ■ The School Health Education Study (**SHES**) was one of the most comprehensive curriculum studies ever conducted. It developed a K-12 study guide.

1980 ■ The **Bureau of Health Education** was established within the Center for Disease Control in the U.S. Department of Health and Human Services. In 1980 a reorganization established a Division of Health Education within the Center of Health Promotion and Health Education.

1980 ■ Representatives of the organizations interested in health education formed a coalition in 1980. One of its tasks was the **Role Delineation Project** to determine the professional requirements for health educators.

1988 ■ The National Commission for Health Education Credentialing was established. Its purpose is to provide a **national registry for health educators.**

SCHOOL HEALTH EDUCATION AND THE FUTURE

At the 1988 annual convention of the American School Health Association, Dr. James Mason, Assistant Secretary of the U. S. Department of Health and Human Services and Director of the Center for Disease Control, urged cooperation among the various agencies concerned with health education. He suggested that improvements in the health status of Americans in the future depends to a large extent on the effectiveness of the various health education programs.

A few years ago, the American Public Health Association adopted a position paper entitled *School Health Education: A Public Health Concern* which emphasized the importance of school health education. Some of the key points of that statement are:

- A health-educated person understands the basic facts concerning health and disease, protects his own health and that of his dependents, and works to improve the health of the community.

- Health is a community affair, and the school, as an ever-present social structure for clustering public activity, provides a convenient central focus in community planning for health.

- Without improved health education, the next generation will be little better equipped to separate "the basic facts concerning health and disease" from the vast amount of misinformation and conflicting counsel that troubles the present generation. Further, the next generation will have even more complex health problems to comprehend and solve if it is to improve the health of the community.

Not only is school health education a logical adjunct of a comprehensive community health program, but one of priority. Problems that stem from misuse of drugs, health quackery, smoking, sexual promiscuity, environmental pollution, and mental illness are already being attacked in a positive fashion where quality school health education programs exist.

There must be assurance that school health education is more than a chance or incidental occurrence during a youth's most impressionable years. Health education must be a planned and systematic process conducted by professionally qualified instructors who are given the time, means, and curriculum structure to be effective in preserving our nation's greatest resource--human health.

STUDY HELPS

PART I

PERIODS OF MEDICINE HISTORY: Indicate the approximate dates.

A. PRIMITIVE MEDICINE __________
B. AMONG EARLY CIVILIZATIONS __________
C. GREEKS AND ROMANS __________
D. HEALTH IN THE MIDDLE AGES __________
E. MEDICINE DURING THE RENAISSANCE __________
F. MEDICINE AND THE AGE OF REASON __________
G. MODERN MEDICINE __________

PART II

Match the following people with the periods listed in Part I.

__ 1. Aesculapius
__ 2. Cooper
__ 3. Dickens
__ 4. Flemming
__ 5. Galen
__ 6. Galileo
__ 7. Hippocrates
__ 8. Hygeia
__ 9. Jenner
__ 10. Lister
__ 11. Morton
__ 12. Moses
__ 13. Newton
__ 14. Pasteur
__ 15. Salk
__ 16. Shattock
__ 17. Simmelweis
__ 18. Thomson
__ 19. Leeuwenhoek

PART III

Indicate the historical events related to health in the following periods.

A. China
B. Arabia
C. India
D. Peru
E. Babylon
F. Mesopotamia
G. Egypt
H. Hebrews
I. Greeks
J. Romans
K. Europeans
L. Americans

Chapter 3

THE SCHOOL HEALTH PROGRAM

A school health program is the health related activities in which a particular school participates. Some schools have very visible and elaborate programs that are administrated in a deliberate manner. Other schools, in contrast, meet only the minimal mandator requirements as unrelated and almost imperceptible occurrences. The programs very f rom state to state and community to community based local laws, perceived needs, and fiscal policies. In the 1930s the Joint School Health Committee of the American Medical Association and the American School Health Association established a three-phased integrated model for coordinating all of the schools' legal and moral responsibilities related to health. That model is still known as the School Health Program. This chapter will explore the School Health Program as a model for coordinating the health-related responsibilities of the school. It will help prospective secondary school teachers understand their future health related depending on local policies and procedures.

School Health Services

School Health Education

Healthy School Environment

> ***What is very clear is that education and health for children are inextricably intertwined.*** *A student who is not healthy. . . is not a student who will profit from the educational process. Likewise, an individual who has not been provided assistance in the shaping of healthy attitudes, beliefs, and habits early in life will be more likely to suffer the consequence of reduced productivity in later years.*
>
> Michael McGinnis, MD, Director,
> Office of Disease Prevention and Health Promotion,
> U.S. Department of Health and Human Services.

LEGAL REQUIREMENTS FOR SCHOOL HEALTH

The government has a responsibility to protect the health of the people. One way it discharges this responsibility is through the schools. The schools, as an arm of government, have the responsibility to not only protect the students while they are attending school, but also to actively promote the health of the students through the means unique to the school.

Health goals are among the goals of education because:

1. Students must be kept safe while they are in attendance at school or involved in school activities.

2. Students must remain healthy in order to take full advantage of the total school program.

3. Students must be prepared to meet their own health-related needs throughout life.

While the primary responsibility for the health of children rests with the parents, the efforts of the health professions, the governmental agencies, and other organizations within the community can utilize the school health program as a valuable medium for promoting the health of not only the students, but eventually the whole community.

THE ROLE OF GOVERNMENT

The health and educational needs of people are a concern of all forms of government. The means used to meet those needs vary depending on the political, economical, and philosophical foundations of the society. In this country, sovereignty or the right to rule rests with the individual, so long as the expression of one person's rights does not interfere with rights of another person. Often the rights of an individual in a community come in conflict with the well-being of the community as a whole. In order to moderate such conflicts, the individuals within a democratic society assign a portion of their sovereignty to the state. The state, therefore, acts in behalf of the people.

In matters pertaining to health and education, according to the Constitution of the United States, the state is sovereign. The federal government possesses only those powers that have been delegated to it by the states. Local governments also derive their power and authority from the state.

The Federal Government

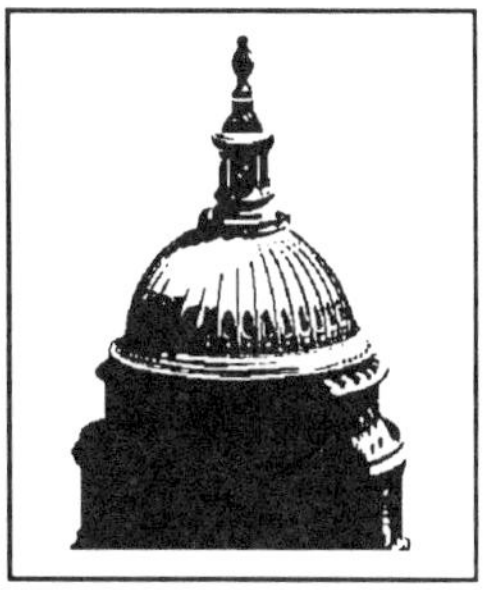

One of the hottest issues in education has been the role of the federal government. Some people favor the traditional interpretation of the Constitution; those powers not vested in the federal government remain within the jurisdiction of the separate states. Others feel however, in view of the increasing mobility of the people and based on the "general welfare," the federal government should take greater responsibility for running the schools.

The role of the federal government in providing health services has been another major issue. Some people would favor some form of comprehensive national health insurance or socialized medicine. Medicare and Medicaid are health insurance programs for the elderly and the indigent. They are examples of moves in that direction. Other people are opposed to expanding the federal involvement in what has been traditionally state, local, and individual responsibilities.

In regard to health services, at first each individual was solely responsible for finding and paying for his own health care. In time, each community and state took care of indigent individuals who were citizens of that city or state. But there was one group, the merchant seamen, who had no place to turn when they became ill or injured in a port in another state. The federal government's first involvement in providing medical care was when it started a hospital program for needy seamen. Since that time, there has been a gradual erosion of the policy of separate powers. Today approximately forty-two percent of the costs for personal health care in this country are paid for by local, state, and federal governments.

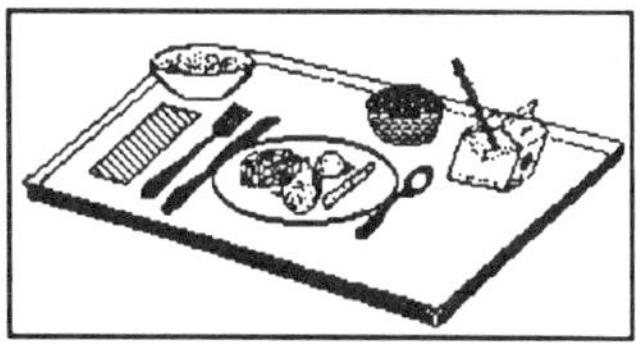

During the depression of the 1930s the federal government helped sponsor a school lunch program. The U.S. Department of Agriculture needed to get rid of the excess food it had on hand, and the school children across the nation were in need of a good school lunch. This was the first time the federal government got directly involved in education. Up to that time, the states had been reluctant to accept any federal assistance, because they were afraid this assistance would come with "strings attached." The people did not want the federal government running the local schools. The school lunch program provided federal assistance without federal control.

Since that time, the federal government has gradually expanded in control over local schools. The federal government has given more and more money to education, and the schools have become more and more dependent. One such program provides education for the handicapped ages 3 to 21. Much federal money has been given to the schools through the National Science Foundation. These programs may be good, but the concern is that too much local control of the schools may be lost. For example, a federal law called "Title Nine" was intended to prevent sexual discrimination in education. This law supported an important principle, but it removed the control for such matters from the local community to the office of a Washington bureau. Any schools which did not comply with the law would not be eligible for federal funding.

Nevertheless, the role of the federal government in education is primarily that of an informational resource service. The United States Department of Education conducts surveys and gathers information, so that the effectiveness of various programs can be analyzed and compared. It attempts to stimulate and assist state and communities with the development of local educational resources.

The U.S. Public Health Service (PHS) is a part of the U.S. Department of Health and Human Services (HHS). The Public Health Service is charged by law to promote and to assure the highest level of health attainable for every person in the United States. Its major functions are to promote the nation's health, control communicable disease, improve the delivery of health services, supervise the distribution of drugs and other potentially dangerous products, conduct and support health research, and assist the states in the development of local health resources.

There are six main operating agencies within the PHS:

Center for Disease Control
Food and Drug Administration
Health Resources Administration
Health Services Administration
National Institutes of Health
Alcohol, Drug Abuse, and Mental Health Administration

International Services

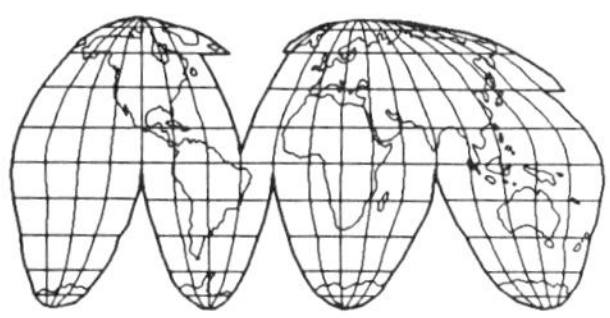

In some parts of the world, international agencies play an important role in promoting health and education. The United Nations Educational, Scientific, and Cultural Organization (UNESCO) encourages educational, cultural, and scientific programs to increase understanding among nations. The World Health Organization (WHO) is the principal agency for dealing with world health problems. WHO's Western Regional Office is the Pan-American Health Organization (PAHO) located in Washington, D.C. Such organizations provide technical assistance to member nations in need of such services. They coordinate programs and encourage member nations to help each other. They collect and disseminate statistical data concerning education and disease prevention.

States

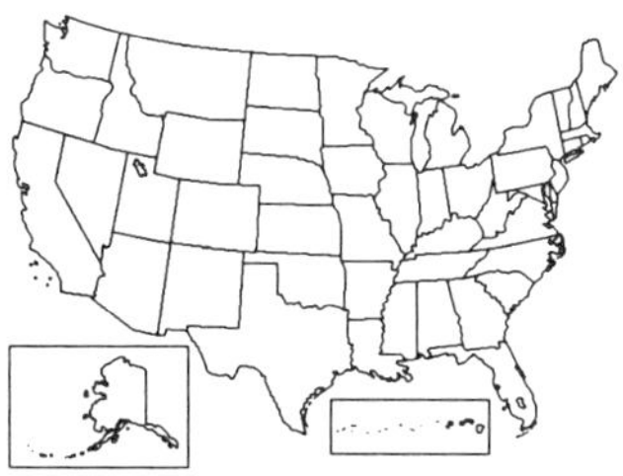

Sovereignty, or ultimate authority rests with the people. The legal basis for the school health program rests with the state legislatures and the laws they pass. Some regulations are in the form of permissive legislation which encourages or permits local schools to follow certain practices. Other laws are mandatory and require local schools to comply with state standards. Failure to comply within a specified time period would disqualify the local school district from receiving certain types of financial aid. For example, in one state the law may be permissive in nature and simply make it possible for a local school to use public school funds to sponsor a certain program. In another state, the law may require the local schools to provide that program.

Most frequently the laws as passed by the state legislature are phrased using *general* terminology. The *specific* interpretation of the laws is delegated to the state Department of Education or the state Department of Health and their respective boards. For example, the state law may require students to receive health instruction on the secondary level, but the specifics such as how many hours of instruction, on what topics, and on what grade level will be left to the state board of education.

Laws and regulations pertaining to school health may involve a dual responsibility. That is, both the State Department of Health and the State Department of Education (or whatever name such departments go by in a particular state) may be involved in making decisions about school health programs.

State boards of education and boards of health represent the people of the state. In some states they are elected, and in other states they are appointed by the governor. Their job is to administer the laws of the state and to make policy as the laws permit. The respective boards direct the activities of the Department of Health and the Department of Education. The boards hire professional administrators to run the departments. The state superintendent of schools is usually a professional educator with a graduate degree and years of experience in educational administration. The state health director is usually a medical doctor with an advanced degree in public health administration. Professional and clerical staff members are hired to do the work of the departments. In practice, the administrators make recommendations to the boards, but the boards are the decision-making bodies.

Local Boards

The local school district is governed by a board elected by the people in the district. The school board hires a superintendent and a staff to run the district. The county or city elects a board of health to govern the health department. The board of health hires a director and a staff to run the local health department. The superintendent or director and the respective staff members may propose programs, but only the board-approved plans and programs have official status. In matters pertaining to school health, there is a close relationship between the board of health and board of education. A good example is the relationship between the school nurse and the county health department. Another example is cooperation in maintaining a safe and sanitary environment within the school.

The members, local boards, and their respective staff members have the responsibility of carrying out the laws passed by the state legislature and the regulations adopted by the state boards. The specific laws and regulations vary from state to state, but examples of areas where they may apply include student health examinations, immunizations, school attendance, exclusion and readmission procedures for communicable disease control, health education requirements, health requirements for student athletes, and health requirements for teachers and other school personnel. Because of permissive legislation and regulations,

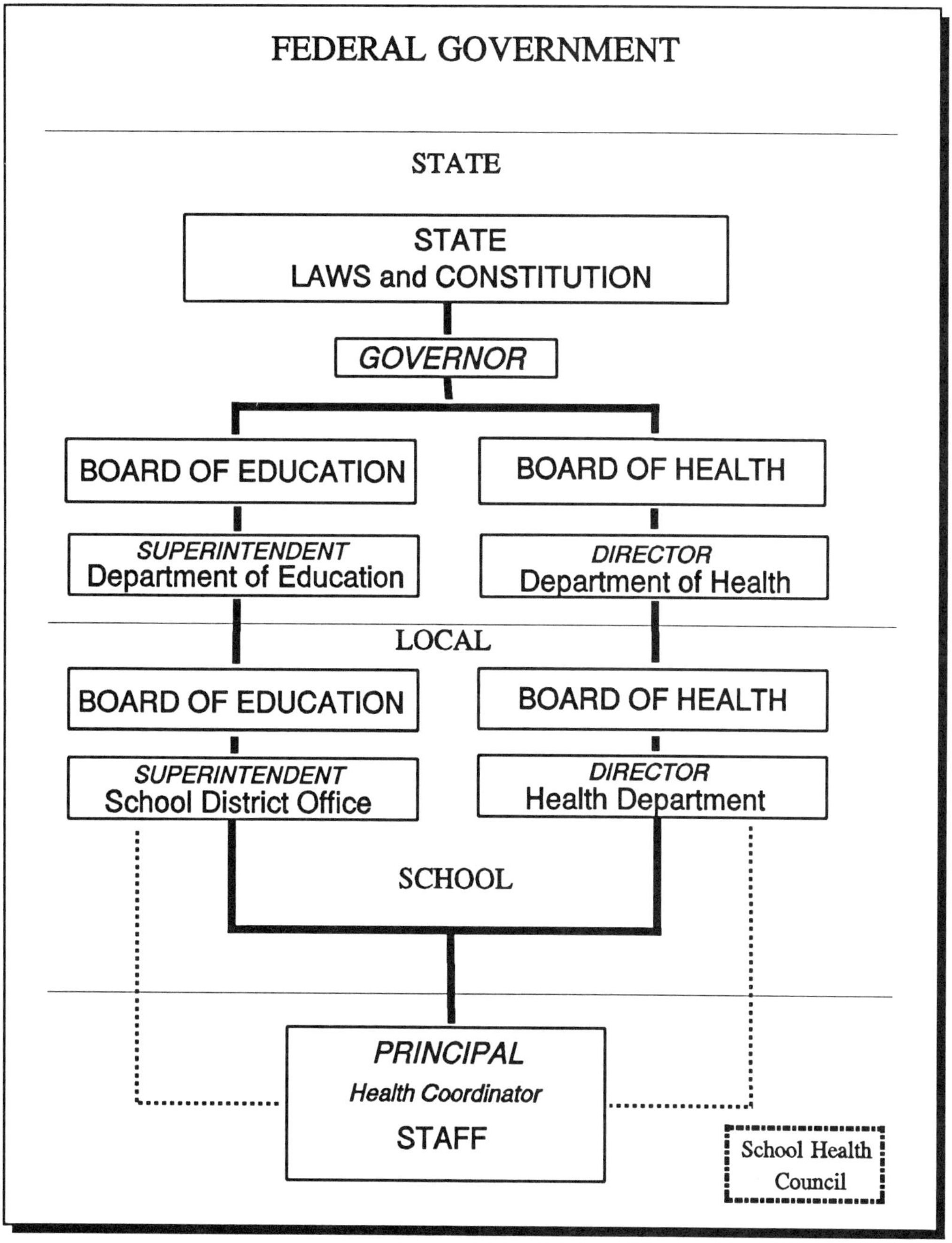
FEDERAL GOVERNMENT
STATE
STATE
LAWS and CONSTITUTION
GOVERNOR
BOARD OF EDUCATION
BOARD OF HEALTH
SUPERINTENDENT
Department of Education
DIRECTOR
Department of Health
LOCAL
BOARD OF EDUCATION
BOARD OF HEALTH
SUPERINTENDENT
School District Office
DIRECTOR
Health Department
SCHOOL
PRINCIPAL
Health Coordinator
STAFF
School Health
Council

there is still considerable opportunity for policy-making and program implementation on a local school level.

Occasionally, one policy seems to come in conflict with another policy. Or, a state regulation may appear to be in conflict with the course that seems to be in the best interest of the local schools or the students within the schools. For example, state attendance policies may be in conflict with what is in the best interest of students who are sick and ought not to be in school. If schools are funded by the state on an Average Daily Attendance (ADA) basis, the schools are motivated to follow questionable attendance policies.

The principal as the school's chief administrator has the primary responsibility for the school health program within the school. If the principal is wise, he or she will make good use of a school health council and a health coordinator to carry out the details of the program. Chapter 4 will provide more details about the school health program and the roles of various people within the school system.

SCHOOL LAWS

A review of state laws concerning school health reveals laws on the following topics:

PHYSICAL AND MENTAL QUALIFICATIONS OF TEACHERS: Some state require pre-employment medical examinations and hearing tests and to be free from physical and psychological disqualifications. The references from college professors, student teaching supervisors, and cooperating teachers as well as interviewers by school officials are used to evaluate the mental health.

HEALTH EDUCATION REQUIREMENTS OF ALL TEACHERS: Certification requirements in some states include a health course. Other states require a health class with specific content areas -- that may be the reason you are reading this book.

TEACHERS DUTY TO OBSERVE STUDENTS' HEALTH: Some state laws indicate that teachers must observe their students for possible health problems.

RELATIONSHIPS WITH LOCAL HEALTH DEPARTMENTS: The responsibility for detecting and correcting safety and sanitation problems may be specified in state laws.

HEALTH SUBJECTS TO BE TAUGHT IN PUBLIC SCHOOLS: Specific health education topics may be listed, for examples: alcohol tobacco and other drugs; sanitation and the cause of disease; safety; and the promotion of qualities of character, honesty, courtesy, respect for the law, and the dignity of honest labor.

COMMON LAW

In addition to the many state laws related to school health, the common law should also be recognized. The common law is a body of standards observed by judges in deciding cases not specifically covered by laws. The common law emerged after many judges decided the same questions in the same way. The decisions reflected what the judges felt most people would think was right. One example of a common law affecting the schools is *in loco parentis* which means *in the place of the parents.* This common law gives the school and teacher the responsibility to do what the parent would normally do if he were present.

Civil laws affecting negligence and liability are also a concern of the schools, the teachers, and other school personnel. The teacher has the responsibility to act as a normal, responsible, and prudent parent would under similar circumstances. A teacher may be found negligent if his or her action, or failure to act, contributes to a student's personal injury. This topic will be discussed in greater detail in lesson 17.

The main concept of this lesson is that laws both permit and mandate certain health-related activities in the school. These activities have become known as the School Health Program. School teachers are involved in these health-related activities daily.

THE SCHOOL HEALTH PROGRAM

Around the turn of the century when public schools became mandatory and attendance became compulsory, the need for programs related to health in the schools became obvious. When groups of children were brought together in cramped quarters, programs were needed to prevent and control communicable disease. The efforts of physicians and nurses to identify and exclude from school those students in danger of infecting others gave birth to the School Health Program.

During the next several decades, our society evolved rapidly. The schools and the students changed, and so have the health problems. In the early 1900s, the major cause of illness and death were pathogens; today the major cause is behavior. The focus of school has changed, but it is still needed, perhaps more than ever.

In the 1930s the Joint School Health Committee of the American Medical Association and the American School Health Association established a three-phased integrated model for coordinating all of the schools' legal and moral responsibilities related to health. That model was the School Health Program. The three phases of the program are health services, health environment, and health education. The Joint Committee published a full sized textbook on each of the three phases. The School Health Program has also been discussed in numerous textbooks, pamphlets, and journals. The *Journal of School Health* published a special issue in December 1987, explaining in detail "The Comprehensive School Health Program." This lesson deals with that model.

Every school has a school health program, at least they do some of the things incorporated into the model. If you were to ask a teacher in a certain school to tell you about the school health program in his school he might say,"I'm sorry. We don't have a school health program". But then, if you were to ask him if his school has a health class, if the buildings and cafeteria are checked for safety and sanitation, if the students are required to have immunizations, (all state requirements), he would answer, "yes." Then you could respond, "You have a school health program." All of those things and many more are part of a school health program. In a particular school, the school health program might not be as organized, as coordinated, as well understood, as well promoted, as it could be; but every school has one.

Schools can do much, perhaps more than any single social agency other than the home, to help young people now--and the adults they will later become--to live healthier, more productive lives. A modern comprehensive School Health Program is the best means of reaching this objective. Such a program includes a school health services component, a school health education component, and a school health environment component.

SCHOOL HEALTH PROGRAM		
SERVICES	**EDUCATION**	**ENVIRONMENT**
APPRAISAL Observation Screening Examinations	H. CLASS	PHYSICAL
RECORDS	INCIDENTAL	EMOTIONAL
COUNSELING		
PREVENTION		
REMEDIAL	Special Programs	Student Behavior
FIRST AID		
Physical Education School Food Services School Counseling		

The *school health services* component promotes the health of students and staff through prevention, identification, intervention, and remediation of specific health problems. Health services provides for first aid for injuries and sudden illness and provides direct health services for handicapped students. Health services should provide health counseling for students, faculty, and staff. Health services are usually coordinated by a professionally prepared school nurse, but includes professional services by physicians, dentists, social workers, psychologists, and speech pathologists. Teacher observation as a means of detecting possible health problems is also an important part of school health services.

The *school health education* component comprises a planned sequential kindergarten thorough twelfth grade health curriculum that addresses the physical, social, emotional, intellectual, and spiritual (moral) dimensions of health. Health education should be provided by a professionally prepared health educator. Health education should be integrated with the other components of the school health program to maximize the opportunities for students to develop and demonstrate increased health knowledge, attitudes, skills, and practices. Every teacher has opportunities to augment the formal health education.

The *school health environment* includes the physical surroundings and the psychological climate in which the students and school personnel study and work. Factors that contribute to the physical environment include the buildings and the surrounding area, biological and chemical agents that may be a threat to health, and physical conditions such as temperature, humidity, lighting, and noise. Psychological factors include emotional and social conditions that affect the well-being and productivity of students and school personnel. The personality traits of teachers, administrators, and other school personnel set a tone for the psychological climate. The school environment is created by combined physical, emotional, and social factors.

The School Health Program is a team effort. The team includes all school personnel--some more than others--but every teacher, administrator, counselor, secretary, resource worker, custodian, bus driver, food service worker, and even every volunteer contribute to the School Health Program. Many school activities have health-related benefits. An effective school health program coordinates the various activities within the school related to health.

Physical education and health education share mutual goals. The physical education class and facilities can serve as a means for developing and maintaining cardiovascular fitness, improving motor performance, providing relief from stress, and providing self-expression and social development.

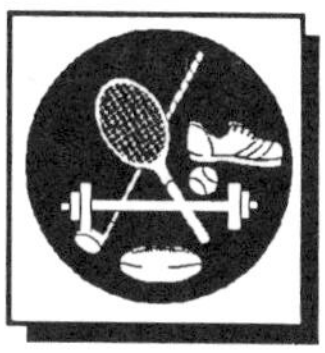

School food services and health education also share some common goals. In addition to serving lunch and breakfast every day (27 million and 3 million respectively), the nation's school food service programs support a nutrition education program. Collaboration between health education and food services can result in a learning experience with practical application.

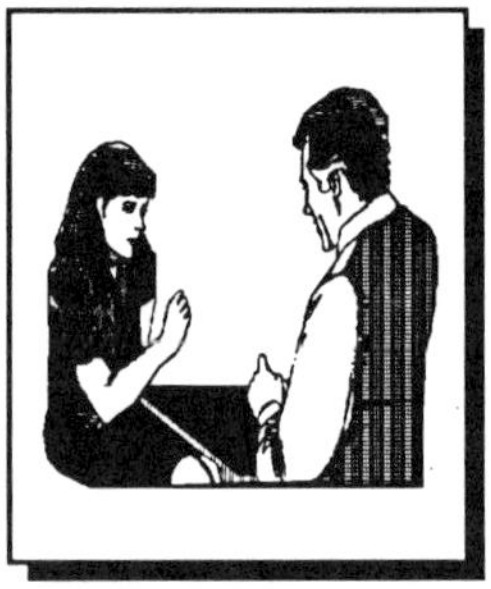

School counseling programs do much more today than provide vocational guidance, as was their original purpose. They provide guidance and intervention programs to promote physical and emotional health. School counseling tries to do for individual students what health education tries to do for the health class. In fact, all teachers and other school personnel try in a limited way to help students develop more self-esteem, become more self-assertive, become more skilled at problem solving, become more adept at dealing with peer pressure, and become more inclined to exercise self-control. School counselors and psychologists can make significant contributions to the School Health Program.

The team even extends beyond the school to parents, community leaders, health workers, health professionals, and others interested in the success of education and the well-being of children and youth. The need for an integrated school and community approach is indisputable. The nature of health problems today makes it necessary for collaboration between health and education professions and coalitions among agencies promoting health. Qualified community representatives are needed to serve on health advisory councils and can help facilitate specific health programs.

SCHOOL HEALTH SERVICES

In the beginning, the role of school health services was well-defined to control infection. In time, many other tasks were added so that today its role is harder to define. School health services are not uniform throughout the nation's schools, they vary from state to state. For example, by law only half of the states require the schools to maintain a health service facility. Although only fifteen states mandate a recorded health history for each student, it is a common practice. A few states mandate a specific nurse to student ratio. Some states require school employees to have routine immunizations, screening tests, and annual physical examinations.

The school's primary purpose is to teach. School health services, whose emphasis is prevention, detection, and referral of health problems, support the process of education. Emergency care in case of injury or sudden illness is also provided. Schools provide rehabilitative services for some students with disabilities and handicaps and maintain student health records. The schools should maintain a health suite that includes an office for the school nurse.

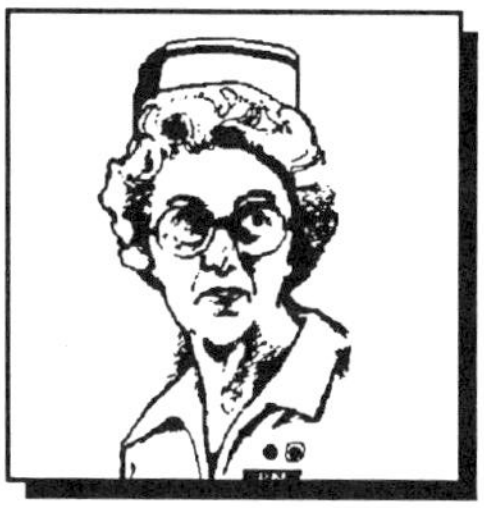

The school nurse is the key person in school health services. Most school nurses are registered nurses (RN) with a baccalaureate degree. Some school nurse practitioners (SNP) have advanced training beyond the RN. The nurse maintains the records, supervises screening tests, provides health counseling, makes medical referrals, and serves as a consultant. The nurse must be able to identify and deal with a variety of minor and occasionally major medical problems. Some minor problems she is able to deal with directly; most problems are dealt with by referral. School personnel depend on the nurse to answer health-related questions. Required examinations, screening tests, and health observations may detect potential health problems among the students. With the help of observant teachers, counselors, and administrators, the nurse is able to recognize and refer students with possible health problems.

Most schools operate under the philosophy that the parent is the primary provider of health services. School health services should play a supplemental role to the parent and personal physician. The nurse's role is to serve as a facilitator. Some school districts employ physicians on a full-time or part-time basis. School physicians may provide direct health services in the schools, but more frequently they serve as managers of the district school health services or as consultants to the school administration.

HEALTH APPRAISAL

Health appraisal is that part of school health services that attempts to evaluate the health of students and sometimes school personnel. The purpose of the evaluation is to detect potential health problems so that steps can be taken to prevent or alleviate any problem that might impinge on the educational process. Health examinations, screening tests, and observations are used to make health appraisals.

Health Examinations

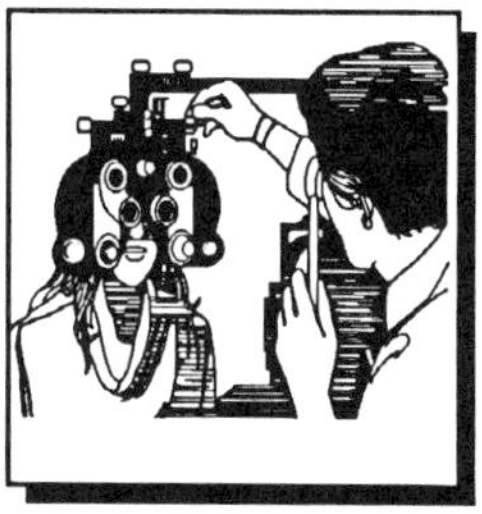

Although health or medical examinations are required by most schools, their frequency and thoroughness vary. Typically, an exam is required before a student enters elementary and secondary school and before participating in athletic events. Usually, the student takes a form supplied by the district to that student's personal physician who will perform the examination and fill out the form, and the student will return the form to the school. Thirty-nine percent of the states require sports physicals, and thirty-three percent of the states require health examinations for other students. Many school districts require health examinations even when they are not required by the state. Eighteen percent of the states require health histories to be taken and filed with the health records.

Screening Tests

Screening tests are a tool for detecting possible health problems among a large group of people. The results are far from conclusive, but they may detect situations that should be referred for a more complete examination. Schools conduct screening tests on a routine basis or in special situations. Some screening tests are conducted by the school nurse, some are conducted by volunteers, and some by teachers. Teachers should be familiar with the screening tests used in the schools and in some cases be prepared to help administer the test. The most frequent screening test is for hearing, sixty-one percent of the states require it. Other required screening tests in some states in descending order are: vision (57%), scoliosis (33%), dental (20%), tuberculosis (18%), speech (16%), height and weight (10%), sickle cell (6%), blood pressure (4%), and lead poisoning (4%). However, many school districts require screening tests even though the state does not require them.

Health Observation

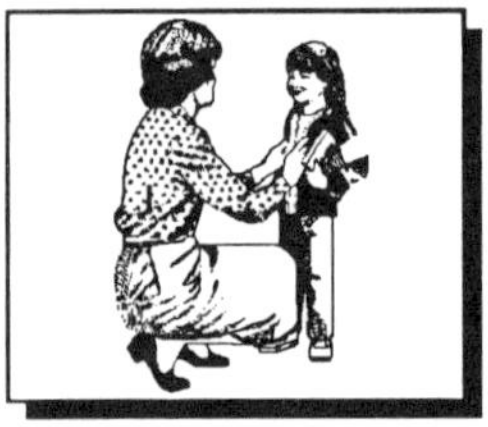

Health observation is an important part of the school health appraisal. Every teacher should carefully observe his or her students for possible departures from normal health. Teachers are not professional health workers, but they should be able to detect possible health problems and make a referral according to the school policies. In some districts, the teacher makes the referral directly to the parent, in some cases to the school administration, but usually to the school nurse. Teachers should try to improve their health observation skills. If a teacher notices that a student may have a health problem, the teacher should refer the possible problem to the school nurse. The nurse should check the student, and if the possibility of a problem is substantiated, the nurse should make a referral to the child's parent or physician or both. The nurse should also do a follow-up to make sure the potential problem was dealt with appropriately. The teacher should also check back with the nurse to get the results of the referral.

HEALTH RECORDS

The school nurse is in charge of maintaining the students' health records. Sometimes the health records may be kept in the main school office in the students' academic file, but it is preferable to have a separate file for health records in the health suite. The file should contain the health examination forms, immunization records, emergency information, and appropriate annotations. The emergency information would include parents' (or guardians') home address and phone number, parents' working address and phone number, the name and phone number of the student's personal physician, the name and phone number of someone to contact in case the parent cannot be reached, and appropriate comments.

REMEDIAL PROGRAMS

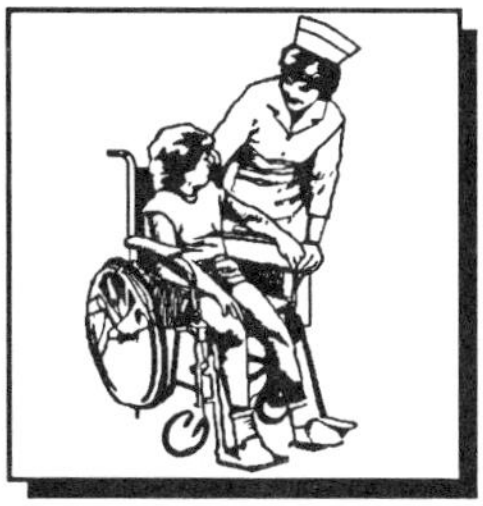

Many schools operate remedial or rehabilitation programs for students with special needs or handicaps. Although these programs may not operate directly under school health services, they frequently require close coordination with the school nurse and other personnel involved. The remedial programs and the regular school programs may be complementary, particularly if a student is part time in both programs. Examples of remedial programs include speech and hearing therapy, adaptive physical education, and special education. The school should be able to provide remedial programs for one or more students with learning disabilities or orthopedic handicaps. Remedial programs should operate under the premise that the program is not to isolate these special students, but to prepare them to return to and profit from regular school activities.

HEALTH COUNSELING

Health counseling is available to students on a number of levels. Professional counseling is available from guidance counselors and the school nurse. Students may also seek counsel or advice from less formal sources such as the regular classroom teacher. Discretion must be exercised by all counselors, but especially by informal counselors. Teachers should not get into situations that are beyond their level of expertise nor into topics that are inappropriate because of legal or moral complications. Yet within these limitations and because of special confidence-developing circumstances, a teacher acting as an informal counselor may be in a position to do much good. Often the best approach is to help bridge the gap between the student and another person better prepared to provide the needed help.

EMERGENCY CARE

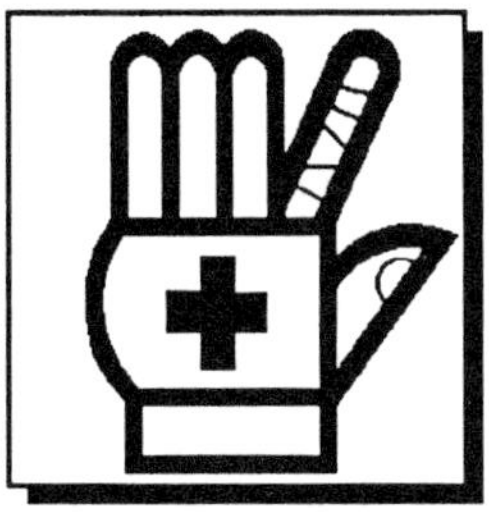

Through the school health services, the school should be prepared to render emergency care in case of an injury or sudden illness. If the school nurse is available, that may be the best source of emergency care, or other arrangements must be made in advance. Emergency care should be delivered according to school policy, not by what seems to be common sense at the moment. Contingency plans for all anticipated emergencies should be made in advance. The plans should be in writing, approved by the school board, and available to all school personnel. Equipment and supplies must be readily available. Student emergency information in the health records must also be accessible.

PREVENTION

Prevention is the primary goal of school health services, and it permeates all components of the School Health Program. Required immunizations and exclusion policies are intended to help prevent communicable diseases. Safety measures are initiated to prevent accidents. Interpersonal relationships that might produce emotional injury are discouraged. Health appraisals are conducted to detect possible health problems early to prevent complications. Care goes into the construction and maintenance of the physical facilities so that environmental problems can be prevented. Prevention is the main purpose of health education and counseling.

ENVIRONMENTAL HEALTH

There are two parts of the school health environment, the physical and the psychological. Buildings and grounds are part of the physical environment. Interpersonal relationships are part of the psychological environment. Sometimes physical items such as decorations and seating arrangements in the classroom contribute to the psychological environment. The concern about the environment is that it is safe and conducive to effective learning.

PHYSICAL ENVIRONMENT

The school district and the Public Health Department are partners in providing a safe and healthful environment. Environmental health is a field of knowledge which enables people to control those factors in the physical environment which may exercise a detrimental effect on health. Environmental health is concerned with the effect of environmental hazards on the quality of human life. Environmental hazards in the school setting include school site location as well as chemical and physical hazards.

Good planning is important in school site selection and building construction, but conditions that were once considered to be safe may be proven hazardous when new information is discovered. One example is school buildings constructed on tailings from mining milling operations. Another more wide-spread example is the asbestos insulation possibly found in over thirty thousands schools. Two federal agencies concerned about environment (including but not limited to schools) are the Environmental Protection Agency (EPA) and the Occupational Safety and Health Administration (OSHA). State and local health departments have personnel with expertise on environmental hazards. Within the school setting potential chemical hazards exist in science laboratories, art studios, industrial arts laboratories, swimming pools, custodial closets, and the parts of the physical plant. Physical hazards such as temperature and humidity, radiation, mechanical vibration, noise, light sources, and atmospheric pressure may cause disease, disability, or death.

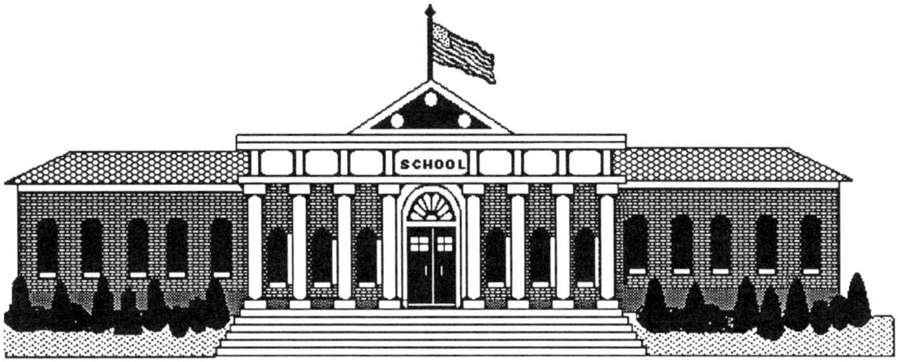

Temperature and humidity are important factors contributing to human performance and in extreme cases may lead to serious health problems. Deaths have resulted from heat-related factors on the athletic field. Thermal comfort within the school environment depends on controlling temperature, humidity, and air movement.

Noise or unwanted sound affects humans both physically and psychologically. Increasing levels of noise may interfere with study and communications, may alter human physiological performance, and may cause hearing loss. To be comfortable in a learning environment, the sound level should not exceed 50 decibels, but some studies have shown that classroom sound levels average 59 to 65 decibels (db). The thresholds for hearing damage are a combination of decibels and time. Exposure to 80 db for sixteen hours, 85 db for eight hours, 90 db for four hours, or 110 db for one-fourth hour could result in hearing loss. Exposure to these high levels of noise could be associated with some school activities. For example, a joiner in a wood shop may produce 96 db and a router 110 db. School administrators and teachers can control noise levels and require ear plugs at school, but they can only counsel students about noise levels outside of school. Rock and country music bands are frequently measured at 110 db.

Lighting systems should be designed to provide the sufficient footcandles of light for proper performance at visual tasks. Other lighting factors such as glare, direction, diffusion, and uniformity affect one's ability to see easily, accurately, and quickly.

The environment also includes potential for injuries. One study reported that within a year there were 6 million injuries to students and adults in and around schools and colleges. Another study reported that 43 percent of the accidental deaths and 57 percent of accidental injuries were associated with school life. The playground, physical education activities, and intramural and interscholastic sports contributed the most to school-associated injuries.

Achieving a healthful and safe school environment requires a team effort by all administrators, teachers, staff, students, and environmental health professionals. Inspections of the buildings and grounds should be conducted routinely. Standards that have been developed in industry also apply to shops, laboratories, food service areas, and classrooms in the school setting. Some of the standards are quite technical, but expertise in these matters is available from professionally prepared environmentalists within the local health department as well as from commercial engineering and architectural firms.

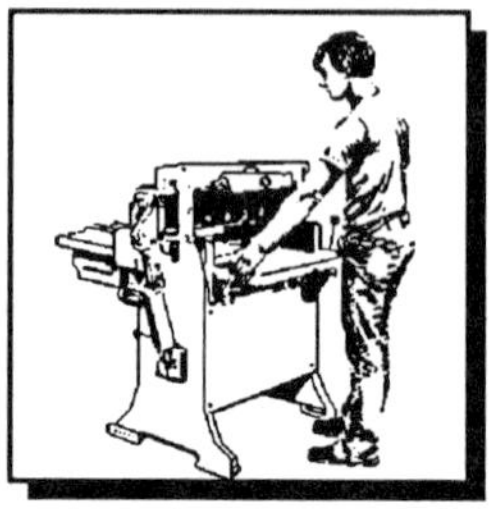

PSYCHOLOGICAL ENVIRONMENT

The psychological or emotional environment in a school reflects the well-being of faculty, staff, administration, and students. When people feel good about themselves, they promote an environment that is conducive to learning. This psychological environment is sometimes called *climate* or *atmosphere.*

Stress is a part of the climate. There are two types of stress, *eustress* which leads to productive and uplifting outcomes, and *dystress* which leads to unproductive and psychologically painful outcomes. What is desired is a school that systematically and consistently strives to promote eustress.

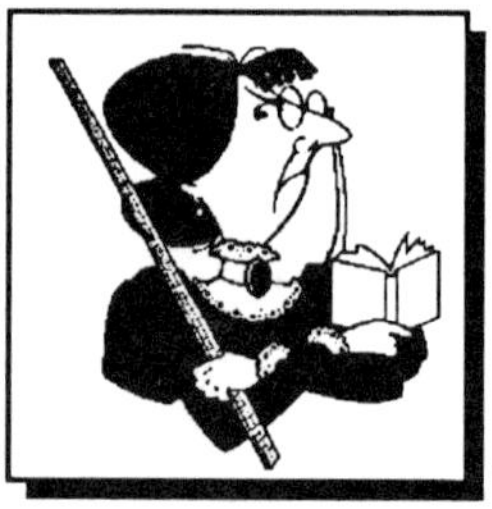

What contributes most to the climate is the quality of the interpersonal relationships. It is important for each person to engage in an open style of communication that values the worth of each participant. Communication should exhibit a spirit of trust, confidence, support, and cooperation. Principles of effective non-verbal communication skills will help develop constructive interpersonal relationships. Such skills as maintaining eye contact and actively listening contribute to a person's sense of worth and security. A healthy school environment is one which nurtures a person's basic needs for safety, belonging, love, and respect.

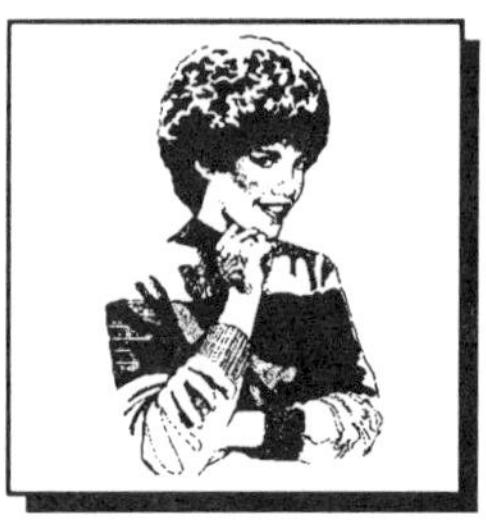

A healthy psychological environment is one where all participants strive to fully know and understand themselves. The conversation is not defensive nor repressive. The question is, can these "life skills" be taught and learned? The answer is yes. Students can learn to share, apologize, negotiate, and deal with pressures. School counselors and special education teachers can teach these skills to individuals and small groups. Effective teachers can promote this atmosphere in larger classes. First and foremost, these skills are taught by example. They can also be learned through demonstrations, discussions, and role playing. Transfer to real life situations is more apt to occur, however, when supported by numerous examples throughout the school environment. Administrative policies and practices have a strong influence on the psychological climate within the school and classroom.

Effective teaching practices can contribute to the school climate. A systematic and consistent approach will help. Daily in-class reviews and previews helps the students remain oriented. Clear presentations, demonstrations, and examples on new material helps the students develop understanding. Time for practice and opportunities for immediate feedback help the students gain confidence. Opportunities for personal application and expression help the students internalize (own) the educational experience.

Discipline in schools and classrooms is a part of the environment. A take-charge "assertive" approach with clear rules and expectations along with rewards and consequences for compliance or noncompliance has its place. It may be useful as a starting place for new teachers. It may be good for a class of difficult students, or teachers who have a problem with classroom control may resort to it. It results in more orderly behavior, but a more democratic approach may do more to promote a healthy teaching-learning climate with positive interactions. The goal is to enhance self-esteem and help students develop problem-solving skills.

Administrators, staff, and especially teachers are in a unique position to influence the emotional health of students. An effective teacher is a model of appropriate health-related behaviors that may inspire students to become more conscious of their own health. Improving the quality of life is the essence of education.

SCHOOL HEALTH EDUCATION

Health education deals with conveying a body of knowledge, cultivating a group of attitudes, and developing a cluster of skills that will result in a set of behaviors that will add quality to life. That means a comprehensive school curriculum that has a formal health class at its center, but which also includes learning from health services, learning from a healthy environment, and learning from the entire school experience. The school nurse, people in food services, the school counselors, and all teachers contribute to the informal health education. There are two levels of health education, the formal class and the informal or incidental learning experience.

COMPREHENSIVE HEALTH INSTRUCTION

Comprehensive health instruction is a planned sequence of courses from kindergarten through twelfth grade. Its content is drawn from biological and behavioral sciences. The curriculum is designed to:

- meet the developing needs of students on each grade level.
- foster physical, social, emotional, intellectual, and spiritual health.
- improve health knowledge, attitudes, and practices.
- promote health maintenance and wellness.
- develop decision-making competencies.

The health instruction areas are:

- Personal Health
- Community Health
- Family Life
- Growth and Development
- Mental Health
- Stress Control
- Interpersonal Relationships
- Drug Use and Abuse
- Alcohol and Tobacco
- Nutritional Health
- Weight Control
- Exercise and Fitness
- Chronic Disease Control
- Infectious Disease Control
- Aging and Death Education
- Consumer Health
- Environmental Health
- Safety and Accident Prevention

INCIDENTAL LEARNING EXPERIENCES

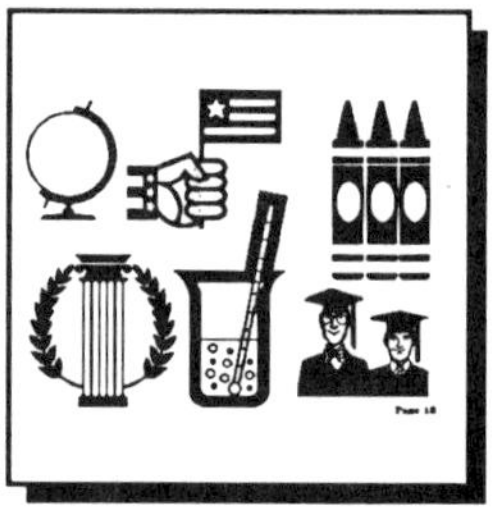

Not every teacher is assigned to teach a health class, but every teacher is a health educator. First, every teacher teaches by example, either a good example or bad example. Second, health concepts can be taught as they come up and are the topic of student interest. Taking advantage of the "teachable moments" sometimes is the most effective way to teach. Third, each teacher has the opportunity to teach health concepts as they fit naturally in his assigned subject. Practical health-related concepts can be found in every school subject. Every teacher can be a practical health educator. A practical health educator is one who has the health facts, who has intimate contact with the potential learner, and who has the ability to put the facts on the learner's level. A teacher should have the health facts, close contact with the students, and the ability to communicate the facts to the students. Every teacher should seek opportunities to teach health on an incidental basis.

CONCLUSION

This chapter should have helped you develop a general concept of the goals and functions of a typical school health program and a more specific understanding of the teacher's role in the program.

The school health program in a given school is whatever that school does to meet its legal and moral responsibilities relating to health. In some school districts, the school health-related activities take place under the coordinated umbrella of a school health program. In other districts, some of the same activities take place in a more haphazard manner. In some districts, the program is very informal; in others, it is very elaborate. Yet whatever a school does in regard to health is that school's health program. Teachers need to be prepared to fill their health-related responsibilities in their school's health program, no matter how modest or complex it might be. They may also use their influence to enhance the program.

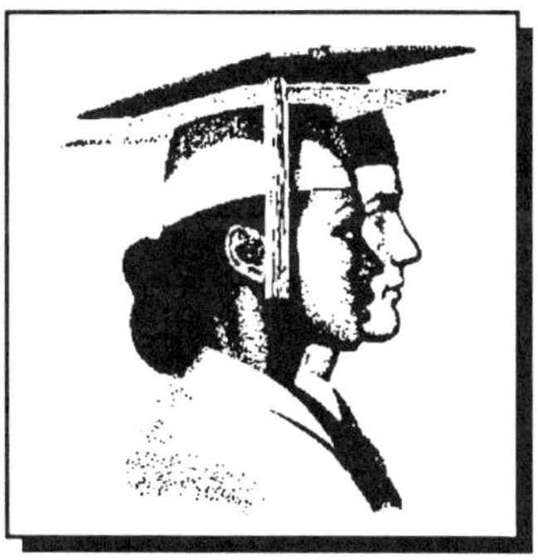

STUDY HELPS

Tell how each of the following school positions can contribute to the school health program.

Staff & Administration
principal
counselor
secretary
resource worker
custodian
bus driver
food service worker
school nurse

Subject Area Teachers
Biological Sciences
Physical Sciences
Social Sciences
Computer Science
Home Economics Ed.
Drivers Education
Physical Education
Health Education
English & Language
Mathematics
Business & Economics
Art & Crafts
Choral & Instrumental Music
Shop & Industrial Arts
Speech & Dramatic Arts

Indicate how each of the following fit into the School Health Program. Also indicate who might be responsible for that phase of the program.

class room atmosphere
chemical hazards
communication
comprehensive health instruction
curriculum (K-12)
decibels
class room discipline
emergency care
environmental health
EPA
health services
health observation
health records
health examinations
health appraisal
health education class
health counseling
health practices
incidental learning
interpersonal relationships
joint committee
life skills
model program
OSHA
physical environment
physical education
psychological environment
remedial programs
school health team
school policies
school food services
school counseling
screening tests
teachable moments

Pay particular attention to the following terms, organizations, etc.

international government
state government
federal government
local government
sovereignty
federal vs. local control
lunch program
Title Nine
permissive legislation
mandatory legislation
general terminology
specific interpretation
common law
in loco parentis
department of health
department of education
boards of education
boards of health
superintendent of schools
health coordinator
health director
school health council
principal or CSA
PTSA

Lesson 4

PROBLEMS AND RESOURCES

This chapter will continue to discuss the organization and operation of the school health program, but first, it will look at some of the health problems experienced by young people. Most of these problems will be considered more extensively in the three remaining units of this course. Then the various resources that might be used to help solve the problems will be discussed. Finally, the discuss lead to the importance of school health policies.

HEALTH PROBLEMS OF ADOLESCENTS

If we look at death rates among adolescents, we would find that accidents and acts of violence are the leading cause of death. Nearly half (48%) of all deaths in this age group are due to accidents. Suicide is usually the second leading cause of death among the youth of this country. It is not uncommon for homicide to rank third. This indicates that many of the health problems of youth are associated with their emotional and social needs.

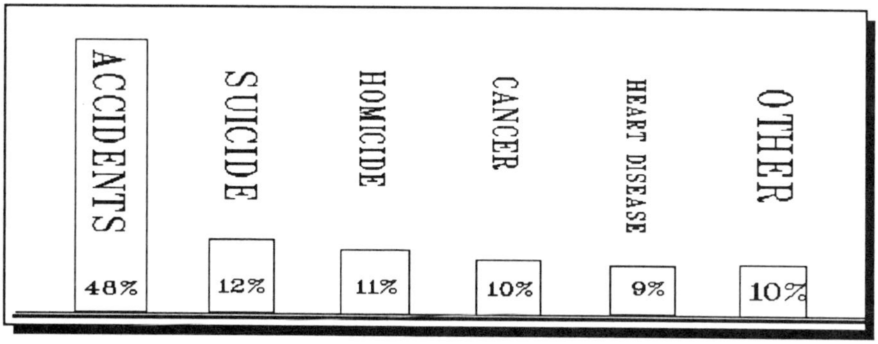

To keep thease figures in perspective we must realize that adolescents are, in some ways, the healthiest group in our society. From the point of view of mortality, the death rate for the high school age group is far less than the general population and considerably less than any other age group. The death rate for the general population is approximately 9.5 per one thousand population, but for teenagers the death rate is only about 1.6 per one thousand population. In spite of their favorable mortality statistics, teenagers have many existing health problems, and their lifestyles may result in more extensive health problems in the future. Many health problems of adolescents are the result of neglected health needs.

The death rate is higher in the childhood years than in adolescence because inherent physical weaknesses and congenital defects take their toll earlier. Furthermore, teenagers rarely have degenerative diseases which occur with increasing frequency later in life. Teenagers are capable of withstanding diseases that are more frequently fatal to the very old and young. Although death rates are an inaccurate index of the health needs of adolescents, they do indicate some problems.

When morbidity or illness rates are used as an index of health needs, we find that teenagers, like other segments of the population, suffer most frequently from the common cold and influenza. Dental health is also a frequent problem. Other typical health problems of adolescents are acne or skin problems, which are partially caused by and contribute to emotional problems; gastrointestinal disorders, which are frequently symptoms of emotional problems; and mental health problems. Being overweight and having other eating disorders are associated with extreme emotional problems. The sexually transmitted disease gonorrhea is the most frequently reportable communicable disease in this country, and the incidence of chlamydia, a non-reportable communicable disease, is even more frequent. The promiscuous behavior that spreads these epidemic diseases is also associated with emotional, social, and moral problems.

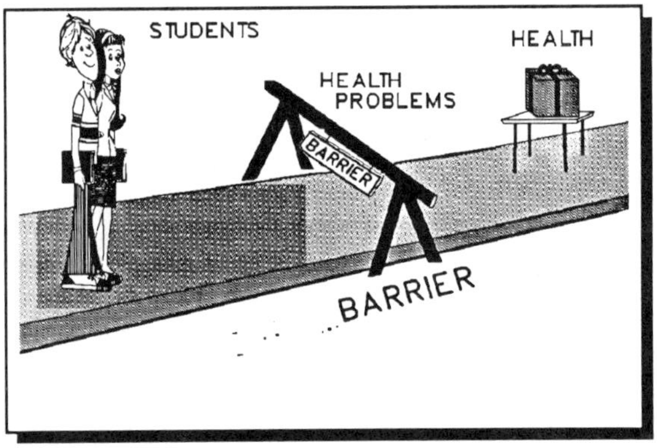

Good health is a **PRODUCT**. The members of a community are the **RECIPIENTS** of the product. Health problems or **BARRIERS** prevent the community from receiving the product. **HEALTH WORKERS** in the community try to remove the barriers so that the recipients can enjoy the benefits of good health, but before they can be removed, the barriers must be identified.

Another aspect of health problems among adolescents is the consequences of their chronic poor health practices. While they may not recognize any immediate effects of poor nutrition, inadequate sleep, and other detrimental practices, these practices will emerge in poor health conditions later in life, after it is too late to do much about it. Although teenagers may not be sick, they may be doing things that will eventually lead to illness.

RECOGNIZING HEALTH PROBLEMS

Identifying health problems is not always easy. What appears to be the problem may not be the real problem, or there may be problems present but not recognized. Many health problems can be compared to an iceberg; often what appears to be the problem is merely a symptom of a deeper and larger underlying problem. For example, some people may view drug abuse as the problem, but others may view drug abuse as a symptom of a larger underlying problem called poor self-esteem. A teacher may not be in a position to deal with the symptoms directly, but a teacher can do much to help students develop a better self-concept. A given symptom may result from one of a number of different basic problems. Also, a basic problem may be manifest by a variety of symptoms. Therefore, it is difficult to look at an apparent illness or overt behavior and tell exactly what the underlying problem is. Problems beneath the surface are obscure.

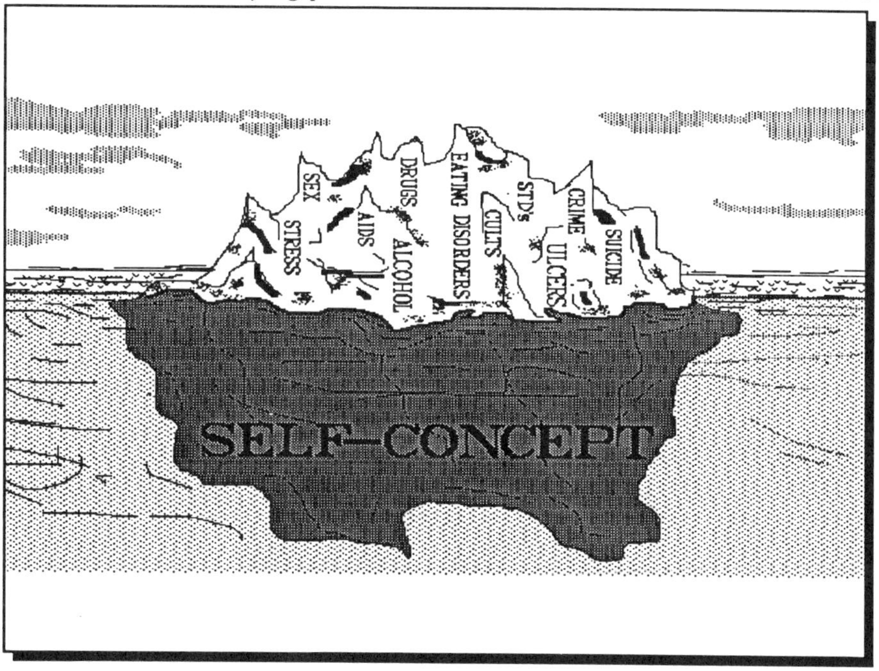

PROBLEM SOLVING SEQUENCE

When community or group action is necessary to solve problems, the process of identifying the problem is even more difficult. The following chart and accompanying discussion may help. In this concept, the word "problem" has a distinct definition. This definition is useful when community action is necessary to solve the problem.

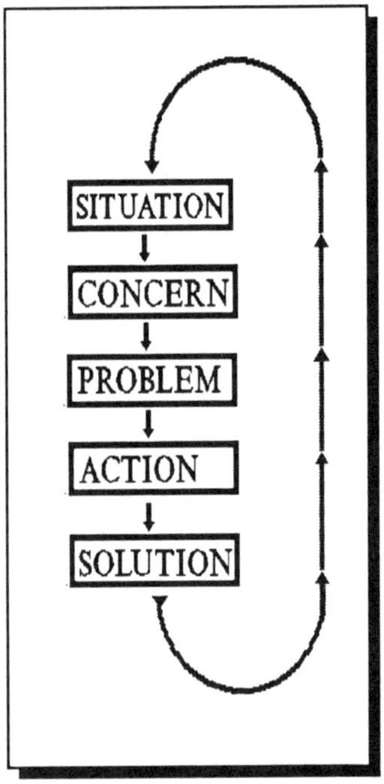

Often an undesirable situation exists without people recognizing it as a problem. The situation is taken for granted.

Then a few concerned people realize that the situation is undesirable, and it does not have to be that way. They campaign to increase public awareness.

When enough of the right people become concerned and recognize it as an undesirable situation, it becomes defined as a problem.

When the community recognizes the problem and is behind an effort to remove it, effective action will take place to try to remove the problem.

With the proper expertise and public backing, a solution will be found. After the mechanics have been established for solving one problem, attention can be focused upon another problem.

Many needless, undesirable situations around us continue, because no one recognizes that there could be a better way. Other times, a few people with social insight recognize the undesirable situation, but because they are unable to solicit the concern of enough of the right (influential) people, the situation continues. For example, for many years a few scientists talked about the dangers of air pollution. Finally, enough people became concerned, the problem was recognized, community action was generated, and some solutions are being found.

Another example of a situation is an intersection used by students on the way to school. A few parents thought it was dangerous and complained to the city, but nothing was done about it. A child from a poorer section of town was even hit by a car, but still nothing was done until the grandchild of an important leader in the community was killed. Action was taken, and a pedestrian overpass was built.

In another example, the frequency of dental cavities among the children of a community was a situation everyone took for granted. A few dentists advocated fluoridation of the water supply, and the proposition was put on the ballot. Because the community did not define the situation as a problem, it failed. A concerned school teacher assigned her English students, with the help of their parents, to write a research paper on fluoridation. The next year the proposition was again put on the ballot, and this time it passed.

A new teacher in an established school for the first time observed a situation that he thought should be changed, but upon talking to and observing other teachers, he realized the administration and faculty was not even able to recognize the situation as a problem, let alone do anything about it. There was not a mood for change, at least at that time for that situation. Since he was familiar with the process of community action, he decided to first attack a situation that they would recognize as a problem. He was successful in mustering the needed support for change, the mechanics for change were installed, and a solution was found. He had to work on their agenda first, but after the mechanics of change were in place he returned to his original agenda. He was able to get others to share in his concern about the original situation. The situation was soon recognized as a problem, appropriate action was taken, and the solution was put into place.

Most people can draw from their own experience and give examples where this problem-solving sequence has taken place. Perhaps you can recall a situation that was serving as a barrier to health until the concern of a few sensitive people caused it to be recognized as a problem and secured sufficient community backing so that appropriate action brought about a solution. Perhaps sometime in the future this problem-solving sequence will help you deal with a health problem in the school setting.

HEALTH PROBLEMS

The purpose of this unit has been to introduce the remaining three units in the course. Although there is considerable overlap, Unit 2 will deal more with problems associated with emotional health, and Unit 3 will deal more with problems associated with physical health. Unit 4 deals with health problems associated with accidents.

A recent article in the *Journal of School Health* (December 1987) provides the following statistics in a summary of the health problems of children and youth. In one study, a sample of tenth grade students in New York City showed that 16% percent of the students smoked, 28% used alcohol, 18% used other drugs, and 32% were sexually active. The article also identified accidents as the leading killer of our youth. Forty percent of all fatal automobile accidents involving youth are alcohol related. Suicide is the second leading cause of death among adolescents. Teenage pregnancy and abortion are continuing problems. Today's children are physically unfit. In addition, it is estimated that about 12% of the children in the U.S. have a chronic disease such as asthma, congenital heart disease, or diabetes which diminishes their ability to fully focus their attention on learning. Another 11% to 16% of the students are defined as handicapped due to hearing, speech, visual, orthopedic, or other health impairment, serious emotional problem, mental retardation, or a specific learning disability.

The first task of the School Health Program is to recognize the health problems of students, and the second task is to mobilize the school and community resources to help deal with the problems.

SCHOOL HEALTH RESOURCES

The School Health program should be organized in such a way as to take advantage of the resources available on the local level. Some resources already exist within the school and among the school patrons. They can be recognized as internal resources. There are also many external resources in the community that are interested in the health of children and youth.

INTERNAL RESOURCES

An effective school health program can do much to prevent health problems and to deal with existing problems. Many people and resources may need to be involved in dealing with health problems. It has to be a team effort, and each classroom teacher is a front line member of that team. Other members of the team include:

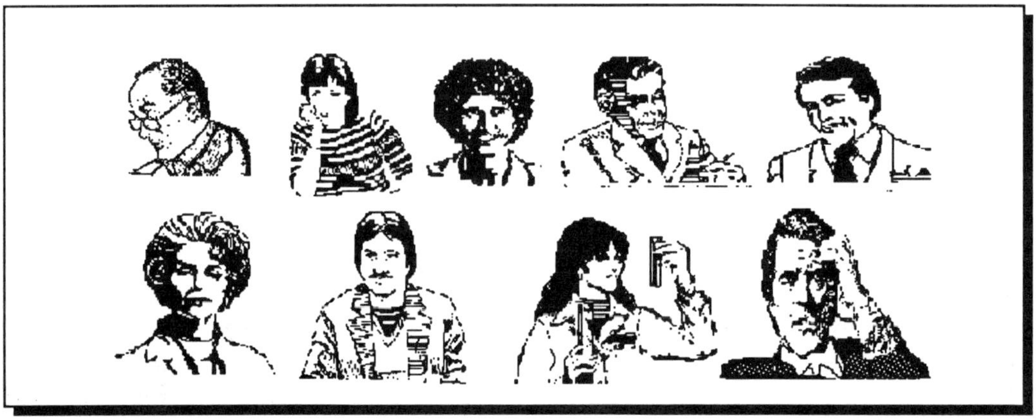

Parents

The parents have the primary responsibility for the health of their children. *The school's role is to help parents recognize and carry out their responsibility.*

School Principal

The principal is responsible for the school's health program.

- Must make sure that the school complies with the state laws and regulations and district policies.
- Initiates programs, policies, and practices to meet the needs of that particular school.
- Provides leadership to ensure that there is a sound health program, qualified personnel, adequate budget, proper facilities, and suitable support from the faculty and staff. A wise principal will appoint a school health coordinator to help carry out the details of the school's health program. He will also organize a school health council to obtain community advice and support on matters pertaining to school health.

Health Coordinator

The health coordinator, working under the direction of the principal, facilitates all phases of the health program within the school.

- Develops effective working relationships among all members of the school health team (internal resources).
- Works cooperatively with and serves as a contact person for the school district, the local health department, and other health programs and agencies in the community (external resources).
- Chairs the school health council, represents the school on the PTSA's (Parent, Teachers, and Students Association) Health and Safety Committee, or works with a health advisory board (if there is any).

School Nurse

The school nurse supervises the health services within the school.

- Receives student health referrals from teachers, administrators, counselors, and other staff members.
- Provides liaison with medical personnel, the local health department, parents, teachers, and students.
- Maintains student health records and counsels students about health problems.
- Serves as a resource to health teachers and may on occasion teach special topics in a health class.

School Staff

Office workers, resource persons, food service workers, bus drivers, custodians, and any other staff are also a part of the school health team.

- Help to make sure the school environment is sanitary, safe, and a pleasant place to live.
- Teach health concepts by example.

Guidance Counselor

School counselors are concerned with health as it relates to effective learning and social and emotional adjustments.

- Seek opportunities to counsel students on behavior and personality traits related to health.
- Recognize possible health problems and make referrals through the school nurse.

Remedial Specialists

The speech therapist and other remedial specialists often work closely with the students.

- Help students correct speech or other remedial defects, thus improving the students' self-concept.
- Counsel students about health when they have the opportunity and make referrals to the school nurse.

Physical Educator

Physical education teachers are in a unique position to influence the health of their students.

- Observe students for possible departures from normal health and make referrals to the school nurse.
- Impress on students the importance of gaining reliable health knowledge, developing desirable health attitudes, and forming appropriate health practices.
- Provide a unique opportunity through sports and dance programs to help students improve self-esteem and develop social and emotional skills as well as physical fitness.

Health Teacher

Because of their dual professional preparation in both health and education, a health educator can be a valuable person in the school health program. The health educator is responsible for the health education component of the school health program.

- Fit the health class into the district's comprehensive health education program and design it to meet the needs and interests of the students.
- Counsel students when given the opportunity about their health and related health problems.

Physician and Dentist

Members of the health professions can make valuable contributions to school health. If they are employed or retained by the district, they are considered to be an external resource.

- Play key roles as they give examinations, correct remedial problems, and encourage preventive programs. Advise the school about any special needs of their student patients.
- Provide advice on curriculum contact and support all phases of the school health program.

All Teachers

Teachers have a number of legal and professional responsibilities associated with school health.

- Observe students for possible health problems and make referrals according to school policy.
- Follow school policies in excluding from the classroom students who exhibit possible signs or symptoms of communicable disease.
- Use information on student health records to enhance their role as a teacher.
- Relate to students with handicaps or learning disabilities in a manner comparable with their needs and complementary to remedial programs.
- Respond to students' health-related questions and provide health counsel in an accurate, ethical, and appropriate manner.
- Maintain a high level of personal health and fitness to enable effective teaching, to set an appropriate example, and to avoid the spread of communicable disease.
- Provide first aid and emergency medical care as needed by students or school personnel and as indicated by school policies.
- Maintain a safe classroom environment by providing safety instructions, giving adequate warnings, and by providing proper supervision.
- Handle any incriminating information relating to students' problems in a manner prescribed by law and in accordance with school policies.
- Maintain a psychological climate in the classroom (including necessary disciplinary action) that promotes self-esteem and is conducive to learning.
- Utilize opportunities for incidental health education as related to students' needs and interests and as related to assigned subjects.
- Seek opportunities to help students develop their full potential in all dimensions.

The principal is responsible for matters pertaining to health within the school, but he or she is already so busy that health may get a low priority. He could assign several health problems and projects to an assistant administrator who handles a variety of unrelated assignments, but then again health tends to get lost in the shuffle. Often health remains a number of fragmented minor concerns rather than a coordinated program. A principal who is really concerned about health will take the suggestion made by national school health advisory organizations and appoint a health coordinator.

THE SCHOOL HEALTH COORDINATOR

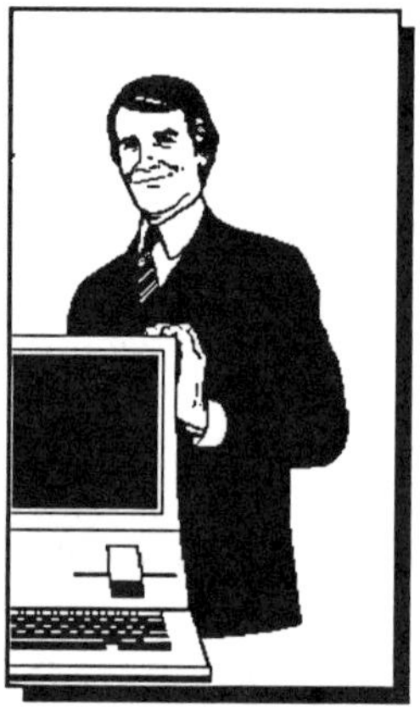

There are advantages of having a school health coordinator. This assignment has grown out of the need for better coordination of school health activities. The appointment of a coordinator can move health from multi-faceted, "haphazard," and minimal performance programs to a unified, orderly, and well-organized program that is at the heart of the school's objectives.

The health coordinator should be a faculty member with a special background, interest, and aptitude in school health, displaying diplomacy, tact, cooperativeness, and a sense of concern. The purpose of the coordinator is to see that students' school-related health needs are met. Teachers and counselors should try to discover why a student is absent or not doing well in school. If the problem is health related, some part of the school health program may be focused on the problem. One goal of the program is to help prevent disease and accidents. Another goal is to educate students in the maintenance of their own health. A number of people in the school and in the community are trying in their respective spheres to do something to help, but without coordination their efforts may be ineffectual. The function of the coordinator is to unify their actions, so that their efforts are more productive. The specific duties of the health coordinator are:

- Stimulate healthful attitudes and practices in the lives of pupils and staff by promoting a positive and dynamic health program.

- Assist the principal in the organization of a school health council.

- See that teacher observations, findings, and recommendations are transmitted to those concerned.

- See that the students' health records are maintained.

- Follow through on physicians' and specialists' recommendations with regard to the placement of pupils in special programs.
- Discuss with the attendance supervisors or registrars the health and educational factors in truancy and poor attendance.
- Cooperate with the health service staff in arrangements for health appraisals.
- Assist in developing and utilizing the health education values and opportunities inherent in the health services program.
- See that the health education subcommittee functions so that duplication and gaps in the health curriculum may be avoided.
- Arrange student health committees for active participation in the health program.

SCHOOL HEALTH COUNCIL

A principal that sees the advantages of a health coordinator may also see the benefit of a service and advisory board relating to the school's health program. Prominent national groups have recommended the use of a school health council for such purposes. A health council consists of both school and community representatives who are interested in the health of students and the School Health Program.

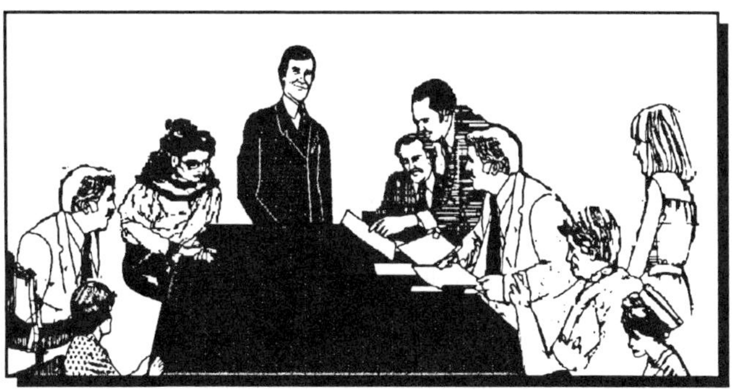

Councils are organized to take advantage of local school and community resources in meeting the health needs of students. Participants on the council drawn from the school may include representatives from the students, the faculty, administration, counselors, dean of students, chief custodian, food service manager, school nurse, and the school health coordinator. Council participants drawn from the community may include representatives from the parents, medical profession, local health department, voluntary health agencies, and business and service organizations in the community.

The council serves an advisory function at the invitation of the school administration and the board of education, and can provide voluntary service to expedite approved plans of action. It can study the needs within the school and community and suggest a course of action. When the school administration approves a plan, the council can coordinate and provide leadership and manpower for the project. When so many of the health problems involve both the school and the community, as is the case today, effective solutions must include several segments of society. National leaders are urging local cooperation, and a school health council is one way of achieving it. A school health council may be concerned with the following:

- Providing the leadership to support the total school health program and suggesting goals, standards, and policies.
- Discovering existing problems and studying the means of solving them.
- Making specific proposals or recommendations to the school administration for approval and action.
- Assisting in health screening projects, health counseling, and other health service projects for students and school staff.
- Encouraging effective student health education by making curriculum recommendations and providing instructional resources and in-service education.
- Encouraging the maintenance of a healthy school environment for students, faculty, staff, and the community.
- Coordinating the work of various agencies involved with the health of students and cooperation in the use of health resources.

<u>Examples of Possible Projects for the School Health Council</u>

- Promote the fluoridization of the community water supply.
- Encourage the addition of a dental hygienist to the school staff.

- Supervise a vision-testing program for seventh grade students.
- Make improvements in the school food services.
- Regulate student traffic and parking problems.
- Improve conduct on school busses.
- Survey health and safety instruction at all grade levels.
- Develop a plan to meet health emergencies during the school day.

COMMUNITY RESOURCES

Many organizations within the community support the School Health Program. Because an effective school health program will help these organizations reach their goals, they are anxious to provide resources to the schools. Probably no curriculum area has more community resources than does health education. A health teacher can obtain a good supply of free audio-visual aids and printed material. The following is a summary of groups within the community who are vitally interested in the health of students:

Parents. Parents are certainly concerned about the health of their children and the health programs within the school. Individually or through organizations such as Parent-Teacher-Student Associations, they can contribute to the School Health Program.

Government agencies. The laws and regulations pertaining to school health were discussed in lesson three. Government agencies also provide valuable resources to school health programs. On the federal level, the Bureau of Health Promotion in the Center for Disease Control and the Food and Drug Administration (FDA) are valuable school health resources. On the local and state levels, the health departments are directly concerned with school health programs.

Professional associations. Professional associations such as the American Medical Association (AMA), the American Dental Association (ADA), and their state and local affiliates are valuable resources. Individual doctors, nurses, dentists, dieticians, pharmacists, etc. are frequently willing to volunteer their time and skills for health service projects or instructional programs. Their advice and counsel is important to planning health programs, and their associations should be represented on the school health council. These associations also provide educational media for health instruction.

Business and industry. Representatives of business and industry also have contributions to make. Although they sometimes have a vested interest, their services are valuable.

For example, while insurance companies are promoting student health, they are also promoting the image of their company and selling policies. Also, if they can improve the health of people generally, they will have to provide fewer benefits. While the American Dairy Council is providing the schools with excellent teaching materials related to health and nutrition, they are also promoting the image of the dairy industry. Nevertheless, if used prudently, they can make a valuable contribution to the school health program.

Voluntary health agencies. A voluntary health agency uses donated time and money to combat a particular health problem or group of related health problems. For example, the American Cancer Society fights cancer, the American Heart Association fights heart disease, and the National Foundation was originally organized to fight polio, but is now working to prevent birth defects. Because health education for teenage girls is one of the best ways of preventing birth defects, the National Foundation provides valuable support for school health education. The funds collected through voluntary contributions are used to 1) conduct research, 2) provide health services, 3) promote health education, and 4) provide administrative expenses. The books, pamphlets, pictures, recordings, and personal services provided by the representatives of voluntary health agencies are valuable resources for a school health program.

Civic groups. Frequently, community-based civic and fraternal groups contribute to a school health program. For example, the Lions Club may buy eyeglasses for a student who needs glasses but can't afford to buy them. Many such groups in a community can be involved in the school health program.

Many of these resources are anxious to get their education resources and other services into the schools. A school health coordinator can serve as a contact person and can help get these materials into the hands of the health teachers and other school health personnel. A school health council may want to review these educational materials and services and facilitate their use in the schools. A teacher should be aware of the resources available in the community.

DEFINITIONS OF TERMS

1. **School health program**. School procedures that contribute to the understanding, maintenance, and improvement of the health of pupils and school personnel are the school health program. Its three divisions are health services, health education, and healthful school living.

2. **School health services**. School procedures that are established to (a) appraise the health status of pupils and school personnel; (b) counsel about findings; (c) encourage the correction of remediable defects; (d) help plan for the health care

and education of handicapped children; (e) help prevent and control disease; and (f) provide emergency care for the sick or injured.

3. Health appraisal. Phase of school health service that seeks to assess the physical, mental, emotional, and social health status of individual pupils and school personnel through such means as health histories, teacher and nurse observations, screening tests, and medical, dental, and psychological examinations.

4. Health observation. A preliminary and informal survey of students in the classroom by the teacher to detect indications of possible health problems. The teacher observes for signs of possible physical defects, abnormalities, disorders, fatigue, worry, or psychological maladjustments. The teacher also checks on the practice or avoidance of health habits. The purpose is to note any early symptoms of illness among children and refer such cases to the proper health authorities.

5. Screening tests. A formal procedure used to detect possible departures from normal health and provide a basis for referral for a professional evaluation. A screening test does not produce a diagnosis. Screening tests most frequently given in the schools are for vision, hearing, growth, and posture. They can be conducted by teachers, nurses, and trained volunteers. Under certain circumstances, screening tests such as blood tests and tuberculosis skin tests may be given by skilled technicians.

6. Health examination. That phase of health service that seeks, through an examination by physicians, dentists, and other qualified specialists, to determine the physical, mental, and emotional health of an individual.

7. Physical examination. A non-diagnostic study by a non-medical examiner to check the appearance, structure, and functional condition of a part or function of the body. The items to be investigated include those that can be seen or measured by some generally acceptable test, and the findings can be recorded as seen or measured. Blood pressure, pulse rate, temperature, and height and weight are examples. They may be observed, described, and measured objectively with no statement as to cause.

8. Medical examination. Diagnostic in nature and performed by physicians who can interpret the nature and cause of conditions. Periodic medical examinations may be required of students at various grade levels and are given to apparently normal and healthy individuals. Special examinations may be required of those who participate in sports and other strenuous activities. Referral examinations are given to check reported possible deviations from normal health that may have been noticed through screening tests, observation, or physical examinations.

9. Dental examination. An appraisal of the present structure, hygiene, and condition of the mouth by the dentist, oral hygienist, and perhaps the orthodontist.

10. Psychological examination. Range from general behavior studies that observe a student's demeanor to extensive psychological examinations. School counselors, psychologists, psychiatrists, physicians, nurses, social workers, teachers, parents, and peers may be involved in a thorough study and therapy program. A variety of tests and procedures are employed to understand a student's thoughts and feelings about himself, other people, and things in his environment.

11. Health records. Include health histories and other information that may be helpful in understanding the student in cases of emergency. It may include previous illnesses, immunizations, operations, accidents, results of appraisals, observations by teachers and nurses, and accounts of current problems. Names and phone numbers of physicians, parents, and those who should be notified in case of an emergency should be included.

12. School health counseling. The procedures by which nurses, teachers, physicians, guidance personnel, and others interpret to pupils and parents the nature and significance of a health program and aid them in formulating a plan of action that will lead to a solution of the problem.

13. Prevention and protection. That phase of health service in which the procedures seek to secure the child's cooperation in health protection and maintenance, improve habits of living, and improve health control through protection from acute and chronic infectious diseases by inoculation and vaccination and prevention of the spread of contagious diseases by isolation and exclusion.

14. School health education. Health education is the process of providing planned learning experiences for the purpose of influencing knowledge, attitudes, and practices relating to individual and community health. A series of well-organized, separate health classes taught by professionally prepared health educators and appropriately placed and emphasized in the curriculum should be required for every student.

    Incidental learning experiences can supplement, but not substitute for planned health education. Incidental learning takes place when teachers of all subjects take advantage of "teachable moments" to develop health-related concepts and attitudes. Incidental instruction also includes integrating health concepts into other school subjects. Occasionally, schools participate in special programs through assemblies, bulletin boards, class discussions, and literature distribution.

These are particularly good when they correspond to community events and interest.

15. <u>School health educator</u>. A person professionally qualified to serve as a teacher, consultant, coordinator, or supervisor of health education in an individual school or school system. The health education classes on the secondary level should be taught by a person who has a major or minor in health education and has the other professional qualifications to be a health educator.

    In the elementary schools, the classroom teacher is responsible for teaching a health class on every grade level. An elementary school teacher should have at least one health education course specifically for teachers in addition to a general college health course.

16. <u>Healthful school living</u>. A term which designates the provision of a safe and healthful environment, the organization of a healthful school day, and the establishment of interpersonal relationships favorable to the best emotional, social, and physical health of pupils.

17. <u>Physical environment</u>. The school site and architecture, lighting, acoustics, heating, ventilation, water supply, toilet facilities, desks, decorations, noise control, cleanliness, sanitation, and safety. It includes the school buildings, playgrounds, lunchrooms, parking lots, and even the areas involved in transportation of the students to and from school.

18. <u>Psychological environment</u>. The climate in and around the school that affects students' social, emotional, and intellectual well-being. The physical environment affects the psychological environment. The health habits of the students and school personnel relating to personal cleanliness and grooming are important. Practices within the school regarding assignments, grading, grouping, and scheduling are also important. One of the teacher's greatest responsibilities is to promote an emotional climate that is conducive to learning.

19. <u>School health council</u>. A representative group of persons organized for the purpose of study, planning and action aimed at the identification and solution of school health problems.

20. <u>Health coordination</u>. The process of developing relationships within the school health program and between school and community health programs that contributes to harmonious action in the solution of problems relating to student health.

POLICIES AND PROCEDURES

The organization and functions of the School Health Program must be guided by official policies and procedures. The local school board is elected by the people and must represent the people in determining the health policies and procedures for the district. Local policies must also conform to state laws and regulations. District policies are made by the school board acting as a body and not by members of the board acting alone.

A policy is a statement of an accepted course of action adopted and followed by an institution or individual. Policies and procedures are needed to delineate responsibilities, give direction, foster understanding, and promote cooperation. Written policies and procedures are needed to protect the people involved so they will know what to do and what not to do under given circumstances. Policies and procedures grow out of experience, and need to be revised occasionally in light of new experience. Their formation should be guided by expert judgment and interagency deliberation and cooperation. They must be approved, adopted, and supported by the administration. They must be circulated to and understood by all individuals involved.

Written policies and procedures are needed for the following areas of the School Health Program:

- Emergency care for injury and sudden illness.
- Communicable disease prevention and control.
- Accident prevention and safety practices.
- Health examinations, screening tests, teacher observation, and referral.
- Health counseling and the use of remedial specialists.
- Maintenance of a healthful environment.
- Health curriculum requirements and scheduling.
- Duties of a school health coordinator.
- Structure and function of a school health council.
- Use of community resources in school health programs.

If the district has no written policies, or if the old policies need revising, the school administration may assign a committee to draft suggestions. The committee should seek the views of the students, parents, teachers, staff, medical professionals, local health department, health agencies, school administration, and all interested groups in the community. After cooperation and deliberation, the proposed policies and procedures should be written and presented to the school board. After thoroughly studying the draft, the board may accept it, reject it, or revise it; but before adopting a policy, the board should be ready to stand behind it.

If the board has not established a set of policies pertaining to school health, some other group such as the teacher's association, the PTA, the local medical society, or the local health department may take the initiative to encourage the board to take action.

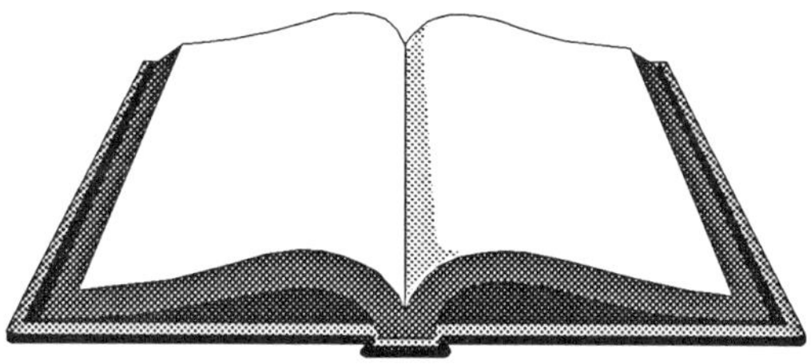

STUDY HELPS

Be able to answer the following questions as they relate to recognizing health problems.

1. What are the leading causes of death and disability among adolescents?

2. Define the following terms as used in this lesson to illustrate health problems: product, recipient, barrier, and health worker.

3. Explain how health problems are compared to an iceberg. What is frequently the underlying cause of the apparent problems?

4. Explain the steps on the problem-solving model.

Understand the following organizations, functions, and services as they apply to health resources.

A. School Health Council
B. School Health Counseling
C. School Health Education
D. School Health Educator
E. School Health Program
F. School Health Services
G. screening tests
H. health appraisal
I. health coordination
J. health observation
K. health records
L. healthful school living
M. health examination
N. physical examination
O. medical examination
P. dental examination
Q. psychological examination
R. physical environment
S. psychological environment
T. policies and procedures
U. internal resources
V. external resources
W. School Health Team
X. parents
Y. school nurse
Z. school staff
AA. guidance counselor
BB. remedial specialists
CC. government agencies
DD. professional associations
EE. business and industry
FF. voluntary health agencies
GG. civic groups

Society is concerned about the behavior of many of today's youth,but teachers are in a position to do something about the problem. As a preview to the next unit, identify some of the problems society is concerned about and consider some of the things that schools and teachers can do to improve the situation. Explain why some of these problems and solutions are school health issues.

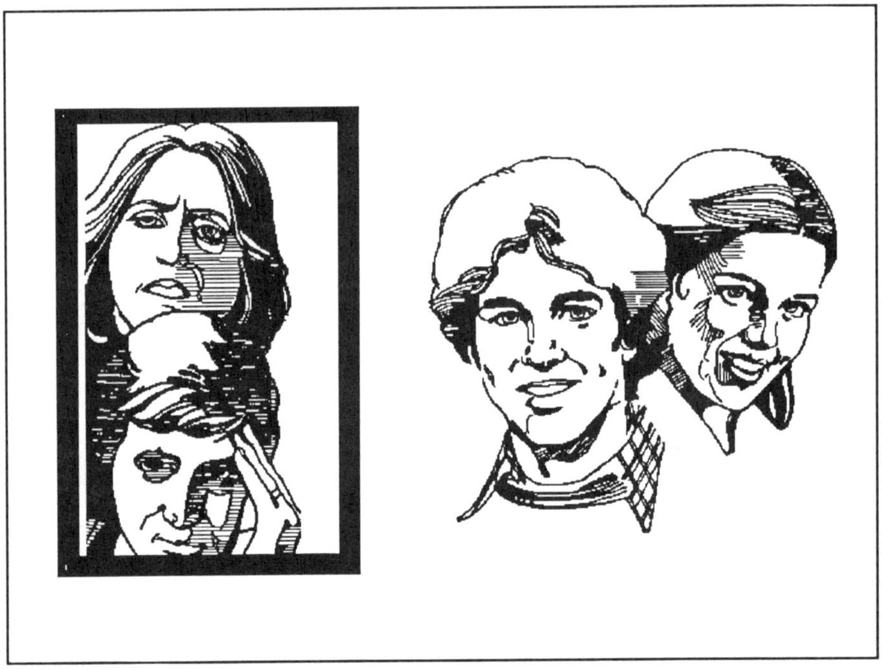

UNIT 2

MENTAL HEALTH AND CONTEMPORARY EMOTIONAL PROBLEMS

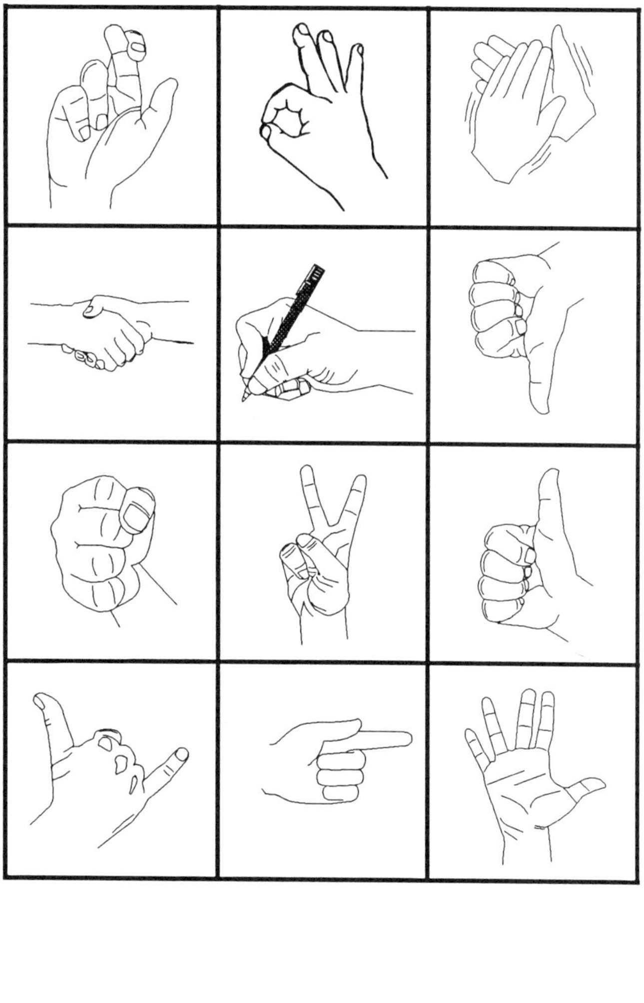

MENTAL HEALTH AND EMOTIONAL PROBLEMS

Perhaps the greatest contribution teachers can make to their students' lives is to help them develop healthy self-concepts.

A teacher's success depends on an understanding of students' mental health. A teacher needs to be aware of the characteristics of normal emotional and intellectual development if he is to set realistic limits and expectations for his students. The teacher must understand students if she is to communicate with them effectively and counsel with them about their intellectual, emotional, social, moral, or physical health problems.

Perhaps the greatest contribution a teacher can make to his students' lives is to help them develop a healthy self-concept. This course is designed to help prospective teachers acquire that fundamental requisite, a sound and practical understanding of their students' mental health.

The teacher is in a unique position to use the subject he teaches as a medium to help his students grow as a total person. A teacher should remember the counsel, "Teach students, not subjects." This is a challenge when every student is on a different level. In some ways, each student may be on several levels, intellectually mature, but socially and emotionally immature.

"Teach students, not subjects."

The school's responsibility is to take each student on whatever levels he or she is on and help him grow from there. The teachers are the key figures in carrying out this school responsibility.

Although some subjects may lend themselves more directly to certain aspects of health, a teacher of any subject can have a positive influence on their students' health. On the other hand, a teacher with poor emotional health can have a negative impact on a student's self-concept.

The concepts and skills discussed in this unit should help you meet the objectives on the following pages.

OBJECTIVES

At the conclusion of this unit, you should be able to meet the following objectives.

1. RECOGNIZE NORMAL MENTAL HEALTH

BE AWARE OF THE CHARACTERISTICS OF NORMAL INTELLECTUAL AND EMOTIONAL HEALTH.

- Explain the main concepts related to the mental function.
- Identify the mental health attributes of adolescents.
- Describe some specific situations that may reflect emotional maturity.

2. RECOGNIZE DEPARTURES FROM NORMAL

IDENTIFY THE MANIFESTATIONS OF UNFULFILLED EMOTIONAL NEEDS.

- Explain how a student's behavior patterns may indicate an emotional problem.
- Indicate the manifestations of unfulfilled emotional needs.
- Suggest ways the teacher may and should respond when a student's behavior indicates a possible emotional problem.

3. CONTEMPORARY EMOTIONAL PROBLEMS

RECOGNIZE AND PROVIDE FORMS OF ASSISTANCE WHEN STUDENTS HAVE EMOTIONAL PROBLEMS.

- Explain how motivation and social problems contribute to emotional problems.
- Describe the approaches in a suicide prevention program.
- Recognize the problems associated with religious cults.
- Explain the relationship between some physical conditions and underlying emotional problems.

4. EMOTIONAL PROBLEMS AND DRUG ABUSE

DISCUSS THE RELATIONSHIP BETWEEN DRUG ABUSE AND ASSOCIATED EMOTIONAL AND PHYSICAL PROBLEMS.

- Describe the scope of the drug problem in this country.
- Explain the motives for drug use, misuse, and abuse.
- Explain the common terms used to describe and classify drugs.
- List the signs and symptoms of drug abuse.
- Compare the approaches that may be used to deal with students who may have a drug problem.

5. MODIFYING EMOTIONAL HEALTH PROBLEMS

EXPLAIN THE EMOTIONAL PRESSURES FACED BY STUDENTS. IDENTIFY BEHAVIOR MODIFICATION TECHNIQUES TO HELP STUDENTS ADJUST.

- Discuss the pressures that can be created by teachers, parents, school policies, and students themselves.
- Discuss ways emotional pressures in school can be relieved.
- Explain the steps a teacher may take in dealing with an emotionally disturbed student.
- List the steps a person should take in dealing with a personal emotional crisis.

6. CONTRIBUTIONS TO POSITIVE MENTAL HEALTH

DISCUSS HOW A TEACHER MAY MAKE A CONTRIBUTION TO THE POSITIVE MENTAL HEALTH OF STUDENTS.

- Suggest ways a teacher can teach love and other positive emotions and traditional values.
- Suggest ways schools can improve the emotional health of teachers.
- Identify the principles and practices involved in Reality Therapy.
- List some suggestions a teacher can give to students to help improve their study habits.
- List some practical approaches to personality improvement.

Chapter 5

THE MENTAL FUNCTION

The material discussed in this chapter will introduce you to one explanation of the mental function. This concept will serve as a backdrop for the emotional health topics and contemporary health problems that will be considered more extensively in the remaining chapters in this unit.

INTRODUCTION TO MENTAL HEALTH

Human behavior is fascinating. It is interesting to contemplate, but it is also immensely complex and abstract. Yet with the increasing emphasis upon the quality of interpersonal relationships, more and more people are recognizing the need for a practical understanding of the mental process. School teachers particularly need to understand the mental function of their students. The discussion which follows is the result of a gradual synthesis of ideas into a concept or model that may help explain the mental function. This model will serve as a backdrop for the emotional health problems encountered among the students in the secondary schools.

From the beginning, man has tried to explain his behavior. He has sought to understand and cope with his mental illness and to find mental health. Mental health problems have been attributed to everything from evil spirits and demons to the influence of subversive political organizations. Cures have been attributed to mysticism, religion, and magic, as well as modern medicine. The misunderstood victims have been treated as witches, criminals, and subhumans.

The medical specialty of psychiatry, which had its beginning in the sixteenth century, made little progress until it brought reason into the study of mental illness early in the twentieth century. But, still today this specialty in many ways lacks the unifying characteristics of a proven discipline. There are many diverse explanations for human behavior and an equally wide variety of contradictory modes of treatment for the mentally ill.

From the earliest time, more has been written about mental illness than about mental health. While the clinical psychologists and psychiatrists have been mainly concerned with the treatment of the ill, others such as social workers, church workers, and educators are becoming more interested in a positive approach to mental health as it relates to the whole person. This lesson should help teachers understand the mental function.

INTELLECTUAL AND EMOTIONAL HEALTH

In the multidimensional concept of health, it is important to recognize the difference between the intellectual and emotional dimensions. Intellectual health may be reflected in the ability to solve problems through the application of memory and logic. It involves the speed and accuracy of perception, memory, and reason. People who are intellectually retarded suffer from disorders in which the central nervous system failed to develop properly because of heredity, metabolic disorders, circulatory interruption, or physical injury. Severe problems of this nature represent a small portion of the mental health problems encountered in the schools.

An ineffective mental function is more frequently due to emotional problems. Emotional health deals with our feelings. Emotions are intense feelings accompanied by body reactions. Emotional problems are functional rather than organic, the individual has lost or has not developed the ability to keep the emotions under control. Fortunately, with proper help a person has a good chance of overcoming his emotional health problems.

Most of the mental health problems encountered in the school setting are emotional rather than intellectual. The problems deal with feelings and attitudes. Within this affective domain there is room for improvement for everyone. That is positive mental health. Hopefully, the following discussion will help teachers contribute to the positive mental health of their students.

The Mental Function concept is not intended to be a scientifically complete or accurate explanation of what takes place on the physiological or psychological level. It is not intended for biologists or psychologists. It is intended to be a model that hopefully will help ordinary people develop a practical understanding of the mental process.

THE MENTAL FUNCTION CONCEPT

The term "Mental Function" is used here to stand for certain human processes used by the individual to facilitate adjustment with the environment. A diagrammatic model is used in Figure 1 to illustrate the concept of the mental function serving as a moderator between the individual and the world in which he or she lives. Doctor William Glasser, in his book *Mental Health or Mental Illness*, used a similar diagram to depict the role of the mental function.

THE MODERATOR

If I were to use a chalkboard to diagram this concept, I would first draw a stick figure to represent an individual. Then, I would draw a large circle around the individual to represent the world or the environment. Next, I would turn the chalk sideways and draw a heavy circle closely surrounding the individual to represent the mental function. This circle would vary in thickness to represent varying strengths in different parts of the mental function. Hopefully, this diagram would illustrate the role of the mental function serving as moderator between the individual and the world.

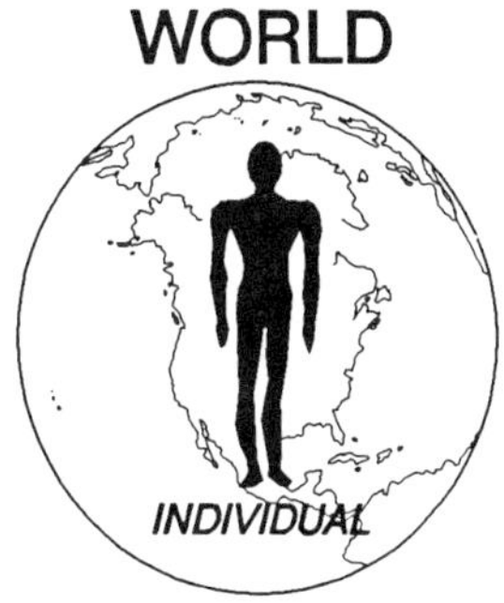

Figure 1

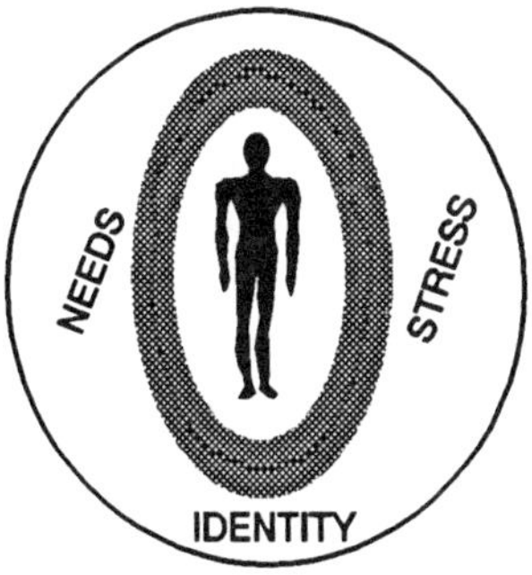

Figure 2

In Figure 2, the three main tasks of the mental function are illustrated. The mental function serving as a moderator between the individual and the world tries to help the individual satisfy his or her needs, defend himself or herself against stress, and gain a sense of identity. The job of the mental function is to 1) satisfy needs, 2) defend against stress, and 3) provide identity.

NEEDS

Every person has the same set of basic needs. The basic needs do not change with age, sex, race, or religion; they remain the same for all levels of mental health. People tend to satisfy their needs in ascending order. As soon as one need is satisfied, they seek to satisfy another. Some needs are more urgent than others; for example, the need for air. If we can't breathe, everything else becomes unimportant.

The well-known psychologist, Maslow, talked about a hierarchy of needs. He depicts man's needs at five levels: physical, safety, love, esteem, and self-actualization. He points out that needs are satisfied in ascending order and satisfaction of higher needs is dependent upon adequate satisfaction of lesser needs. There are exceptions, however. Sometimes people who have experienced life only on a lesser level are content to continue existing on that level. Also, some people reverse the hierarchy and are willing to give up much for a particular ideal.

Generally, the mental function satisfies our basic physical needs without any awareness on our part. Vital functions such as breathing, digesting, regulating of blood pressure, and activating the immune system take place on an unconscious level. As the environmental temperature changes, the mental function makes adjustments by causing the body to sweat or shiver.

The psychological needs are much more complex and less urgent, but nevertheless common to all humans. Sometimes they work together, and sometimes they are in conflict. People are usually aware of their mental functions attempts to satisfy psychological needs. In his book, *Reality Therapy*, William Glasser brought the psychological needs together into two needs: (1) the need to love and be loved, and (2) the need to feel worthwhile to ourselves and to others. He emphasized that these needs are only fulfilled through involvement with other psychologically-healthy people. In a more recent book, *Control Theory*, Doctor Glasser listed the psychological needs as 1) the need to belong, 2) the need for power, 3) the need for freedom, and 4) the need for fun.

Another point of view suggested by Ashley Montage in *Direction of the Human Species* involves various classes of needs. Some are vital, basic needs that an individual requires to survive--such as oxygen, food, activity, rest, and avoidance of pain. Emotional basic needs are necessary to develop and maintain adequate mental health. These are love, communication, and involvement with others. Derived needs become socially necessary for the maintenance of mental health such as adequate clothing and shelter. Acquired needs grow out of the derived needs and are not usually necessary for the maintenance of mental health. The need to avoid pain is a vital, basic need, the avoidance of the pain of cold by the use of clothing or shelter is a derived need, and the need for fashionable clothing or to decorate a home in a particular style is an acquired need. Basic needs are common to all.

Derived needs are quite similar in a culture or subculture, and acquired needs are individual and personal. Satisfaction of needs contributes to mental health; frustration contributes to mental disorders, whether the needs are basic, derived, or acquired.

STRESS

People not only must learn to satisfy needs, but they must also learn to defend against stress. A healthy mental function will defend against physical stress such as heat, cold, fatigue, poisons, pollution, etc. It must also defend against the psychological and emotional stresses present in this complex world. Emotional stress may be related to people and things in one's external and internal environments.

IDENTITY

Another mental function is to provide identity or self-concept. Identity means we know who we are in relation to the world in which we live. It gives us a clear, positive feeling of "I am I." If placed in a different situation where things are unfamiliar, we try first of all to establish who we are and how we fit into the new setting. We try to identify ourselves with reference to elements that are familiar. When we are unable to establish identity, we suffer what is probably the most upsetting of all human experience--we become frustrated, anxious, and often immobilized. The lack of sense of identity is related to many of the psychiatric problems in our society.

A healthy mental function gives people a sense of identity. They have a definite picture of themselves; they accept their body and their sex; they have a well-established set of values; and they remain unshaken by changes. They feel secure in themselves and able to relate to others effectively. They know who they are and where they are.

Anytime a person faces significant changes in their life their mental function faces a challenge in providing a sense of identity. A healthy mental function will facilitate that adjustment. Appropriate and consistent feedback from people who are important to the individual is vital to the development of a sense of identity.

Each person has a self-concept, a mental blueprint, a picture of himself which guides his or her behavior. Our self-concept is built from our beliefs about our past successes and failures and our interpretation of others' reactions. A person's self-concept may be vague and not even consciously recognized, but it guides his or her behavior. Even when a person's self-concept is based on false images, a person may act consistently with it just as if it were true. What a person believes is true is more important than what is true. A girl's actions, feelings, behavior, and abilities are consistent with her self-image. A boy acts like the sort of person he conceives himself to be.

The person who conceives himself to be a failure-type person will find, perhaps unconsciously, some way to fail, and thus prove that his self-image is correct. Self-concept is the key to human personality. Change the self-image, and you change the behavior of an individual. One's present self-concept is the result of what has been experienced in the past. A self-image can be changed by different experiences. One can learn to function successfully by experiencing success. Since all people have the same needs and encounter approximately the same stresses, one may wonder what makes the difference. It is the attitude that makes the difference. The emotionally healthy person has a healthy self-concept and a positive attitude.

CENSOR

We have defined the mental function as a moderator between the individual and the world. The mental function also serves as the censor between the conscious and the subconscious.

In a model of the mental function acting as a censor, a large circle represents all that we know. A smaller circle in the center represents what we are currently aware of, and we call this the *conscious*. At a given moment we are aware of only a few things. The rest of the area inside of the large circle represents everything we know but are not currently aware of. It is called the *subconscious*. Information can flow back and forth between the conscious and the subconscious. As you receive new information, you may be consciously aware of it for a moment, and then you file it somewhere in the subconscious for future reference. As you remember, you bring information from the subconscious to the conscious.

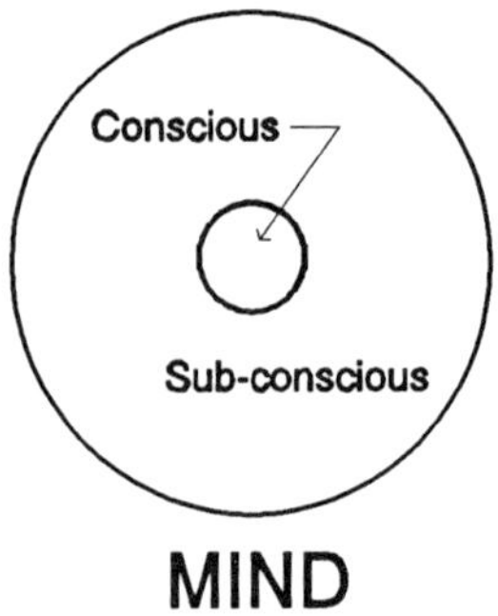

Figure 3

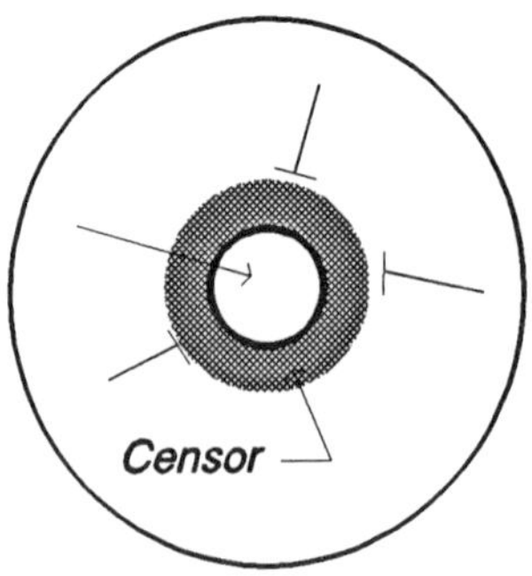

Figure 4

Reasoning is the process of relating new information to previously known information. Some information is filed near the surface of awareness and is readily available to enter the conscious, but other information is filed at a deeper level of the subconscious, and it takes a stronger clue to jog the memory and bring it into awareness.

The mental function, acting as a censor, regulates the flow of information between the conscious and subconscious. If too much information or inappropriate information enters the conscious, the person's ability to concentrate is impaired. If a person is unable to recall known information, his ability to reason may be limited. A mental function acting as a censor regulates the flow of information between the conscious and the subconscious. This allows the person to concentrate. This also reduces excessive worrying. It facilitates the flow of information, so that people can reason and solve problems.

When the mental function is healthy, it exercises appropriate censorship. But when it is unhealthy it lets information through that is not in the best interest of the individual and blocks information that is needed for the individual to function successfully.

When a person is under stress or in a state of anxiety, his censor becomes less effective. When the mental function becomes so involved in maneuvers to defend the self-concept, it cannot perform its censor functions effectively. The greater the anxiety level, the less effective is the censor. Under stress, some people's mental function acting as a censor is not able to perform its tasks as effectively as it can normally. People who have a good self-concept are less apt to be affected adversely by stress.

In an educational setting, most students do not perform up to their capacity in an emotionally stressful situation, at least until they have had the opportunity to strengthen their self-concept. Constructive criticism is most fruitful in an atmosphere of peace, after the anxiety has subsided, when there is a free two-way flow of information, and when there is a compatible relationship between the conscious and subconscious.

The mental function mediates all contact between the person and his world. The mental function also censors the flow of information between the conscious and the subconscious. A healthy mental function uses normal means to satisfy needs, defend against stress, and provide identities. A person with an ineffective mental function will turn to abnormal, ineffective, or inappropriate means to try to satisfy their needs. These attempts also meet with failure, so they resort to even less appropriate means. Other people consider their behavior to be strange. Perhaps one person in ten suffers from an inadequately developed mental function.

DEVELOPING THE MENTAL FUNCTION

At first, an infant does not have the ability to satisfy its own needs, defend itself against life's stresses, or to gain an accurate recognition of its own identity. It could not survive on its own. It is totally dependent upon its parents or other adults who share their mental function with the infant.

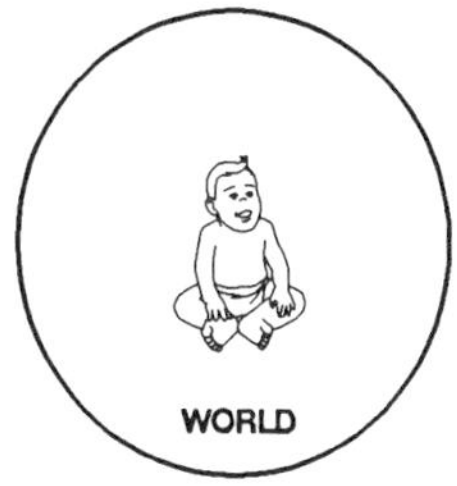

Figure 5

In time, the infant starts to develop its own mental function. Perhaps the first exercise of a beginning mental function is a cry for help. When the infant experiences the stress of a wet diaper, it

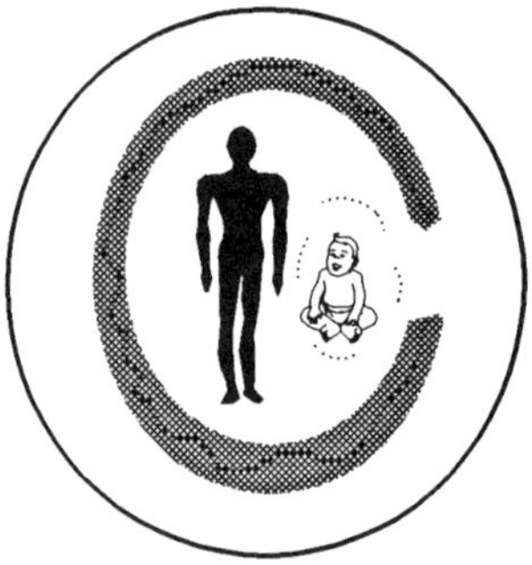

Figure 6

cries. Someone hears the cry and changes the diaper. When the infant experiences the need for food, it cries and someone gives it a bottle. From there on, it begins to further manipulate its environment and make adjustments to the world in which it lives. At first, the infant cannot distinguish between itself, others, and the world. When the infant realizes that he or she is a person different from other people, mental function begins to provide a sense of identity. Gradually the relationships which were at first a one-way relationship become a two-way relationship. The mental function is developing.

This process occurs gradually throughout childhood. The child learns that its parents' mental functions will continue to serve it much of the time, but not all of the time. A challenge for parents is to know when to share and when to withhold their mental functions from the child. The child should not be left unprotected too early or too much, but it does need opportunities to develop and exercise its own mental function; either extreme can hamper the development of the child's mental function. Parents with effective mental functions will know when and how to extend and withhold their help.

In order for a child to learn how to fulfill needs, it must be involved with other responsible people, usually parents and teachers. People with healthy mental functions recognize the difference between satisfying a child's needs and helping the child learn how to satisfy its own needs. Learning to fulfill one's needs should begin in infancy and continue throughout life. If a person fails to learn to fill his or her needs, he or she will suffer. Such suffering will drive the person to unsuccessful and unacceptable need-filling behaviors.

At all times throughout life, a person needs to love and be loved. Also, throughout life a person needs to feel a sense of worth. In order to fulfill these needs, a person must be involved with other people. A person who does not learn as a child to give and receive love or recognize his or her own worth may spend the rest of his or her life unsuccessfully trying to meet these needs. The younger and more thoroughly a person learns to fulfill these needs, the more satisfactory his life will be.

Parents with effective mental functions tend to rear children with effective mental functions. Likewise, parents with defective mental functions tend to rear children with defective mental functions, and the chain goes on. Sometimes when the parents fail, someone else along the way--a teacher, a friend, a church leader, a counselor, or a psychiatrist--becomes involved in a meaningful relationship that enables the child's mental function to develop and become stronger. The mental function develops best in an atmosphere where needs are met, where someone cares, where people appreciate each others' worth, in an atmosphere where love is exchanged. Love is sharing mental functions and deriving satisfaction from seeing each other's needs fulfilled. Mental functions develop best in two-way relationships with an atmosphere of consistency and acceptance.

Doctor Glasser emphasized in his book, *Reality Therapy*, the importance of three principles in developing a healthy mental function. These three R's of Reality Therapy are responsibility, right and wrong, and reality.

The following discussion about the role of parents also applies to the role of teachers.

RESPONSIBILITY

Responsibility is taught through the proper combination of love and discipline. Responsibility can be learned at any age, but it is easier learned at an early age, before the person has to overcome previous bad learning. For some children, the learning of responsibility does not come easy. From infancy, they struggle against learning how to fulfill their own needs. When they are older, they test their parents with irresponsible behavior to see if what they have been taught is valid.

Through discipline tempered with love, parents must teach their children responsibility. Thereby the child learns that the parents really care. Children somehow realize that parents who really love them will make them do what is good for them, not merely indulge them. Parents who are willing to suffer the pains of the child's intense anger by firmly holding the child to the responsible course are teaching a valuable lesson. Parents must understand that taking the responsible course will never permanently alienate the child.

The parents must not only hold the child to the correct course of action, but they must also show by example that they are capable of taking the responsible course. Parents who have no self-discipline cannot successfully discipline a child. When discipline is responsible and has with it the element of love, and when the parents' own behavior is consistent with their demands on the child, he will love and respect them even though on the surface he might not show it. Ultimately however, responsibility means accepting the responsibility for one's own actions and imposing self-discipline accordingly.

RIGHT OR WRONG

All society is based on morality, and if the parents and other important people in a young person's life do not discuss whether behavior is right or wrong, there will be no basis for feeling self-worth. If there is a disparity between one's values and one's behavior, there will be an absence of the feeling of worth.

REALITY

Reality refers to the ultimate consequence of a particular behavior. A person must learn to accept the consequences of his own behavior. If he wants different consequences, he must change his behavior.

STRENGTH OF THE MENTAL FUNCTION

The diagram of the mental function in this model can be altered to illustrate various degrees of strength and weakness. For a normal healthy adult, the diagram of the mental function would surround the individual completely, indicating that it deals effectively with all areas of life. It would be thick enough to suggest sufficient strength to accomplish its tasks. It would be wavy with varying thicknesses to suggest flexibility, changing degrees of effectiveness depending on the circumstances.

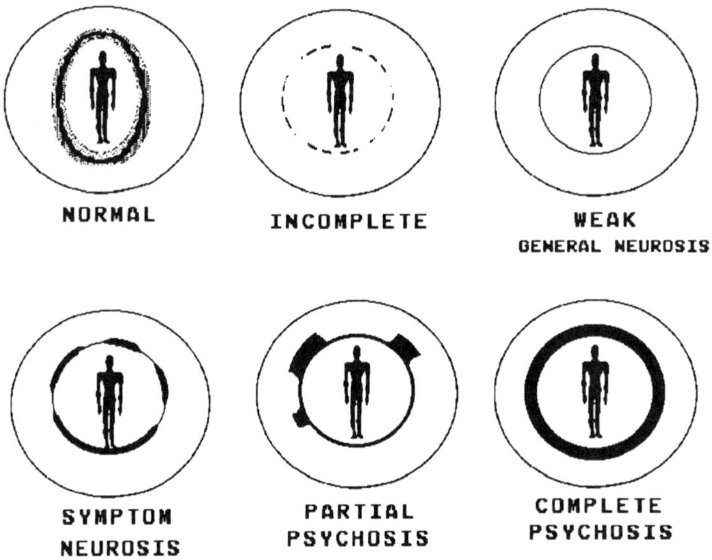

Few people have a mental function that is completely effective at all times. From time to time, most people have minor and transient emotional disturbances. A person may be a functioning member of society and still have minor weaknesses. The mentally healthy person keeps his defects within bounds. Under stress, however, minor defects can get out of bounds and become major problems.

At first, an infant has no mental function, but as it matures, a few thin scattered segments of the line appear to represent very limited mental function. As the child's mental function develops, the circle becomes more complete and segments of the line become a little thicker. A thin or weak mental function is appropriate for a child; but unfortunately, some people reach the age and physical size of adults without the mental function developing beyond that of a child.

A normal teenager's mental function could be diagrammed to show that it completely encircles the person but with some areas represented as being strong and other areas weak. In some areas of life, teenagers typically function in mature ways, but in other areas their behavior is immature. By adult standards they seem unpredictable, but this is normal for teenagers. The teen years are in-between years. In some ways they are like an adult, but in other ways they are like a child. These are difficult years for the youth, their parents, and their teachers. They are in the process of developing their mental function. They are testing the world, trying to personally fill their needs and to gain identity. Throughout this time, they need to be involved with adults who have mature emotions and healthy mental functions.

A weak mental function is diagrammed with an incomplete circle. The mental function has not fully developed. This is normal in a child, but in a teenager this may be associated with juvenile delinquency, and in an adult it may be described as a character disorder. The failure of the mental function to develop may be associated with the absence of any meaningful relationships with other mentally healthy people.

In an adult, a mental function illustrated by a thin line indicates some form of neurosis. If the diagram illustrates a mental function that is generally effective, but with weakness confined to specific areas, it may indicate specific symptoms such as phobias and compulsions. A case where there is generalized weakness of nearly the whole mental function can be illustrated with a complete, but thin, line. This represents neurosis which is marked by considerable anxiety. No one is completely free from weakness in the mental function, but the difference between the normal and the neurotic depends on how the person has learned to handle anxiety.

A thick line in the diagram of the mental function can be used to illustrate a break from reality known as psychosis. A psychotic mental function could be diagrammed as very thick, rigid, and impenetrable. In psychosis, the mental function serves not as a moderator between the individual and the outside world, but as a barrier to shut out the person's awareness of the outside world. In psychosis, the world exists in the mind; perceptions come in the form of hallucinations. Although the person's needs remain unfilled in the real world, they may be completely filled within his mind. A diagram of a completely psychotic person's mental function would show a very thick line completely surrounding him, but this is rare. Usually psychosis occurs only in limited segments of the mental function, and the person retains an otherwise normal relationship with his environment.

PHASES OF THE MENTAL FUNCTION

The mental function serves as the moderator between the individual and the environment. It operates in three phases: receiving, reasoning, and responding. It receives information; it uses that information to reason and make decisions; based on those decisions, the individual responds. Perception is the product of the receiving phase, judgment is the product of the reasoning phase, and action is the product of the responding phase.

PHASES OF THE MENTAL FUNCTION

RECEIVING⇒	REASONING⇒	RESPONDING
PERCEPTION	COGNITION	ACTION
sight *sound* *smell* *taste* *touch*	*memory* *knowledge* *understanding* *comprehension* *translation* *analysis* *synthesis* *evaluation*	*passive* *assertive* *aggressive*
Real or Imagined? Complete or Incomplete?	Logical or Emotional? Objective or Prejudiced?	Act or React?

RECEIVING

In the receiving phase, the individual perceives the sensations such as sight, sound, smell, taste, and touch from the environment. The success of a person's adjustment depends to a great extent on the accuracy of the receiving phase. A person with a healthy mental function has developed the skills of observation. This is important in satisfying needs, defending against stress, and establishing identity. A person's background affects his or her perception for people tend to see only that which they have been prepared to see. The information a person receives may be either real or imagined, or may be complete or incomplete. Incomplete or imagined information may lead to faulty adjustments. Perception is an important phase of the mental function.

REASONING

In the reasoning phase, the individual processes the information obtained in the receiving phase. New information, as well as stored information, is processed on various cognitive levels. Some information is merely stored in the memory for future use. Simply knowing facts is a lower cognitive level. Understanding, comprehension, translation, analysis, synthesis, and evaluation are increasingly higher cognitive levels. A mentally healthy person has functional skills on all cognitive levels. He or she is able to recall information, understand and comprehend facts, translate concepts into different levels or situations, analyze concepts by breaking them down into smaller components for purposes of comparison, synthesize several lesser ideas into new and larger concepts, and evaluate information to arrive at decisions. Reasoning can proceed along logical and objective lines, or it can be based on prejudices and emotions. The mentally healthy person tends to rely more on a rational and objective form of logic and less on emotions and prejudices. Generally poor reasoning leads to faulty judgment and poor adjustment.

RESPONDING

The information obtained in the receiving phase and the decisions made in the reasoning phase result in the behavior observed in the responding phase. We cannot observe what is taking place in another person's receiving or reasoning phases; all we can see is the behavior in the responding phase. Yet poor adjustments are often the result of faulty perception or reasoning. Conversely, people can have good receiving and reasoning skills, but weak responding skills. Extremes in the responding phase may range from complete passiveness to excessive aggressiveness. Either extreme is a sign of emotional health problems.

Assertive Behavior

In the model, appropriate behavior rests between the passive and aggressive extremes and is called assertiveness. It reflects effective receiving and reasoning and is the follow-through behavior required to achieve and maintain adjustments. An assertive person is able to do what needs to be done. A certain amount of passiveness is necessary occasionally to allow time for conditions to cool off or settle down so that wise judgments can be made. On the other hand, at times a certain amount of aggressiveness is necessary to provide protection and to meet the demands of life.

Passive Behavior

People whose mental function has not developed properly are frequently too passive. They can make decisions but do not have enough strength in their mental function to carry out the actions. Passiveness ranges from occasional procrastination to complete physical immobilization. Sometimes we see overly passive students in our classrooms; they are quiet, unobtrusive, and withdrawn from any effort to adjust. They do not draw attention to their problems and often go unnoticed and are not referred for help. Those who are apathetic soon become prey to the stresses of life and may have to be protected by society.

Aggressive Behavior

On the other extreme, overly aggressive students may also be observed in the classroom. They usually draw attention to themselves and are therefore more likely to get psychological counseling. Although a certain amount of aggressiveness is necessary for survival, a strong aggressive quality coupled with inadequate information or poor judgment may lead to inappropriate and excessive behavior. Most laws and rules have been established to regulate extremes in aggressive action. The over-aggressive often run afoul of the law and must be controlled by confinement in jails or mental hospitals or other forms of reprisals.

Frequently, problems in the responding phase occur when people learn to react rather than to act. In this model, when people act, their response is based on effective receiving and reasoning. When people act, their behavior is a follow-through on well-planned decisions corresponding to their personal goals and purposes. When people react, their behavior is motivated more by pressures, circumstances, and the actions of others than by their own decisions. Their receiving and reasoning phases are short-circuited. They follow the crowd; they take the course of least resistance. Sometimes a group of people will do something no one in the group wanted to do just because they all thought the others wanted to do it. They don't think or reason; they merely react. A person with an unhealthy mental function is more apt to react.

ADJUSTMENTS AND MALADJUSTMENTS

Our emotions are a powerful means of communication. The mental function uses emotions in its role as a moderator and a censor. The emotions tell us how we feel about ourselves and whether we are effective or defective. When the mental function is effective in defending against stress, satisfying needs, and providing a sense of identity, it produces positive emotions. When it is defective, it produces negative emotions.

Positive emotions may be described as warm and comfortable feelings and a sense of well-being. The positive emotions reinforce the successful behavior and lead us to develop mentally healthy characteristics such as maturity, happiness, autonomy, integration, productivity, and self-actualization. Negative emotions serve as warning signals, indicating a weakness in the mental function. The model can be diagrammed to illustrate this weakness. The weaknesses are due to underdevelopment rather than illness. Whenever an individual attempts to use this part of his mental function, he experiences negative emotions

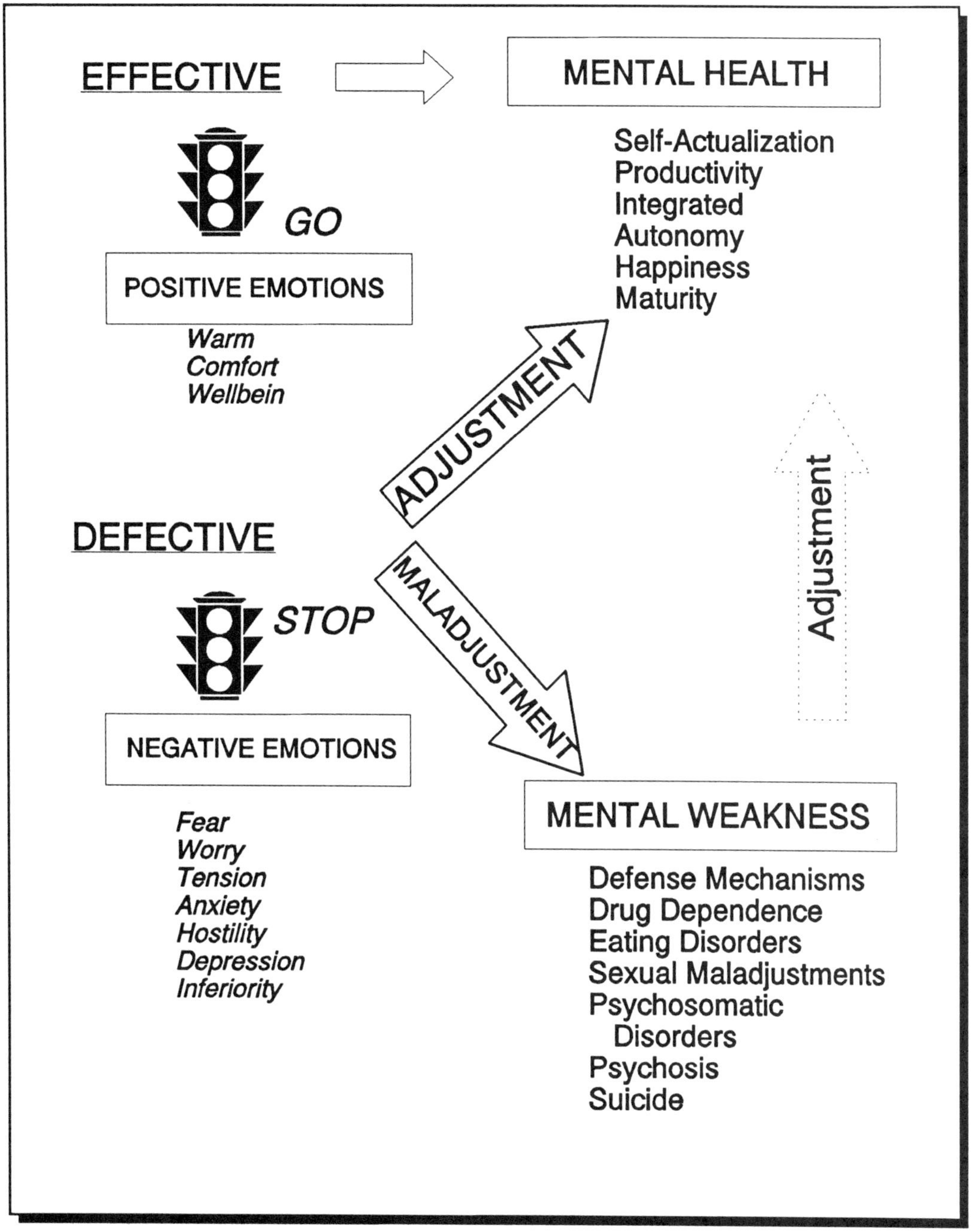
EFFECTIVE
MENTAL HEALTH
Self-Actualization
Productivity
Integrated
Autonomy
Happiness
Maturity
GO
POSITIVE EMOTIONS
Warm
Comfort
Wellbein
ADJUSTMENT
Adjustment
DEFECTIVE
MALADJUSTMENT
STOP
NEGATIVE EMOTIONS
MENTAL WEAKNESS
Fear
Worry
Tension
Anxiety
Hostility
Depression
Inferiority
Defense Mechanisms
Drug Dependence
Eating Disorders
Sexual Maladjustments
Psychosomatic
Disorders
Psychosis
Suicide

such as uncomfortable feelings of uneasiness, tension, worry, fear, hostility, depression, emptiness, boredom, inferiority, and other forms of anxiety. The negative emotions are forms of psychological pain that may range from mild to extreme. We do not like to live with this pain, so we try to make an adjustment or maladjustment.

Adjustment is the process of strengthening the mental function. It is a learning process that requires sufficient time and appropriate circumstances. These circumstances were discussed earlier in this lesson under the heading "Development of the Mental Function." Adjustments can be thought of as learning or strengthening experiences rather than a healing process. No mental function is strong enough to be completely successful all of the time; therefore, negative emotions are common to all of us. Growth comes through overcoming temporary weaknesses. We all face about the same problems, but the people who are successful are those who have learned how to make adjustments.

When there is not enough time, opportunity, or strength in the mental function to make adjustments, the person will either have to live with the pain of the negative emotions or resort to some form of maladjustment. We all have to turn to maladjustments occasionally. Sometimes the maladjustment is temporary until time and circumstances permit adjustment.

Maladjustments are processes employed by a person to overcome emotional pain by hiding his inadequacies from himself. When the mental function does not have sufficient strength to adjust, the person's pain is compounded. He continues to suffer because the original needs are not met, and he also suffers an insult because he is unable to adjust. Maladjustments are defensive maneuvers employed by the mental function to hide its inadequacies from itself. They take place on the subconscious level. In the model, the maladjustment may be diagrammed as a curtain to hide the weak part of the mental function.

Defense mechanisms are the mildest and most commonly used maladjustments. Everyone uses them occasionally. They are unconscious reactions which free the mental function from the pain of negative emotions and allow it to concentrate on major functions. They may be used to temporarily protect the self-image until adjustments can be made. Some types of defense mechanisms are healthier than others, depending on the intensity and frequency of use. Defense mechanisms that emphasize substitutions are healthier than those that involve denial. They become more harmful when they inhibit normal adjustment. Examples of defense mechanisms include rationalization, fantasy, compensation, sublimation, substitution, identification, projection, repression, regression, and withdrawal.

Defense mechanisms may be compared to the application of a bandage to protect a wound, but the bandage is not left on permanently. Bandages are applied consciously, but defense mechanisms take place subconsciously. If we are not aware we are using them, it may be difficult to stop. The use of defense mechanisms may also be compared to taking a pain pill for an ankle injury. If the injury is a simple sprain, it may be all right to take the pill for pain, but if the injury is a fracture, taking the pill may delay proper treatment or contribute to further injury.

Drug dependence is another form of maladjustment. Sometimes people use alcohol and other drugs to blot out negative emotions, hide a sense of inadequacy, or act as a crutch to bolster a defective mental function. Not only do they drink or use drugs because of mental health problems, but the use of drugs or alcohol also contributes to situations which may cause additional mental problems. Alcoholics usually hate alcohol, but they hate reality more. They drink to blot out their inadequacies, yet in that state they develop more inadequacies. When people take drugs to hide their problem, they are unlikely to take the steps to solve their problem.

Eating disorders have recently been added to the list of maladjustments. People may engage in overeating, anorexia, and bulimic behaviors to hide their inadequate feelings. Overeating may be a substitute for unmet emotional needs. Anorexia is associated with an inadequate self-concept.

Deviant sexual activity is often a form of maladjustment associated with a poor self-concept. People who engage in inappropriate sexual behavior often do so to try to prove something about their identity.

Psychosomatic disorders are conditions where a psychological or mental problem results in physical illness. Psychosomatic disorders (*psycho* meaning mind and *soma* meaning body) occur when mental problems result in physical problems. Emotions that are not expressed outwardly are discharged inwardly and channeled to a vulnerable organ. The difficulty in understanding psychosomatic disorders is that the psychological problems remain on the subconscious level. Medicine can treat the physical problems, but it is difficult to identify and effectively treat the responsible emotional problems. Usually the person's mental function is having difficulty meeting his needs, defending against stress, or providing a healthy identity. More and more medical disorders (perhaps 70%) are being diagnosed as psychosomatic. Ulcers, colitis, asthma, hives, headaches, and muscular aches and pains are often, but not always, psychosomatic. Psychosomatic diseases are serious and can be fatal, but effective treatment involves not only treating the physical problem, but also the mental problem.

Psychotic behavior is manifest in a wide variety of ways, but most often it involves an extreme departure from reality. In order to avoid having to deal with life and the world as it really is, the mental function shuts out its awareness of the real world and makes a world of its own. Psychotic behavior may occur in large or small segments of a person's life. People may be mildly psychotic or deeply psychotic. They may move into and out of psychotic behavior patterns with surprising ease. Their psychosis may be manifest by a defect in the way they relate with other people. Usually the person who uses this ego reaction has been unable since early in life to form close, warm, loving relationships. They are frequently distant to the point of isolation. Often as children they seemed good, self-sufficient, and preferring solitary amusements. They continue to be unable to respond emotionally, to withdraw from other people, to be preoccupied with their own inner world, and to find gratification in fantasy rather than reality.

Most patients in mental hospitals are classified as undifferentiated psychotics. They may at times demonstrate behavior that fits into one of the following categories. Psychosis which begins in the teenage years is called *dementia praecox* or early (precocious) mental illness (dementia). *Schizophrenia* (split-mind) may indicate that part of a person's mental function is in contact with reality and part of it is not. This can occur at any age. The *paranoid* person may think that someone wants to hurt him and, in self-protection, becomes dangerous. The *catatonic* person shows both mental and physical symptoms and may become mute, inactive, and even assume a bizarre posture for hours. The person exhibiting *mania* may be excessively elated, happy (he may laugh inappropriately at everything), and hyperactive; but his behavior is extremely disorganized. The *manic-depressive* person has moods that swing from mania to deep depression. Depression may exist in all degrees of severity from mild to severe psychotic depression. *Insanity* is the legal term for people who are psychotic. They are considered dangerous (although they rarely are) and can be put in a mental hospital.

Neurosis or psychoneurosis refers to a very weak mental function. It is not a form of maladjustment, for a neurotic person's mental function has insufficient strength to adjust or not to adjust. People who are neurotic may have quit trying. Their needs remain unsatisfied. They continue to live in a state of emotional pain. They are continually fearful, miserable, and ineffective. This type of person preys on others and makes them suffer. They create situations which tend to produce neurosis in their children and other people they associate with, especially those with weak mental functions. They try to maneuver situations so they always end up looking bad. They try to manipulate people and make others appear responsible. They have built in excuses for their problems, and they conjure up situations that will invoke sympathy and pity. Neurosis breeds neurosis.

Neurosis may be expressed as a form of *depression*. Depression results from the inability of the mental function to handle emotions such as anger satisfactorily. In depression, the person is unable to discharge anger for fear of retaliation or the loss of love and respect. As a result, the anger remains and envelops and immobilizes the mental function. The life of people suffering from neurosis may be characterized by irrational fears (*phobias*) attached to particular people, places, or situations. They may be unable to avoid certain thoughts (*obsessions*). They may feel driven to exhibit certain behavior (*compulsions*). Their emotions such as anger or guilt may be transformed into some physical or mental defects such as blindness, paralysis, or amnesia (*conversions*).

Suicide is an extreme form of maladjustment. It is the ultimate way of hiding inadequacies, denying reality, and escaping emotional pain. The mental function may first attempt alternatives to suicide. In suicide a person kills himself physically; in psychosis a person kills himself emotionally. If his mental function will not allow the departures from reality necessary to be successful in becoming psychotic, he may resort to suicide. At this point, with the bizarre logic of a psychotic, he may commit suicide physically.

MENTAL HEALTH

We all use maladjustments, particularly during a crisis. Perhaps most normal people are occasionally a little neurotic and occasionally a little psychotic. The difference between normal and abnormal is not what people do, but how much they do it, and when they do it. It is a matter of degree. We can all find ways to improve the quality of our mental health. It is a matter of finding the opportunities to strengthen the mental function, so it can help us make the appropriate adjustments. That is the positive approach to mental health.

People who are generally mentally healthy exhibit the following characteristics:

Maturity. Maturity is the ability to satisfy needs, defend against stress, and gain a sense of identity. Maturity is relative. Behavior that might be considered mature for a child may be immature for an adult.

Happiness. People who are mentally healthy are generally happy, not always, but generally. We all occasionally encounter situations that should make us genuinely sad, but mentally healthy people are able to rebound. Happiness is a by-product of effective living. Perhaps the best single indicator of mental health is the answer to the question, "Are you happy?"

Autonomy. Autonomy means independence and sovereignty. People who are autonomous are generally able to run their own life. We never achieve complete independence. We have to rely on other people sometimes for some things. Normal mentally healthy people are autonomous. They accept responsibility for their own behavior.

Integration. When people are integrated, all parts of their life are compatible. Their behaviors are synchronized, and one interest does not conflict excessively with another. Mentally health people have got their lives together.

Productivity. Mentally healthy people make a contribution. They are not afraid of hard work; they are creative and can come up with original ideas. These people use their skills, strengths, and talents to benefit other individuals, groups, and causes. They do more than carry their own load; they get the job done and then some.

Self-actualization. Self-actualization is the process of becoming what you are capable of becoming. It is reaching your potential. It is the highest level of mental health. Self-actualization occurs by degrees, not all at once. For example, a student can do the best he can and reach his potential as a freshman, but as a senior his potential will be much greater. Or a student can reach her potential in mathematics, but may fall short of her potential in geography. We become self-actualized one level at a time until eventually, given enough time, we may become fully self-actualized.

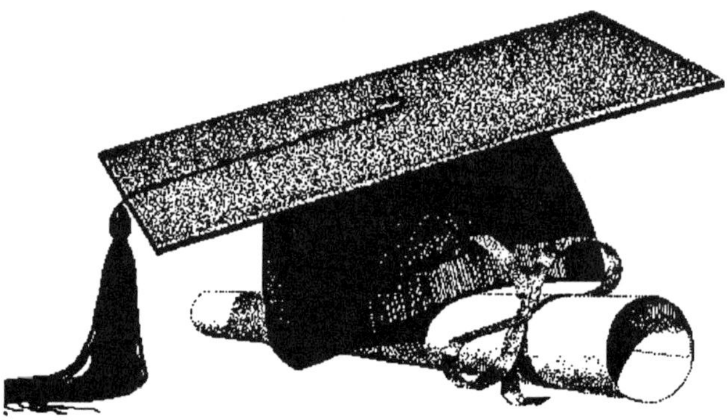

STUDY HELPS

Fill in the blanks.

SUMMARY OF THE MENTAL FUNCTION

This discussion of the Mental Function concept has been presented to help prospective teachers better understand ____________, their future ________, and others they encounter in their personal and professional pursuits. This model provides a ______ ______ for the remaining lessons in this unit dealing with various emotional health problems and approaches to positive mental health. It may be well to review it often.

The mental function has been defined as a __________ between the individual and the world. It also has been defined as a ________ between the conscious and subconscious. The mental function has three major tasks: to satisfy our ___________, to defend against ______, and to provide a sense of ____________. The mental function operates in three phases, ____, ____________, and _________. Healthy mental functions develop over time as a learning process through association with others who have a __________ ________ _________. People with healthy mental functions try to distinguish between what is real and what is _____ and try to get the full picture before responding. They try to be objective rather than ______and try to differentiate between right and wrong, to act rather than _ ______, and then, to take responsibility for their own behavior. Positive emotions ______ _____ successful behavior and contribute to the characteristics of a mentally healthy person: maturity, happiness, autonomy, integration, productivity, and self-actualization. Negative emotions are painful feelings which motivate either adjustment or _________________.

Adjustments are a process of overcoming negative emotions by ______ the mental function. Maladjustments are a process of ___________ the pain of negative emotions without strengthening the mental function. Some of the common maladjustments are the use of defense mechanisms, the use of drugs, deviant sexual behavior, eating disorders, psychosomatic conditions, psychosis, and suicide. Many of the emotional problems and deviant behavior expressed by secondary students are maladjustments. The teenage years are important times for the mental function to mature and become healthy and distinguish between adjustment and maladjustment. The _____________ ___________ play an important role in facilitating this process.

Words that have special meanings as used in this lesson.

adjustment
aggressive
assertive
autonomy
defense mechanisms
deviant sexual activity
drug dependence
eating disorders
emotional
happiness
identity
integration
intellectual
maladjustments
maturity
mental health
mental illness
moderator
needs
negative emotions
neurosis
passive
positive emotions
productivity
psychosis
psychosomatic disorders
psychotic behavior
reality
reasoning
receiving
responding
responsibility
right or wrong
self-actualization
stress
suicide

Chapter 6

MENTAL HEALTH PROBLEMS

The material discussed in this chapter will help you recognize possible departures from normal mental health among your students so that if needed appropriate help can be provided.

RECOGNIZING DEPARTURES FROM NORMAL MENTAL HEALTH

In an imperfect world there are many circumstances that may motivate a person to exhibit unusual behavior. Acts that may be very peculiar in one set of circumstances may be quite predictable in another set of circumstances. This makes it very difficult to recognize departures from normal mental health. Nevertheless, there are some key indicators that this lesson will consider.

Because emotions are highly complex and subjective, they are very difficult to understand and often impossible to explain. However, a teacher should be alert enough to recognize some behavior patterns that may suggest the possibility of a problem and refer the student to someone who can help.

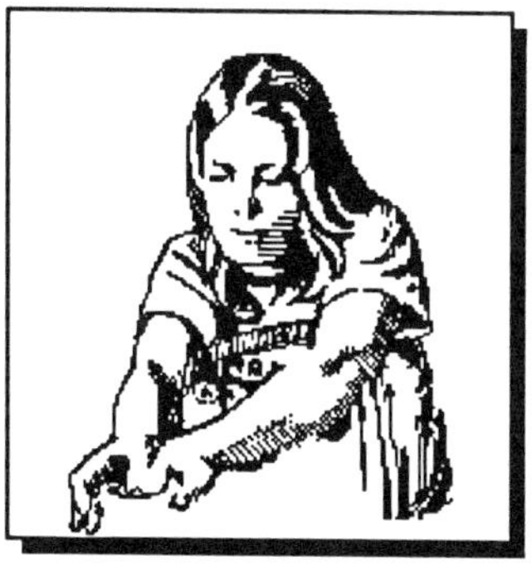

Departures from normal emotional health may range from mild disruptions in the mental function to serious disorientation of the personality. Departures from normal emotional health differ not so much in types as in degree. Most departures are quite tolerable if they occur only occasionally, but more frequent manifestations of the behavior may indicate a serious problem. For example, it is natural for a student to come to class depressed or discouraged once in awhile, but if the behavior continues for one or two weeks, something is wrong. The teacher should refer the student to a school counselor, school nurse, or an appropriate person who may be able to discuss the source of the depression and be in a better position to tell if professional help is needed.

Few people can meet the standards of good mental health at all times; we all fall short occasionally. The question is, "How can we tell when a person has reached the point where he or she needs help?" We recognize that mentally healthy people are generally happy, but there are many circumstances that ought to make people unhappy. A false, unrealistic, unwarranted optimism is considered abnormal and is known as *pollyannaism.* The opposite extreme is excessive *pessimism.* When unhappiness or depression begins to interfere with people's normal activities, schoolwork, job, relationships with family and friends, ability to sleep, or capacity for enjoyment, then they may need help.

No one should be embarrassed to seek help for his emotional difficulties. The question is, "Where can we find help?" Help may first come from talking it over with someone--parents, a friend, a teacher, a school counselor, a school nurse, or a clergyman. Talking it out often gives some relief from pent-up feelings and may help provide a new point of view. After that, it may be easier to seek help from a physician, social worker, psychologist, or psychiatrist if necessary.

Often teachers will be able to recognize minor departures from normal mental health and implement practices to help the student make meaningful adjustments. When teachers observe more severe departures, they should make sure the student receives the necessary help before extreme forms of behavior develop.

ADOLESCENT DEVELOPMENT

As adolescents enter this time of rapid growth and development, they often exhibit characteristics that are not normal for the general population but are quite normal for teenagers. Someone said, "For teenagers to be normal is abnormal." While this statement is an exaggeration, it illustrates a point.

In contrast to adults, teenagers more frequently exhibit the following:

1. They have more energy, drive, and vitality. This may be channelled into constructive, destructive, or meaningless directions.

2. They have heightened sensory awareness and perception. They may be attracted to or annoyed by sounds, tastes, smells, sights, and textures that are not noticed by others.

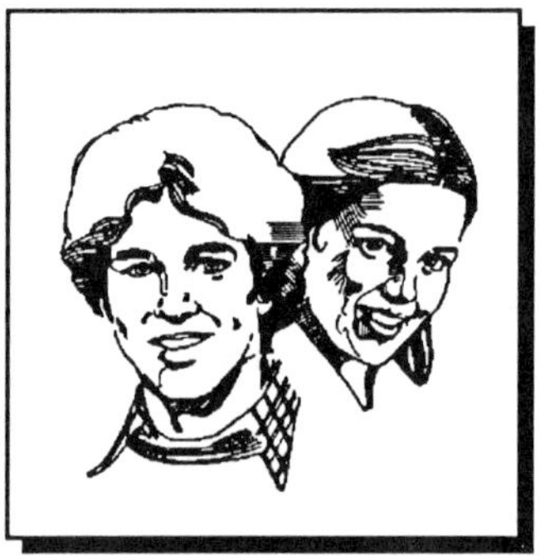

3. They have a strong sense of fairness, and they dislike intolerance. They have a sensitivity and awareness of other people's feelings. They exhibit more loyalty.

4. They have a concern for the future of the country and the world. They tend to be idealistic and to question contemporary values. They often think seriously and deeply.

5. They are flexible and adapt to change readily. They are usually open, frank, honest, and have an optimistic and positive outlook on life.

6. They have a feeling of independence. They are courageous and willing to take risks.

7. They have a sense of humor that often finds expression. They find humor in situations that are not at all funny to adults.

8. They are engaged in a sincere and ongoing search for identity, and they strive more for self-improvement.

These are strengths generally found among adolescents. They will continue to build upon them unless they are thwarted. If they become frustrated, they may turn in the opposite direction. Teachers and other adults should strive to reflect back to their youth. They should reflect on young people's strengths, and not to their weaknesses. Young people will then carry these strengths into adulthood. An individual with good mental health will generally exhibit the following traits:

- Has a high level of self-esteem and self-respect.
- Has a reasonable amount of security.
- Feels reasonably confident in himself.
- Has the ability to concentrate on a task.
- Has the ability to keep his emotions under control.
- Recovers quickly from disturbing experiences.
- Has a perception of humor and can laugh at himself.
- Can take disappointments in stride.
- Gains satisfaction from day-to-day pleasures.

- Accurately estimates his own abilities.
- Is tolerant towards himself and others.
- Moods fluctuate within a relatively narrow range.
- Is sincerely interested in others.
- Can obtain self-gratification through socially approved means.
- Considers others' interests as important as his own.
- Has satisfying and lasting interpersonal relationships.
- Trusts others and feels he is trusted by them.
- Likes others and can feel that he is a part of a group.
- Feels a sense of responsibility to his fellowmen.
- Respects new ideas, experiences, and can meet new situations.
- Meets life's demands and can handle problems as they arise.
- Is able to think and make independent decisions.
- Is productive, creative, and makes a contribution of value.
- Is integrated; his interests are orderly and complimentary.
- Is generally happy and enjoys life.

PROBLEMS FACED BY ADOLESCENTS

Breaking ties. Teenagers are in the process of breaking former ties with parents, brothers and sisters, and friends. Advancing from elementary school to middle school or junior high school, and from there to high school, signals a time for making new associations and diminishing former alliances. This may be accompanied by considerable ambivalence. Even though they live in the same home and neighborhood, they begin to experience a psychological separation from those they have learned to rely on for approval, guidance, and sympathy. They are not sure how to react. They may feel suspended uncom-fortably

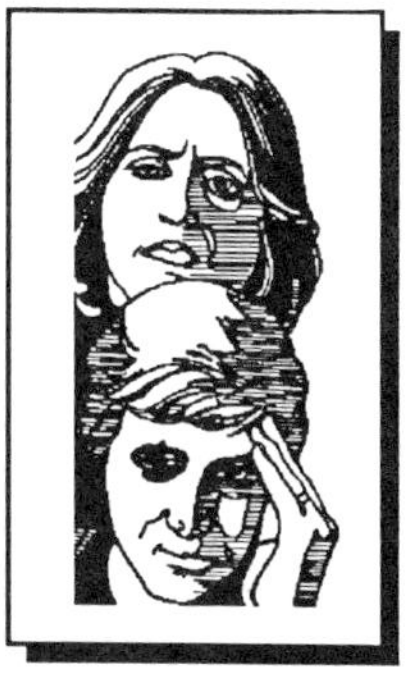

between the past and the future. Some oscillation and experimentation between a marked break and clinging to former ties is normal.

Self-esteem. Praise and acceptance from former associates was almost automatic. The family loved them because of who they were, and elementary school teachers passed out praise freely. Now their worth is measured by what they do, and there is more and more competition for good grades, popular friends, dates, positions on teams, and parts in the play. They must discover their worth for themselves.

Self-direction. Teenagers are in a position to start making more choices for themselves. Teenagers exercise significant purchasing power in today's marketplace, and advertisers direct their commercials to this vulnerable audience. Prior to this time, there were few options in the choice of friends. Now they are faced with real choices. They also face a greater choice in how they spend their time.

Value conflicts. Teenagers are exposed to new knowledge, ideas, and attitudes. New philosophies, morals, standards, and values challenge the old ones. At the same time, they are experiencing newly discovered sex drives. They encounter new problems arising from dating and other current boy-girl relationships as well as sex-role conflicts for the future.

With this in mind, a teacher cannot expect their students to behave entirely like adults. Even new teachers who may have been out of high school for only five years may have forgotten what it was like to be seventeen, much less thirteen. Textbooks cannot tell prospective teachers what teenagers are really like; that must come from observation and experience. But books and college classes combined with observation and student teaching experiences can help. Teachers should be able to recognize the manifestations of unfulfilled emotional needs and perhaps take steps to remedy the situation.

A variety of phrases have been used to describe adolescence. Garbowsky said "They are a study of contrasts." Hoffer called them "Temporary Misfits." Fetro and Vitello referred to adolescence as "no man's land," and Rogers called this time "a period of storm and stress . . . a state of internal civil war." They are experimenting with their own identities. However, most experienced teachers would probably feel that these phrases overstate the problem. New teachers should be aware of the unusual characteristics of adolescents, but also recognize that in many ways most teenagers are very normal. It would be unfortunate if this lesson caused new teachers to walk into the classroom with a lot of false preconceptions and stereotyped ideas about the youth they will teach. They should, however, be able to recognize the occasional departures from normal emotional health.

MANIFESTATIONS OF UNFULFILLED NEEDS

Unfulfilled emotional needs may be manifest through physical and emotional behavioral acts and through unusual speech patterns.

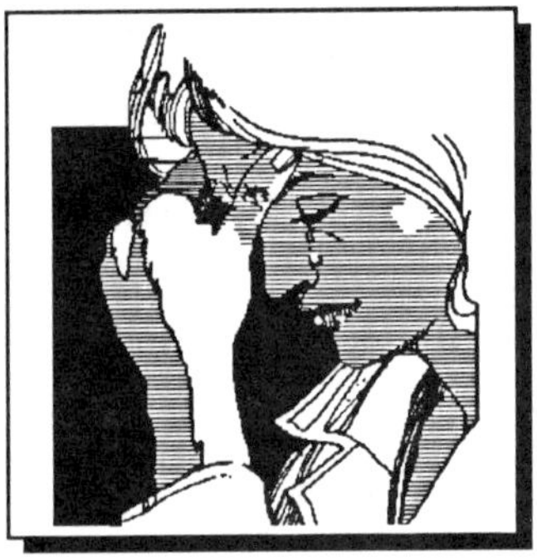

Physical manifestations. Sudden, drastic changes in weight may indicate that something is wrong emotionally. Sometimes emotional turmoil will cause twitches, hyperactivity, hypochondria, or psychosomatic illnesses in the individual. Abnormal dress may manifest that the individual is suffering from emotional disturbances that make him unable to worry about appearance.

Emotional manifestations. Emotional manifestations of unfulfilled needs may include crying, pouting, and depression. The individual may also show signs of neurotic or psychotic emotional behavior.

Behavioral manifestations. Individuals who suffer from unfulfilled emotional needs often manifest abnormal behavior. They may be severely withdrawn, violent, or argumentative. Delinquency, promiscuity, or other forms of attention-getting behavior may also serve as manifestations of unmet inner needs.

Speech manifestations. Sometimes unfulfilled emotional needs will interfere with the individual's ability to communicate. Stuttering, the use of baby talk, or profanity may be signs of emotional needs. Individuals whose speech patterns fall into these categories may be crying out for emotional satisfaction.

BEHAVIORAL PATTERNS RELATED TO EMOTIONAL PROBLEMS

Changes in behavior may be desirable if they are improvements, but sudden changes for the worse can be signs of emotional disturbance. Students who call attention to themselves, neglect their appearance, become preoccupied with sex, manifest aggressive behavior, or daydream excessively may be showing signs of inner emotional turmoil. Other signs may include excessive nervousness, over-talkativeness, abnormal sensitivity toward the opinions of others, unusual pleasantness, fidgeting, or acute anxiety. The following may also be signs of emotional immaturity or departures from normal emotional health.

1. **Fear** is natural in dangerous situations; however, fears that are not based on reality are abnormal. Those types of fears indicate something is emotionally out of order. Worry is an imaginary fear of the future. This emotion is not positive, and it should be controlled.

2. **Fatigue** is helpful in maintaining a regular schedule of sleep; but when fatigue is constant and sleep doesn't seem to help, emotional strains may be causing the problem.

3. A **shy** person may be a lonely person. It may be an indication of an inferior feeling, a fear of failure, or a form of embarrassment. It may simply be a lack of ability to interact with students of the same age. A teacher can help the student overcome this behavior by trying to involve the student in a group activity, and/or expressing high regard for him.

4. A student who is a **loner** and seeks to do everything by himself may be hiding a feeling of inferiority, or perhaps he's just never had to work with others. To deal with this, a teacher can involve the individual in group activity, or try to put him in a situation where he can feel important.

5. The **restless** student may simply be tired. However, it may be a feeling of inadequacy or a lack of success which leads to disinterest. The teacher should try to create activities to allow this student to find success and to bolster his interests.

6. **Daydreaming** may be a sign of escape into a fantasy world. It may mean there is a feeling of lack of success. Students who get self-gratification entirely in a dream world must be brought back to reality through assigned tasks that require their attention to be focused away from themselves.

7. The student who shows signs of **anxiety**, tension, and apprehension, may have a fear of censorship, punishment, or failure. The teacher can make himself a close friend to the student. Perhaps the teacher working closely with the student on a special project would develop a better attitude.

8. A student who **must be coaxed** is usually seeking attention. The teacher should try to draw the uninvolved student into the activities as naturally as possible.

9. A student who displays **hysteria** is highly unstable. This person may have a tendency for explosive conduct. A person may become unconscious or semi-conscious with an absence of physical sensitivity. A temporary functional paralysis may result. The person's greatest need is to get insight into his real motives, with guidance in learning to adjust wholesomely to frustrations and conflicts.

10. A **belligerent**, quarrelsome student may be putting up a defense which hides a feeling of inferiority, rejection, or defensiveness. This may be because of lack of status or even the result of brain damage. In such a case, a physician's help might be advisable.

11. The **suspicious** student distrusts others, even to the extent that he feels everyone is taking advantage of him. This is a defense mechanism and may express a feeling of extreme insecurity or inadequacy. By being friendly to the student, a teacher may help him to better adjust to people.

12. A **selfish** student who lacks consideration for others and their belongings or public property may have a feeling of self-contempt or hatred of self. The teacher should emphasize respect and consideration for property, not only in word but in action.

13. A **depressed** student may reflect his home life. He may also doubt his capability to succeed. He may become emotionally insensitive or feel a lack of self-worth. This may lead to suicide or drugs to escape life's problems. The teacher can help the student overcome his problems, but it may require the teacher's helping him each step of the way.

14. A student desiring to escape a stressful situation or get sympathy may **accentuating physical illnesses** to achieve his ends. The teacher may refer the student to a physician for treatment.

RECOGNIZING EMOTIONAL ILLNESS

There are no clear definite means of recognizing emotional illness, but there are some signs which may lead one to suspect emotional difficulties. Seldom do we see the extreme signs such as hysteria, but we see other signs quite frequently. *Depression* is a common symptom, but we all get depressed at times. Prolonged, severe, frequent depression or despair may be a sign. The American Medical Association estimates that 15 to 25 percent of the total population will experience sometime in their lives at least one period of depression severe enough to require medical assistance. Classical symptoms of depression include apathy, loss of interest in eating, loss of interest in other normal pursuits, headaches, indigestion, sleep disorders, etc.

Fear is another symptom, not the fear that is necessary for survival, but unexplained or displaced fear or panic. Excessive *nervousness* expressed by fidgeting or over-talkativeness may also suggest a problem. *Immobilization* for a long period is often a symptom. When a person becomes immobilized for a long period of time or is unable to continue doing whatever he or she does normally, that person may be suffering from some kind of emotional disturbance. Another symptom may be *anxiety*. Acute anxiety may include stomachaches, vomiting, diarrhea, or urinary urgency. Feelings of *fatigue* may be due to either physical or psychological problems, but in either case complaints of constantly feeling tired should be checked out by a physician.

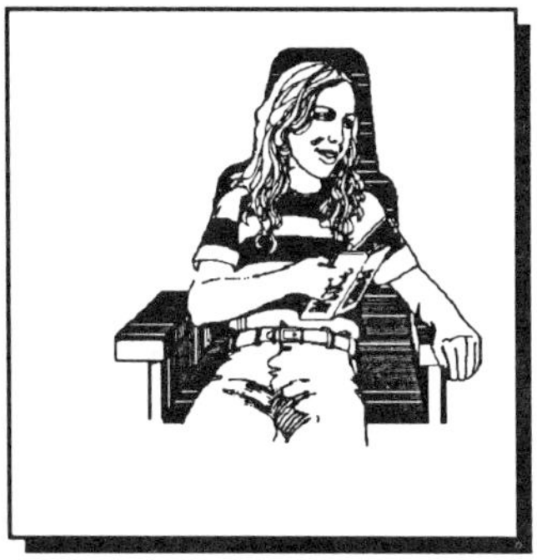

Involvement in organized or spontaneous student demonstrations may be an outlet for frustration. Resentment and loss of respect for parents, the school administration, the government, or other authority figures may be at the roots of student discontent, protests, and rebellion. Feelings of *alienation* expressed by such words as noninvolvement, isolation, separation, estrangement or detachment are often indications of the instability of teenagers. Feelings of alienation seem to be the forerunners for teenage drug abuse, pregnancy, eating disorders, runaways, involvement in cults, and suicide. School programs designed to prevent or intervene in such feelings may help reduce the incidence of such problems.

Personality disorganization such as disassociation, compulsive behavior, obsessions, or motor-sensory dysfunction are also symptoms of emotional disturbances. A more extreme sign might be a form of *hysteria*. This may show up as uncontrolled laughter or crying, alternating spells of laughing and crying, or even screaming. Underlying fright, panic, rage, or grief may have been pent up until the emotions overwhelm the individual's controls, and he bursts out with violent hysteria.

BEHAVIOR PATTERNS AND EMOTIONAL PROBLEMS

Of all of the symptoms a teacher might observe, a sudden change in behavior is the most common and most important indicator of emotional disturbance. The change may be to either extreme. It is not the behavior, but the sudden change that is significant. Here are a few examples:

- **Exhibitionism** or behavior that calls attention to the person such as clowning around or wise-cracking may be symptomatic.

- **Appearance** may change. A person may become neglectful or overconcerned about their looks.

- **Behavior toward others** may change becoming either harsh, non-cooperative, and without concern for the rights of others; or becoming over-anxious to secure approval by being unusually pleasant, conforming, and docile.

- **Interest in sex** may become abnormal. There may be either a compulsive preoccupation with sex or a complete lack of interest.

- **Escape mechanisms** such as fantasies and daydreaming may be turned to with sudden frequency.

Any of these, or similar changes, should not be ignored; they should be carefully monitored. Since one teacher cannot do this alone, it may be wise to have a conference with other teachers, counselors, or perhaps parents. Remember it is not the behavior, and not necessarily the sudden change, but the reason for the change that might be the cause of some concern.

EMOTIONAL MATURITY

Although basic maturity means that a person can meet the demands of life through socially accepted means, there are various levels of maturity, and most people can continue to grow and develop in one area or another. Teachers too can improve their emotional health. Stress is an occupational hazard of the teaching profession, and teachers ought to occasionally evaluate their own emotional stability. The following questions may help a person evaluate emotional maturity. A "yes" answer shows past achievement and a "no" answer indicates an area that needs improvement.

1. Even though you want something very much, can you still weigh various courses of action objectively?

2. Can you feel satisfied to make important decisions without having them approved by some person important to you?

3. Have you developed a consistent philosophy of human values which you use in making right-wrong decisions?

4. Are you willing to put controls on yourself to avoid advantage-taking, rather than requiring the other person to draw the line, e.g., satisfying sexual desires, sharing the work, spending money?

5. Do you judge a person on his qualities of character rather than by some predetermined quality, e.g., skin color, height, place of residence?

6. Are you able to talk without embarrassment or being disturbed about emotionally charged subjects, e.g., death, sex, racial membership, religion?

7. Are you usually able and willing to say whether you are or are not capable and well-qualified to do something you are asked to do?

8. If you believe in a principle, are you willing to say this even though you may meet disagreement or disapproval?

9. Are you able to say what your values are and which are more important to you than others?

10. Do you refrain from using sarcasm, anger, or hurt feelings to get your way or to punish others?

11. Can you accept a situation in which you have been in error without trying to excuse or justify yourself?

12. Can you be relaxed and confident when you are thrown with people who are older or younger than yourself?

13. Are you quite sure of what to say or do when meeting an uncommon situation, e.g., a crippled person, a person who is bereaved?

14. Can you account for the amount of anger or despair you feel?

15. Are you generally happy in your work?

If a teacher feels he is on the verge or in the midst of a personal emotional crisis, there are some things he can do.

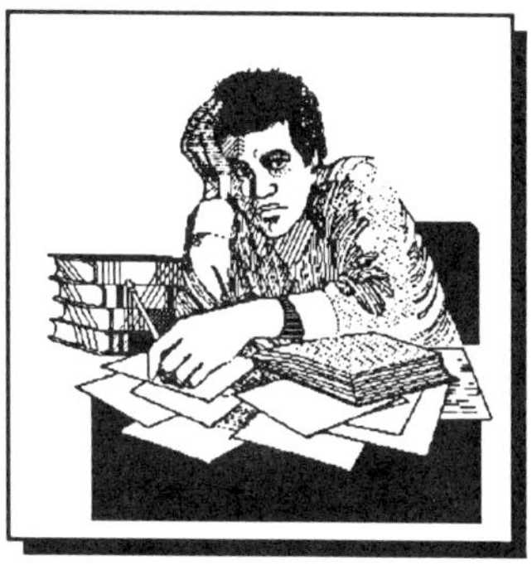

- __Take a breather__. It may be hazardous to make an important decision during an emotional turmoil, so a cooling-off period may be wise. Turn your attention to something else for a little while. After you have settled down, it may be easier to give some thought to your decision.

- __Talk it out__. In a crisis situation, a person needs a friend to talk to. Talking it out, or even writing it out, usually gives a new slant on the situation. Don't expect your listener to solve your problem, but talking about it will make you feel better.

- __Attack one point at a time__. Break the problem down into parts so that the big dilemma consists of a number of small, not too difficult problems. Taking them one at a time seems less frightening and easier to handle.

- **Stay healthy**. At a time of crisis, more than any other time, it is important to guard your health. Make sure that you eat sensibly, get some exercise, and get enough sleep. Illness at this time will complicate the problem. A healthy, rested body will give psychological strength.

- **Exercise courage**. If you have an accurate estimate of your capabilities, you will have greater courage during a time of crisis. If you know your true worth, you will be able to work within those bounds.

If you keep the above suggestions in mind, it will be easier to weather the crisis. If teachers are not emotionally healthy themselves, they will not be able to assist their students who may need help with an emotional problem.

FINDING WAYS TO HELP

Remember that emotional problems might be recognized not by what you do, but by where and when and how much you do. There is a range in which behavior is considered normal; if behavior exceeds that range so that it interferes with a person's own effectiveness or if it interferes with the rights of others, something should be done.

In a school setting, the right thing to do depends on the policies and practices of the school. In some cases, the observed abnormality merely suggests some changes the teacher might incorporate into the classroom procedures. In other cases, a referral along school policy lines may be necessary.

In the meantime, here are a few suggestions on how to help someone with emotional problems. Everyone at one time or another has the opportunity to help someone else who is anxious or upset emotionally. The most important key to helping is being a good listener. There is a correct way to listen, but few people understand this principle of human relationships. Here are some guides to listening.

- **Don't talk, listen**. The listening process is disrupted when the listener blames, criticizes, pities, or offers logic. To try to explain to someone why he or she is upset is dangerous.

- **Don't belittle the problem**. Sometimes the problem may seem trivial, but the person may react negatively to attempts to minimize it. Besides, there may be more than meets the eye. The problem the person speaks about may just be leading up to the bigger problem, if the listener is willing to listen.

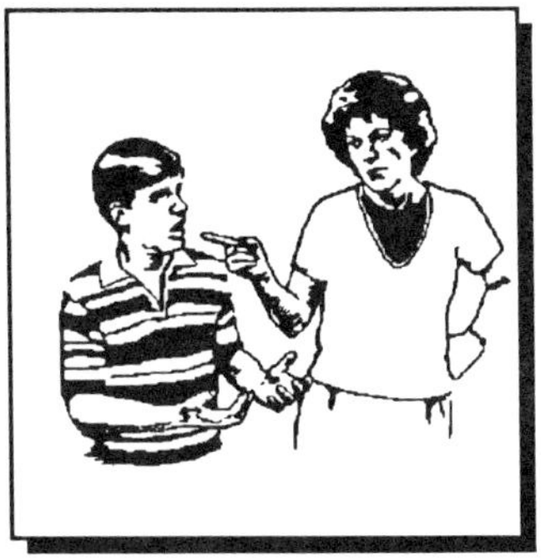

- **Don't be impatient.** People have difficulty expressing themselves when they are in distress. The listener must be willing to tolerate considerable repetition, delays, and vagueness from the troubled person. Listening takes time.

- **Don't provide the answers.** The person must come to his own decisions. The role of the listener is to either serve as a sounding board for the expression of feeling or to bring into view possible alternatives.

- **Don't try to treat the problem yourself.** Get professional advice. Call a family doctor, a mental health clinic, or a hospital.

- **Don't become anxious yourself.** If the person is at all hysterical, try to remain calm; show you are in control. This is not easy, because emotional outbursts are often contagious. Nervous attempts to calm a hysterical person usually intensify the problem. The following acts are apt to be viewed as acts of desperation and make the situation worse.

- **Don't shout.** Shouting conveys anxiety and loss of control on your part. Speak quietly, but firmly. Try to remain calm and listen.

- **Don't scold.** This is not the time to scold, argue with, or criticize the person. Don't tell the person all he has to do is snap out of it.

- **Don't slap.** Even though you may see it in the movies, don't slap or throw water on a hysterical person. These physical approaches may work, but they are more apt to make the situation worse.

Listening is a form of emergency first aid for emotional wounds. It may bring relief, but the troubled person should also be referred to a source of professional help.

STUDY HELPS

Be familiar with the following terms as used in this lesson.

alienation
anxiety
behavioral manifestations
belligerence
breaking ties
daydreaming
depression
disorganization
emotional crisis
emotional manifestations
escape mechanisms
exhibitionism
fatigue
fear
hyperactivity
hysteria
immobilization
isolation
lack of involvement
moodiness
nervousness
pessimism
physical manifestations
"Pollyannaism"
restlessness
self-direction
self-esteem
selfishness
shyness
speech manifestations
suspicion
unfulfilled emotional needs
value conflicts

True or False

1. Acts that may be very peculiar in one set of circumstances may be quite predictable in another set of circumstances.

2. We recognize that mentally healthy people are always happy. There are no circumstances that ought to make people unhappy.

3. When unhappiness or depression begins to interfere with people's normal activities, then they may need help.

4. Adolescents often exhibit characteristics that are not normal for the general population, but are quite normal for teenagers.

5. Sudden changes in behavior, even if normal, may be a sign of emotional disturbance.

6. Emotional problems might be recognized, not by what you do, but by where, when, and how much you do.

Fill in the Blanks

1. Departures from normal emotional health may range from __________ ________ __ in the mental function to ____________________ ____________ personality disorientation.

2. Of all of the symptoms a teacher might observe, ____________________________ __________________is the most common and most important indicator of emotional disturbance.

3. Everyone at one time or another has the opportunity to help someone else who is anxious or upset emotionally. The most important key to helping is being ______ a ________.

Short Answer Questions

1. All people occasionally experience unhappiness or depression, but how can one tell when they need help with their unhappiness and depression?

2. How may students show signs of inner emotional turmoil?

3. There are no clear definite means of recognizing emotional illness, but there are some signs which may lead one to suspect emotional difficulties. What are they?

4. What are some guides to being a good listener?

5. Rate yourself when you were a teenager on the characteristics listed on page 141-142.

6. In contrast to adults, what traits are exhibited by teenagers?

7. How are unfulfilled emotional needs often manifested?

8. If a teacher feels that he or she is on the verge or in the midst of a personal emotional crisis, what can he or she do?

Many people talk about the contemporary emotional problems faced by our youth, but teachers are in a position do something about them.

When we are inclined to focus on the weaknesses in our educational system, perhaps it is time to recognize that its successes are un-calculable. It is difficult to count the problems that never happen.

Teachers should be held in highest honor. They are the allies of legislators and physicians; they are the prime agency in the prevention of crime and illness.

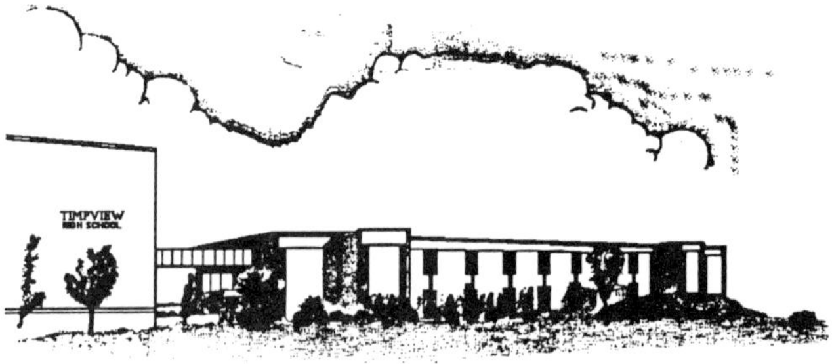

Chapter 7

CONTEMPORARY EMOTIONAL PROBLEMS

There are many contemporary problems in our society and our schools today which are symptomatic of underlying emotional problems. Some of the contemporary emotional problems will be discussed in this chapter, while others such as drug abuse, eating disorders, indiscriminate sexual behavior, child abuse, and sexually transmitted diseases will be dealt with in later chapters.

CONTEMPORARY EMOTIONAL PROBLEMS

Emotional problems are psychological barriers to health. Emotional problems are associated with feelings, obsessions, and compulsions that interfere with accurate perception and appropriate reasoning. Contemporary problems include those which persist from the past as well as those which are distinctively associated with the present.

Many emotional problems are a result of social problems, and many social problems are a result of technological changes in the society. Teachers need to understand how social problems contribute to the emotional problems of their students.

SOCIAL PROBLEMS

Social problems occur in any community, but in some communities they are more apparent than in others. Three social conditions are almost always found together: poor health, poverty, and inadequate education. Each negatively contributes to the other, and improvement in one is followed by improvement in the other two. A reciprocal relationship also exists between social health and emotional health. Many of the situations society considers to be problems are really symptoms of greater, more complex, underlying problems.

Scientific progress is not all good. Science contributes to industrial and technological progress, but this results in changes that sometimes contribute to social upheaval. For example:

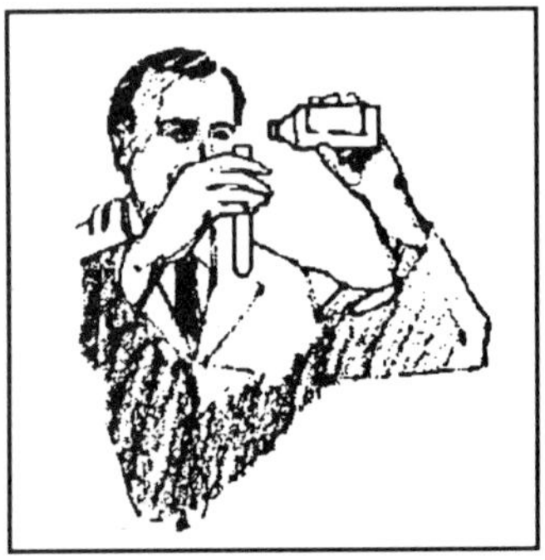

- Society sometimes suffers from a "cultural lag." There may be a gap between the discoveries produced through scientific research and their useful social application.
- Automation is one outcome of technology. Automation increases production efficiency, but replaces manual labor. This results in job obsolescence and unemployment. Unemployment and shorter work weeks result in boredom and destructive free-time pursuits.
- Scientific advancement has created a new demand for highly intelligent and carefully prepared personnel. This trend places pressure on schools and students. Specialization may tend to dehumanize people and make them slaves to science.
- Dynamic changes in social attitudes and practices are predicted outcomes of scientific advancement. There is a danger of people losing their identity. Traditional social institutions such as the family and religion may be disrupted.
- Economic fluctuation is considered to be a constant threat. Recession, depression, inflation, wage spiral, over-production, shortages, inadequate earning power, and fixed income are frequently expressed problems.

Urbanization, arising as an out-growth of scientific technology and industrial expansion, constitutes a whole new problem for society. Population displacement from farm to city and from city centers to suburban areas results in overcrowding in some areas and inefficient use of public facilities in other areas. Urban renewal projects attempt to relocate entire neighborhoods. This also contributes to a sense of alienation and social disruption. This impersonal climate results in a transient community of superfluous people who are unable to serve a useful function and who impose a burden on society.

The role of the family in transmitting traditional values is eroded as work obligations pull individuals away from the family. Values and interests are determined more by peer influences than by parents.

Overcrowding and robot-like factory conditions contribute to a kind of mass culture. Such a culture is marked by poor taste, lack of personal responsibility, an urgent need for self-gratification, and an "anything goes" society. When people are forced into identical "molds," they lose the sense of individuality and personal identity.

Industrial and urban developments have also given new perspective to conservation. The housing boom has destroyed rural settings; freeways threaten to carve up cities and to disrupt established communities. The rapidly increasing population requires more public recreational facilities. Pollution and contamination of air, water, land, and foodstuffs are inherent dangers.

Social problems contribute drastically to detrimental social practices. Behavior that was previously inappropriate either becomes acceptable to society or is tolerated because society finds itself powerless to prevent it. A climate of violence appears to stem from confused values and a lack of family guidance. A shifting quicksand of moral and ethical foundation may be indicated by scandal, dishonesty, malfeasance of duty, and crimes of every description. Obscenity and pornography are licensed under the cloak of literary and artistic expression.

Large segments of the population have come to rely on various forms of "escape from the responsibilities of life": alcohol, narcotics, tobacco, pills, gambling, sexual deviation, anti-social activities, and bizarre forms of self-expression. Personality and deep mental disturbances appear to relate to the fast urban pace, confused social roles, and overemphasis on social status.

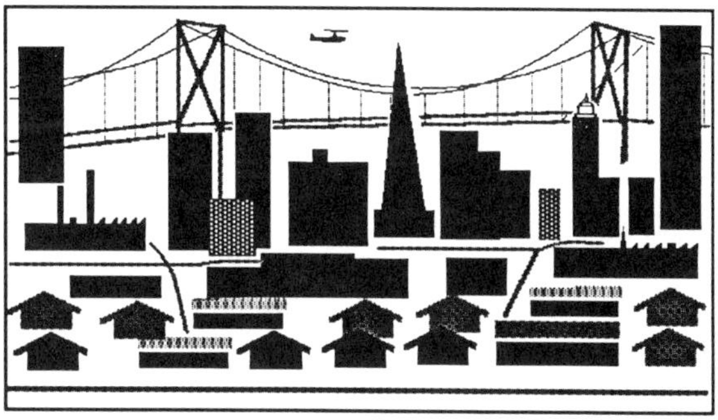

The common problem of poor physical conditioning is also accompanied by emotional and ethical flabbiness. Society suffers from a sense of noncombatance and softness of willpower. The failure to follow responsible safety precautions seems to reflect emotional instability. There is an extreme rise in venereal disease and pregnancy. Social welfare programs fail to rehabilitate and are subject to misuse. Concepts of law and order are frequently under attack from both sides: one side argues that the rights of the accused must be protected from "police state tactics"; and the other side argues that the public, and particularly potential victims of crime, deserve reasonable protection from the criminal through an effective system of law and order.

It would be unfair to blame all of our social problems on the rapidly changing industrial-technology complex, but society's inability to effectively adjust to these changes contributes significantly to the emotional problems of today's youth. Not only are the teacher and the school faced with dealing with the consequences of these problems every day, but they also hold the greatest promise for improving the situation.

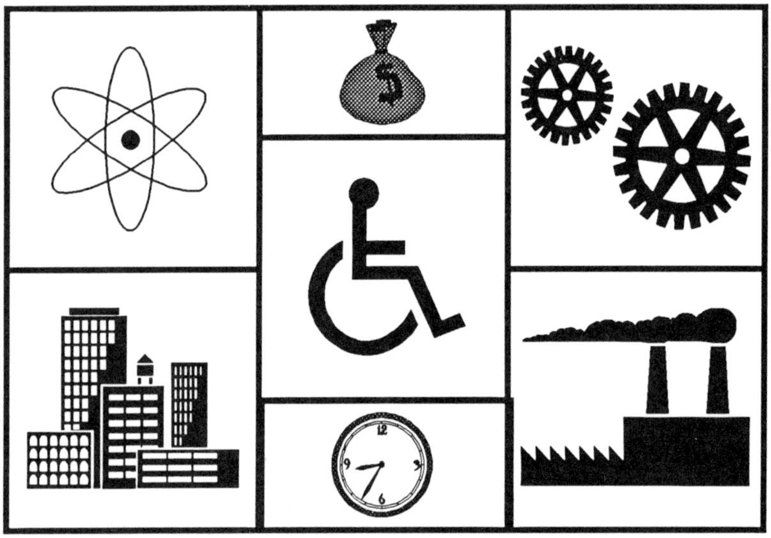

EMOTIONAL PROBLEMS

Parents, teachers, social workers, religious leaders, police officers, and other community leaders are concerned about the emotional problems of today's youth. They worry about the rebellious activities, self-destructive behavior patterns, and extremes in attitudes exhibited by many adolescents. While adults are concerned about the *consequences* of such behavior (addiction, suicide, pregnancy, AIDS), young people are concerned about the *motivation* (popularity, acceptance, self-expression, and appearance).

While adults generally are merely concerned about the problems, teachers are in a position to do something about the cause of the problems. But in order to make a difference, teachers need to understand what motivates the behavior of young people.

Motivation

The news media has exploited the emotional problems of some youth and has helped create a distorted image of adolescents. While the behavior of most youth does not fit this image, some youth fail to take an independent stand, follow the crowd, and continue to adhere to this distorted idea of normal adolescent behavior.

Commercial interests in our society have used the advertising media to exploit the teenage image and perpetuate the fallacy that "everybody is doing it." Advertisers are not selling products; they are selling emotional illusions. Youthful consumers are not purchasing products; they are buying dreams.

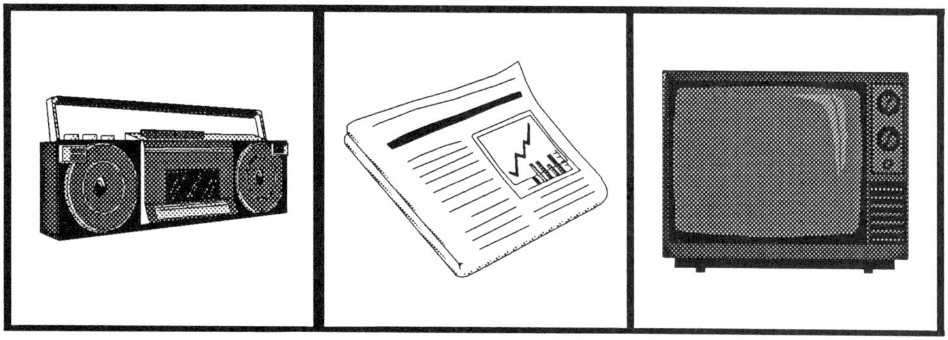

Until recently, the cigarette and alcohol advertisements illustrated this point. When a young person purchased a cigarette, he or she was buying the feeling depicted in the advertisement--strength, freedom, excitement, and masculinity or femininity. If a young person relies upon the cigarette to generate the desired feeling, he or she also becomes dependent upon it as a drug. Then after the youth matures and no longer needs the cigarette to generate the feeling, he or she still needs the drug. If a boy smokes a cigarette to prove he is a man, how will he discover he could have become a man without smoking?

Of course not all illusions are perpetuated by the media; society also passes counterfeit measures of success from one generation to the next. If a child's swearing and vulgar language seems to get him the attention he wants, how will he be motivated to learn to get attention through more socially accepted means? If a girl engages in sexual activity to gain popularity, how will she be motivated to develop her personality in ways that will earn her genuine pleasure and lasting popularity? Until they learn better, it is characteristic of youth to try to take shortcuts. But the shortcuts may interfere with the growth and development necessary to learn to handle emotion. Youth need to learn how to deal with their complex motivations.

We cannot always interpret a person's motivation from observing his behavior. Identical motivations may lead different people to quite different behavior. Conversely, identical behavior may result from quite diverse motivations. It follows that if different people do something for different reasons, different approaches may be needed to persuade them to change that behavior.

The situation is further complicated by the fact that behavior is usually influenced by more than one motive. Health may be a motive, but health motives are often less compelling than other conflicting motives. Young people, like the rest of us, do not always regulate their lives according to their best knowledge and understanding of the facts. To a large extent, young people are rational beings, but often they are influenced more by their emotions. Their actions are influenced by their desires, aspirations, uncertainties, ambitions, worries, and fears. Emotions also reduce a person's ability and willingness to learn and accept new facts. When emotions get out of control, they can lead youth into a number of contemporary emotional problems.

NEGATIVE SELF-CONCEPT

Ideally, children grow up feeling good about themselves. Based on positive experiences, they develop a sense of being loved and being able to give love. They also develop a sense of worth and a positive self-concept. But as children mature, they encounter situations that challenge their self-concept. They have disappointing experiences which may contribute to a negative self-concept.

There is a distinct difference in the way people react when something goes wrong and they fail to meet their goals. People with a positive self-concept will acknowledge that something went wrong, make adjustments, and try again. People with a less healthy self-concept may try to preserve their self-concept by denying that anything went wrong or by transferring the blame to someone or something else. A worse reaction is to develop a negative self-concept. People with a negative self-concept feel demoralized, unloved, and ineffective. They tend to think in the negative and to see the black, not the white or the shades of gray. They just give up. They get into a vicious self-destructive cycle where failure leads to poor self-concept and poor self-concept leads to failure.

A negative self-concept is almost universally associated with the contemporary emotional problems discussed later in this lesson and in several of the subsequent lessons. Teachers have a unique opportunity to intervene in the destructive cycle. Methods that can be used by the teacher to improve self-esteem will be discussed in lessons eleven and twelve.

DEPRESSION

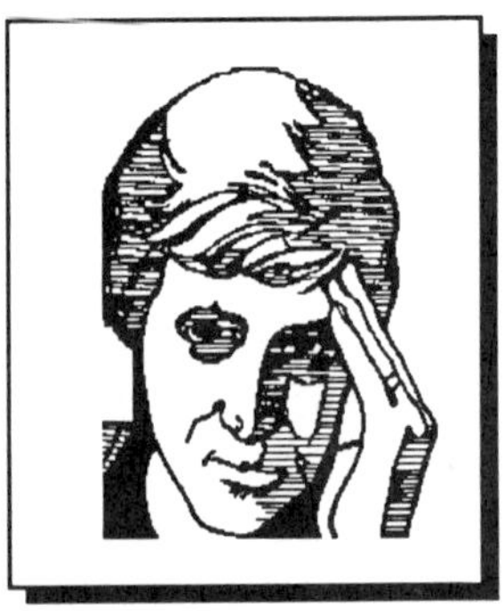

Depression is the most common emotional disorder in the United States. Approximately 15 percent of the population are apt to experience at least one bout of depression in their lifetime severe enough to require medical help. Nearly two out of every three cases of depression occur among females. Adolescence, middle age, and the years after retirement are the periods in life when people are particularly susceptible to depression.

There are several kinds and degrees of depression. Most people have occasional bouts of "the blues," but depression lasts longer and is more severe. The difference between being depressed and having the mental illness known as depression is that people who are severely depressed are unable to lift themselves out of their misery.

Chemical depression. Some types of depression are associated with a chemical or hormonal imbalance in the body. Women tend to become temporarily depressed during the weeks following the birth of a baby. Certain illnesses are often followed by depression. Alcohol, drugs, and medications may cause depression.

Distressing event. Depression may be associated with a failure or a significant loss. A distressing event such as the death of a loved one, a divorce or separation, loss of a job, being cut from the team, or failing to be selected for a part in the play can lead to depression.

Psychological. The most common form of depression is of psychological origin. A negative self-concept is usually associated with this type of depression.

Depression will include several of the following:

- A feeling of sadness, helplessness, and hopelessness
- A loss of interest in or pleasure from usual activities
- A poor appetite or eating too much
- Insomnia or sleeping too much
- Restlessness or lethargy
- Fatigue
- Inability to concentrate
- A feeling of worthlessness or guilt
- Thoughts of death or suicide

The presence of any five of these characteristics indicates some depression. The more characteristics, the more severe the depression.

People in mild depression can still meet their obligations and things appear to be normal, but there is no joy in life. A person may experience a loss of pleasure and interest in activities that are usually enjoyable and appealing. The person may feel that normal activities require greater effort and are less rewarding.

More severe depression may include deep despondency, gloom, and despair. The most severe consequence of deep depression is the high incidence of suicide. Severe depression is treated through medications, psychotherapy, and suicide prevention. A person is at greatest risk for suicide not while in deep depression, but when they start to feel better. In deep depression, people do not have the psychological strength to commit suicide, but as they start to come out of their depression they may gain enough strength to carry out the act. Also, when they finally decide to commit suicide and start to make definite plans they appear to feel better. People who are monitoring their condition may start to relax, but that is the most dangerous time.

SUICIDE

In the United States, suicide is generally recognized as the second leading cause of death for young people of high school and college age. In this age group, the suicide rate per 100,000 rose from 8.8 in 1970 to 39.8 in 1980, an alarming 287 percent. The United States was not alone; of 29 nations reporting to the World Health Organization, 26 experienced an increase. A 1987 report from the National Institute of Mental Health (NIMH) estimated that up to 5,000 adolescents per year commit suicide in the U.S. and another 500,000 attempt suicide. A study conducted among 2,200 youth in Minnesota found that 3 out of every 100 youth had attempted suicide in the period of one month. The National Committee on Youth Suicide Prevention estimates that one out of every two teens consider suicide by the time he or she finishes high school. Suicide data is often inaccurate, for in many instances completed suicides are recorded as accidents to save the surviving family from embarrassment.

Adolescents are very vulnerable to suicide due to the many changes taking place in their lives. These changes may foster both positive and negative feelings. Biologically, the process of growth and sexual maturation is a totally new and volatile experience. It is also a time for determining one's individuality. The role changes may make them feel like they are out of control. They may ask, "Who am I? Am I normal? Am I alone?" Moving toward becoming adults may be alarming and distressing, particularly if they have little regard for adults. If early efforts to adapt into the adult role fail, they may try to defend themselves by attempting a variety of coping behaviors. At first, they may withdraw or rebel; later, they may take drugs; and finally they may even attempt suicide.

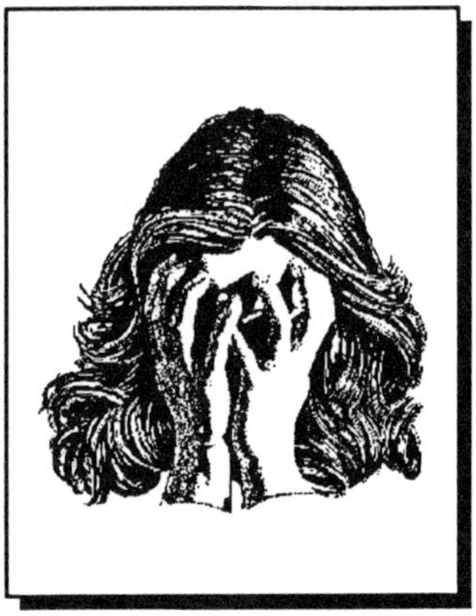

There are many theories to help explain suicide, but no theory alone is sufficient. A 1984 pamphlet published by the U.S. Department of Health and Human Services, *Adolescence and Depression*, listed the following:

- The *psychodynamic* theory explains that suicidal behavior may develop from deprivation, rejection, and the loss of love.

- The *developmental* theory recognizes that suicide may be an impulsive overreaction to a long standing sense of entrapment.

- In the *cognitive* theory, it is believed that the adolescent's perspective is limited by incomplete intellectual development. The teenager sees himself as immortal or that death is reversible.

- The *social* theory relates suicide to alienation, isolation, withdrawal, and the loss of social contacts and guidelines.

- The *biological* theory correlates suicide to a deficiency of serotonin or other chemical abnormalities.

One of the highest risks factors associated with suicide is depression. Low self-esteem is one of the chief indicators of depression. The number of teenage suicides could probably be reduced significantly if the signs of depression were recognized and if appropriate actions were taken.

Another risk factor for suicide is poor family relations. Family violence or the loss of a parent through death, divorce, or a marital separation can cause a sense of helplessness and vulnerability. One report in the *Journal of Adolescent Health* (Mehr et al., 1981) indicated that nearly three-quarters of suicide attempters reported family problems, including substance abuse, physical abuse, lack of support, and instability of the family structure. It is estimated that over sixty percent of today's youth will live for at least a part of their school age years in a single parent family.

Teens face a fast-paced life that is full of pressures and that is very competitive. They see examples of violent solutions to problems on both the news and the entertainment portions of television constantly. People who are shocked to learn that suicide is the second leading cause of death among teenagers are even more shocked to learn that homicide ranks third. A violent expression of emotion is also associated with many accidents, the number one cause of death among teenagers.

It appears that many young people are not prepared to handle the emotional situations they encounter. There are fewer opportunities for young people to assimilate social values today. In many homes, the traditional family meal is often replaced by quick meals prepared by individuals. The discussions that once took place around the family dining table were important times for transmitting social values from one generation to the next, but that time is often replaced in today's society by time in front of the T.V. and other individual activities that take members of the family out of the home. Society also places less emphasis on religious instruction and other value clarification activities.

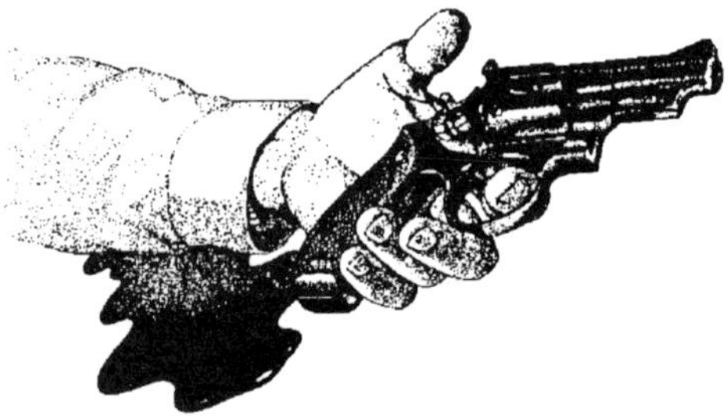

The risk of suicide is increased when teenagers abuse drugs. Alcohol and then marihuana are the most frequently abused drugs. Drugs frequently complicate the life of the adolescent and make him more prone to suicide. Adolescents under the influence of drugs are more apt to act impulsively. The same drugs that may precipitate suicide may be the mechanism used by teenagers to commit suicide.

A number of other factors are associated with suicide. Girls attempt suicide three times more frequently than do boys, but the boys commit suicide twice as frequently as girls. One of the reasons for this is the choice of weapons; boys tend to use the more deadly weapons. For example, there is a much greater chance for someone to intercept the effect of pills than a bullet from a gun.

A wide variety of circumstances precipitate the suicide. Often teenagers who are anticipating some form of discipline attempt suicide. Suicide may follow the loss of someone important to them. Being rejected by someone may also trigger suicide. A dispute with a friend, teacher, sibling, or parent may be a provocation for suicide. Loss of security, failure in school, an unwanted pregnancy, or even the thoughts of moving to a new neighborhood may be associated with a suicide. Teenagers who get involved in cults have a higher incidence of suicide. Suicide is more common among adolescents whose parents or siblings have attempted or committed suicide.

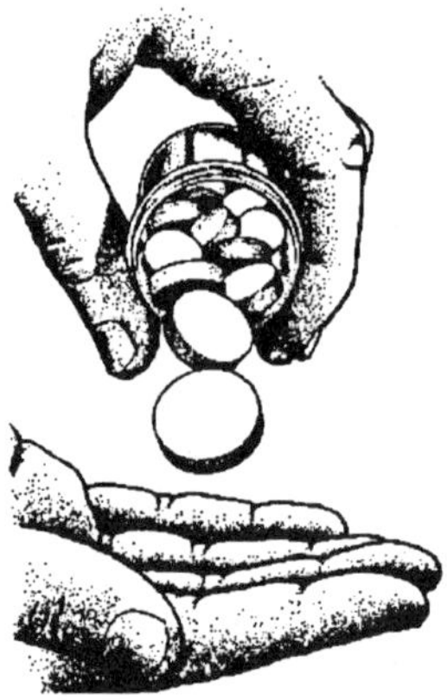

MYTHS ABOUT SUICIDE

There are many myths regarding suicide, and teachers should be able to separate the facts from the fiction and dispel the prevailing myths. Following are some of these myths which apply to the student suicide problem.

"The Student Who Talks About Suicide Won't Commit Suicide."

Anyone talking about suicide should be taken seriously. Of all the people who have committed suicide, up to 80 percent of them talked about it or communicated the idea in some way. Sometimes this communication is very straightforward: "There isn't anything in this life that's worth living for." Other times comments made about committing suicide are vague and covered up or hidden within the comment: "How about one last date together?" The teacher must learn to listen carefully and be able to interpret what the student is actually saying. Those who talk about suicide are, in fact, crying for help. They need to talk to someone who will be willing to listen, be patient, and not criticize them.

Suicide Happens Without Warning.

This is simply not true. Most students will either communicate the idea of suicide (whether it be straightforward or ambiguous), or their behavior will change along with an increase in feelings of depression, isolation, and/or obvious signs of mental illness.

Talking About Suicide Will Help Plant Ideas in Someone's Head.

It is a myth that if you are concerned that a student is considering suicide, and you ask him about it, you are planting the idea in his head. If something has happened that makes you think the student might consider suicide, he already has the idea. Bringing up the subject may open the doors for further conversation to help him with his problem.

Suicide and Attempted Suicide Are the Same Class of Behavior.

This myth is apparently not true. Nine out of ten people who attempt suicide do not go on to commit the act. This supports the idea that young people who attempt suicide are asking or begging for help.

Suicides Occur More Among the Poor.

One universal myth is that "good circumstances" will prevent suicide, or that suicide occurs more often among the poor. Suicides can and do occur among different economic levels. There is no correlation at all between economic levels and suicide rates. It is true, however, that families which are constantly operating under stress produce suicidal youth.

Suicide Is an Act Committed by the Insane.

Suicide is not an act committed only by the mentally ill. It's true that the mentally ill are more apt to commit suicide if the right circumstances are present, but many students who are not mentally ill commit suicide.

Once a Person Attempts Suicide He or She Is Suicidal Forever.

This is probably the worst myth of all, because one attempt may brand a person for life. The fact is that most persons who are considered suicidal are actually only suicidal for a short duration of time. They may have become extremely depressed, and at that particular moment could feel no hope at all, their only recourse being suicide. However, having people around can help stop the risk of another attempt. If the person is fortunate and the elements in his life change for the better, he may never attempt suicide again. Never reject anyone who has tried to commit suicide.

People Who Attempt Suicide Really Want to Die.

This is not true. Some students do it to get attention and sympathy from people, to change something, to regain a lost relationship, to rebuild self-esteem, or to escape from an overpowering situation. Even up to the last moment, the individual has a desire to be rescued, to go on living, and to find a better way of life.

Suicide Is Inherited.

This is erroneous. It is a fact that the tendency for suicide is not biologically passed on from parent to child. If a child commits suicide, that doesn't mean all the children in that family will.

CLUES AND WARNING SIGNS OF SUICIDE

Sometimes a teacher may be able to observe some clues that may help identify a suicide-susceptible student. Some of these clues may include observable changes in behavior such as the following:

- Sudden and unexplainable neglect of school work. Inability to concentrate, increasing tardiness and absence, messy school work, and lower grades should be explored by the teacher.
- Decreased communication. Less class participation, aloofness, or inability to communicate. Non-communication is a communication of need.
- Changes in social behavior. Decreased concern about appearance, social withdrawal, dropping out of extracurricular activities, quitting part-time work, and isolation are behavioral clues to suicide.
- Changes in eating and sleeping patterns. Eating too much or too little, sleeping too much or too little, sudden weight change, or insomnia point to a need for help.
- Changes in the student's emotional life. Low self-esteem, depression, crying for no apparent reason, apathy, irritability, rebelliousness, risky behavior, violent outbursts, or increased use or abuse of drugs or alcohol may be warning signs.

More specific warning signs or clues may include:

- Sudden threats or statements revealing a desire to die.
- Making final arrangements such as giving away possessions, paying debts, apologizing for old arguments.
- Paying attention to death such as writing or circling the words of songs and poetry dealing with death.
- Buying such things as a gun, rope, or pills.
- Sudden dramatic improvement for no apparent reason after a period of depression.

These clues and warnings are particularly significant when they are accompanied by a feeling of isolation from emotional involvement with parents, peers, and teachers.

SUICIDE CLUSTERS

Sometimes suicides occur in groups or clusters. A *suicide cluster* is defined as a group of suicides or suicide attempts which occur closer together in time and space than would normally be expected in a given community. Recently, several suicide clusters have received national attention. Many people are becoming concerned about the possibility of a suicide cluster occurring in their community. Much more research is needed to determine what the relationship is, if any, among the suicides and suicide attempts in a cluster, but many people believe that there is a sort of "contagious" relationship between the early suicides and the later suicides in a cluster.

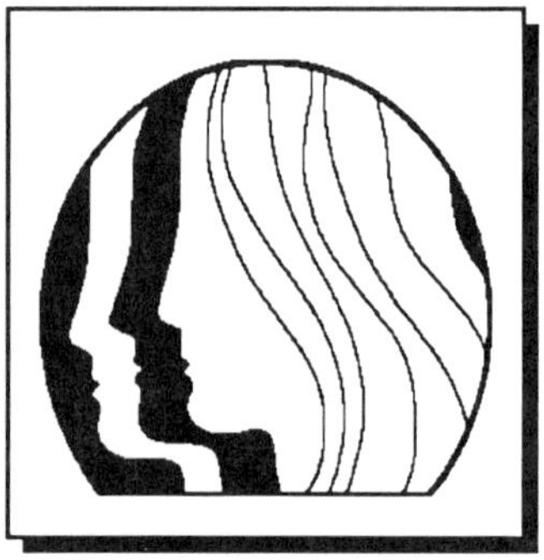

The Center for Disease Control (CDC) has developed a list of recommendations to help communities develop a response plan for dealing with cluster suicides. The first step is the planning stage. Each community should review the CDC recommendations and make necessary adjustments. The planning would involve all concerned sectors of the community and identify all relevant resources. Educators are key resources. Teachers, counselors, administrators, and other school personnel should be trained in their respective roles. The plan requires coordination among various agencies within the community. The plan could be implemented when a suicide, a suicide attempt, or a traumatic death occurs among teenagers and the members of the coordinating committee think it may potentially influence others to attempt or complete suicide.

If the plan is implemented, the first step is to inform the various resources so they can fulfill their assigned tasks. A single spokesman to the media should be identified. Every effort should be made to minimize any sensationalism about the incident and to avoid glorifying the victim. Care should also be taken to avoid vilifying the victim either. Nor should there be an attempt to whitewash the event. Sometimes schools have erected parks or established scholarships in memory of a student who has committed suicide. Although these efforts are well meant, they are inappropriate. Neither is it advisable to allow funeral services to unnecessarily disrupt the regular school activities.

Giving too much attention to the suicide or to its motivation might increase the likelihood that someone who identifies with the victim or who may be contemplating suicide might also attempt suicide.

Persons who might be at risk should be identified and screened by trained counselors. The advisability of establishing a hotline or a walk-in crisis center should be considered. The school may be the best place to set up a counseling center. It may be necessary to bring in trained counselors. If it is necessary to announce the suicidal death of a student, it should be done in a manner that will provide maximum support for the students while minimizing the likelihood of hysteria. The deaths should be announced privately to those students who are most likely to be deeply affected by the tragedy.

Long term efforts to prevent suicides should be addressed. If particular methods or sites have been used in previous suicides, they should be identified and dealt with. A suicide surveillance system may be put into place. A three-phased approach should be implemented. Prevention is a plan of education. Intervention is a course of action in dealing with a possible suicide risk. Postvention involves working with individuals who have attempted suicide.

PREVENTION

Teachers should have an understanding of their role in suicide prevention. Prevention is simply a plan for educating both the student and society at large. It must deal with myths surrounding suicide as well as helping individuals to recognize the existence of possible suicidal tendencies. Discussing suicide can be extremely helpful in prevention. First, a discussion of suicide inherently includes the topic of individual feelings and emotion as well as the underlying factors behind these feelings. Secondly, as students talk about suicide, they come to realize that other students experience the same feelings they do and that they are not alone in the concerns they have. Finding this out can release a lot of pressure that adolescents experience.

The best time to discuss suicide in the classroom is after an attempt has been made. At this time, feelings will be intense, and it would be good to bring these feelings into the open.

Educators want to help their students, but they are sometimes afraid that talking about it might suggest it. For that reason, schools steer away from suicide prevention programs. Sometimes individual teachers take it upon themselves to lead a discussion in class about suicide. This may be good, but it has some risks. It is much better if it is organized on a school and community wide basis. It is good to have a course available for all students that deals with suicide and other topics that require coping skills. If schools have a comprehensive health education program, the health course should meet this need. It should be taught by a well- qualified instructor who will effectively utilize community resources.

Here are a few guidelines for school activities related to a suicide prevention program. First, it should have broad community support including the school administrator. It should be implemented before, not after a suicide has occurred, and it should not glamorize suicide victims. It should teach students that suicide is not a way to solve problems, and it is not a courageous act. The program should encourage students to ask for help and provide information on where they can get help. It should dispel the myths about suicide. It should help students recognize the warning signs of suicide and understand what to do for someone who is suicidal.

Parents should also be aware of the school's suicide prevention activities. A means should be provided to discretely omit students should their parents object to their children being involved in those suicide prevention activities. Hopefully, both school administrators and parents will give strong support to a well-organized suicide prevention program.

One of the most important ways of preventing suicide is by helping students build self-esteem. This can and should be the goal of every teacher. Teachers can help students improve their self-esteem only when the teacher's self-esteem is also high. Although a teacher might be brilliant academically, if he or she rips students apart emotionally, it does not help build self-esteem and confidence.

INTERVENTION

Intervention is the course of action taken once a person has been identified as a possible suicide risk. The teacher can do one of three things. First, he can consult the student directly, not with the idea to solve the problem, but just to let the student know that he is aware that there is a problem. This act alone shows the student that there is at least one person who cares. The second thing a teacher can do is get together with the family. This can be a delicate situation and requires thought and tact. It is important that the teacher not come right out and tell the family their child is suicidal. It is better to simply let the family know that a significant change has occurred in their child's behavior at school. Thirdly, a teacher may take his concern to the administration of the school or to the family physician or clergyman. This last recourse is available mainly in situations when talking to the family may not produce results. The main purpose of intervention is to provide the student with someone whom he would feel comfortable enough with to talk openly and honestly about his feelings.

Whenever a suicide occurs among teenagers, there is a chance that the cluster effect may take place. The schools should move to prevent this potential. Each school should already have a crisis team established and additional trained counselors on call. Teachers should have already been trained to know their role and to deal with the emotional responses of students. They should know what to say and what not to say. They should know where to refer students who are most upset. When a crisis occurs, the principal may call a special meeting of the staff to inform them of the event and to allow the school psychologist to review possible student reactions and appropriate staff response. A crisis center may be set up for a few days so that students might walk in and talk with counselors.

High-risk students should be identified and their parents contacted so that prevention strategies can be discussed.

POSTVENTION

Postvention is for the student who has attempted suicide. The teacher must try to reduce his or her isolation by reestablishing lines of communication with the student. The student must be integrated into the classroom. It may help to hold a class discussion before the student returns. It is not wise to pretend that nothing has happened. This discussion should not give excessive attention to the method used by the student as a cry for help or in any way glamorize the student. The discussion might focus on the impact the suicide attempt had on their lives and help them deal with the accompanying feelings without ignorance and fear. The discussion may help prepare them to accept the student back as a normal member of the class.

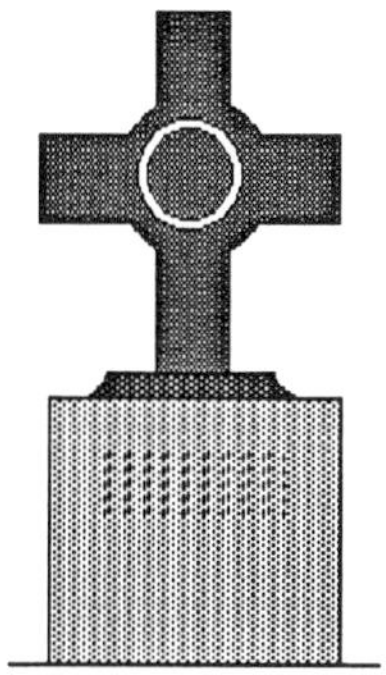

COPING WITH DEATH AND DYING

Death is a part of life's experience. Whether it be one's own death or the death of another, the emotions associated with it are individual and personal. It is a concept that many people are not comfortable with. A brief discussion here about death and dying may help you, as a teacher, better deal with death in the school setting.

The death of young people seems tragic, particularly when the events surrounding it are questionable. Usually the death of young people is violent and sudden. Students can become quite emotional when a fellow student dies, and you will need to know how to deal with these feelings in the classroom. You may also have a student in your class who is mourning the death of a close loved one and your response may really help. On a rare occasion, you may have a student attending your class with an incurable disease. In all of these situations you may be puzzled about the best way to help.

It is not easy to know how to help a person in these situations, because their responses can be so varied. People usually respond to the news of a death by sequentially moving through a series of psychological stages. The stages are the same when a person learns they are dying themselves, or when they learn about the death of a close family member or friend. The length of time required to pass through each stage varies with the person and the situation. The appropriate way to respond to a person depends on the psychological stage they are in. Therefore, the most important thing to do is be alert and sensitive to the clues the person gives and respond accordingly. It is well to have a variety of responses in mind, so that you are ready to use the one that is most appropriate.

PSYCHOLOGICAL STAGES OF DEATH AND BEREAVEMENT

There are psychological stages that a person may experience in adjusting to the idea that he or she is approaching death. The person who is terminally ill or the person who loses someone they care for may experience the same psychological stages. A psychiatrist, Dr. Elizabeth Kubler-Ross, has studied extensively the reactions of terminally ill patients and has identified five psychological stages that people often pass through.

Denial. Denial is generally the first stage of adjustment. They psychologically reject the idea. They may try to go on as though nothing has happened. By refusing to accept the truth, people in this stage are trying to gain time to adjust to it. They will not want to talk about it. A person may pass through this stage in just a few moments or may remain in this stage for an extended period of time. In trying to help a person in this stage, accept their behavior and give them time. Do not try to contradict them or take away their hope.

Anger. When denial is no longer effective, a feeling of anger may arise. The person may feel they are being treated unfairly or cheated. The dying person may blame other people. The person who has lost a loved one may feel anger toward the deceased. Their anger may not be at all logical, and their blame may be misdirected. Not being able to find an appropriate target, they may lash out at anyone, even others who are suffering as they are. Unfortunately, this may result in some unpleasant and regrettable last memories. Those who appear to be the targets should realize that the anger is not really directed at them. Encouraging the dying or bereaved person to express his or her feelings may bring some relief from the anger. They should be allowed to cry and air their feelings.

Bargaining. A bargaining stage often follows denial and anger. This may be a reversion to childhood when we learned that if we want something we can sometimes trade something else for it. Here again the logic may be clouded. The dying person may try to bargain for time, for forgiveness, or for reassurance that their life was worthwhile. The bereaved person may be negotiating to be freed in their own mind of any blame associated with the death. Those trying to give help should try to understand and give support during this stage.

Depression. When a person has exhausted their energies in denial, anger, and bargaining; depression may set in. Reactive depression is associated with memories of past and lost opportunities. Preparatory depression is associated with preparing for the future. Both kinds of depression involve gloominess and general low spirits. People in depression may not appreciate lengthy discussions. Those who are trying to help should listen and provide encouragement and reassurance. They should follow the dying or bereaved person's lead. Grief is such a powerful emotion it can cause physical aches and pains. The process of bereaved people sharing their feelings and experiences as they adjust to the death of someone close is called mourning. The sharing of their feelings will make the situation much more bearable.

Acceptance. Given sufficient time, the dying and the bereaved person will reach a stage in which the death is accepted. For the dying person, this stage is neither happy nor sad, but peaceful without much feeling. It is not a time for much conversation, but it is comforting to have close friends and family members near. For the bereaved, this stage marks the time when they are able to get on with life without as much pain. There may still be intermittent returns to any of the five stages, but gradually they will diminish in frequency and effect.

How a teacher responds to a bereaved student depends not only on the psychological stage of the student, but also on the prior relationships between the teacher and the student. Hopefully, there will be a bond that will permit the teacher to be helpful. Teachers should feel fairly comfortable about the situation and know what to do. Sometimes people are so afraid of saying or doing the wrong thing that they do nothing. They ignore it or avoid it, and this is usually the worst thing they could do. Teachers should at least acknowledge the situation in some way to let the student know that they know and care. After that, they should look for clues from the student as to what to do. Often in times like this, nonverbal communication is more effective than cautiously selected words.

CULTS

The participation of young people in cults is another social trend that has many educational leaders concerned. It seems that adolescents get involved in cults for the same reasons they become depressed, attempt suicide, or get involved with drugs. Young people who are unable to satisfy their needs in normal healthy ways turn to dangerous alternatives. Some withdraw from society physically, and others withdraw psychologically.

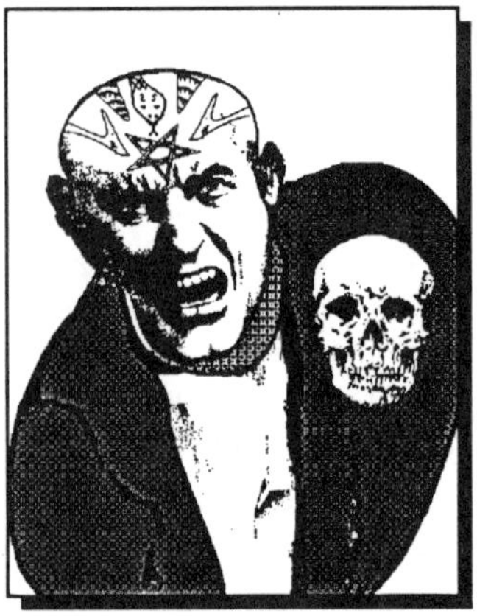

Cults are religious type movements which break with the traditional religions of the culture. Religious sects emphasize their ties with the past. They are reformed versions of the faith from which they split. Religious cults emphasize their newness, difference, or irreligious nature. Cults are strongest in regions where conventional religion is eroded.

Some of the characteristics of cults include:

- Complete subservience to one individual who is a messenger of deity.
- Separation from society except to proselyte or to raise money.
- Distrust of parents, organized religion, government, and civic groups.
- Destructive behavior-modification techniques such as Pavlovian conditioning.
- Discourages education and self-development.
- Not concerned with the physical body; only the soul is important.
- Organization claims all material possessions; members do not own anything.
- Uses physical restraints and psychological fears to keep members from leaving.

Sociologists who have studied cults do not always agree on which organizations should be regarded as cults. Some are large, well-organized, and nationally well-known; others are small and loosely organized. Most cults are antagonistic toward families, community, and some traditional social values.

Why do young people join cults? Cults offer a channel for rebellion, a chance to discard routine concerns, the appeal of a drama of struggle and danger, and a sense of community in a closely knit subculture. The conversion process exploits individuals who are socially and psychologically vulnerable.

Over a million young Americans have become involved in recent years with the estimated 100 religious cults. Many of America's young people, most of them middle class, and most of them reared in traditional Christian and Jewish faiths, are moving towards radically different religious cults. Teachers of American youth need to understand what is behind this fascination with cults and what the consequences may be.

Why are parents, educators, social workers, religious leaders, and community leaders concerned when young people become involved with cults? Membership in the cults often brings a total break from past friends, jobs, studies, and family. Defectors have told how their religious activities follow a strict routine and how their lives become completely dominated by the cult. They lose their individuality and become subservient to the cult leaders. Some of the most frightening cults are the so-called Satan worshippers who desecrate animals as a form of sacrifice.

Parents who have lost their children to the cults are concerned, frustrated, and broken-hearted. They charge that the cults have changed their children into zombies, robots, or puppets. Psychologists assume the cults have used mind manipulation which takes away the young person's personality. Rehabilitation or deprograming is very difficult, and many young people, even when they want to, find it difficult to return to normal life. Prevention is the best hope.

Parents and other concerned groups, for the most part, have not been successful in using legal channels for help in regaining their lost children. Ex-members have had little success in their legal charges that they have been exploited. Government officials remain leery of any action that might tamper with the nation's tradition of religious freedom. Some people would say that any form of religion involves some brainwashing, so how can the government say that one religion is more valid or safe than another?

Converts to religious cults can be seen roaming the streets and corridors of U.S. cities and airports selling oriental incense, singing gospel hymns, and taking up collections. Millions of dollars are collected through work and begging by the cultists. Young people are invited to weekend retreats and while there, are attracted to the smiling and affectionate members. After long hours of work and indoctrination, a process sometimes called "psychological kidnapping" or "brainwashing," the young people join the cult. Perhaps the situations of our time have made the young people susceptible to the philosophies of the cults. Many youth today have a feeling of anxiety and guilt, often caused by being brought up with so many material possessions. They also lack a sense of direction. For these young people, cults seem to fill the void.

PSYCHOSOMATIC PROBLEMS

Few physical health problems are without some associated emotional problem. Likewise, emotional health problems result in some physical problems. Sometimes these associations are understood, but more often this relationship is very obscure. Modern medicine has acknowledged that many physical health problems have a psychosomatic basis. The word psychosomatic, is a combination of the words *psycho,* meaning mind, and *soma,* meaning body. It means a physical problem with an emotional basis.

Psychosomatic illnesses are not imaginary, they are real; but their origin is emotional rather than organic. Among the illnesses which may be, but are not always emotional in origin, are: chronic diarrhea or constipation, colitis, ulcers, headaches, insomnia, skin rashes, and asthma.

Another word, *somatopsychic*, means that a physical problem is accompanied by an emotional disturbance. Diabetes, acne, obesity, and orthopedic problems are a few examples where students may have both a physical and emotional problem. A student may use his physical problem to secure sympathy and special favors. Sometimes the problem becomes cyclic, and each side makes the problem worse in this reciprocal relationship.

ADDICTIVE BEHAVIORS

In Roman law, the Latin word *addictus* meant a debtor awarded as a slave to his creditors. Today the word addict means one who is a slave to a habit. Instead of the courts making us a slave, we put ourselves in bondage to a substance or a behavior.

There are several components of the addiction scenario. There is the addictive substance or behavior that may be either good or bad, depending on how it is combined with the other ingredients. There is the addict. There are also benefits and consequences, both good and bad, which motivate the behavior. Overindulgence has undesirable consequences such as dependence, compulsion, and the loss of control. The Roman *addictus* probably originally obtained something of considerable value, but the price he ultimately had to pay, his own freedom, was too great.

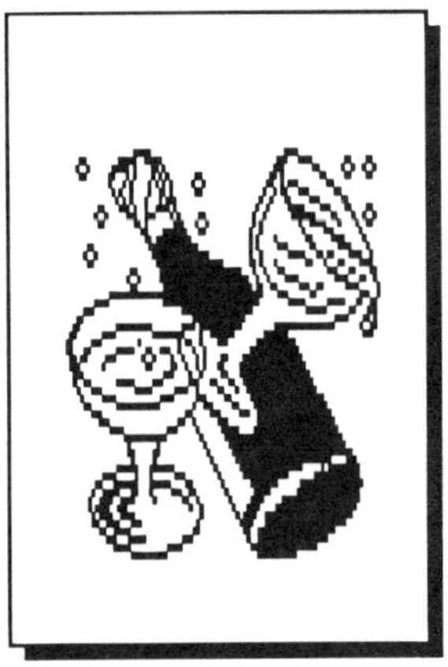

There are other components of the problem. There are the promoters who profit from the slavery. And, unfortunately, there are also the innocent victims; family members who are deprived of more than physical needs--affection, attention, and a proper role model. Neighbors and friends are sometimes victims of crime and violence, and the whole community suffers.

People frequently visualize these consequences when associated with drug abuse, but may not be aware of the consequence of overindulgence in behaviors that are normally acceptable and sometimes highly regarded. However, most people can find something they need to work on. It might even be something that others--such as friends, teachers, or counselors--can help them with.

WHY PEOPLE BECOME ADDICTS

Addiction may be the result of a person attempting to use alternative methods of meeting needs. Some of the factors leading to addiction are on the following page:

Needs. People have certain basic needs, and when those needs are not met in normal ways, people attempt alternative methods of meeting those needs. Often those needs are linked to a sense of worth and a sense of belonging: finding love, affection, and acceptance; being adequate, understood, and appreciated; becoming what we are to become. These needs are normally met through effective interpersonal relationships. But when other people are not available, or when we lack the skills to facilitate interpersonal relationships, we begin to suffer. So when our esteem needs are not met in the normal ways, we may attempt alternative methods of meeting those needs. Frequently, our alternative behaviors are considered by others to be strange, bizarre, or weird, and we feel even less accepted. In frustration, we may try even more diverse alternatives until something seems to work, and to that we become addicted.

Stress. Stress is a physiological response to a perceived threat. When our safety and security is threatened, we feel stressed. Various forms of pressures--whether self-imposed or from others--also create stress. With stress, we feel very uncomfortable; we experience painful negative emotions. Some behaviors or substances may provide a false sense of relief from the stress and pressure. We begin to depend on these maladjustment techniques and become addicted to them.

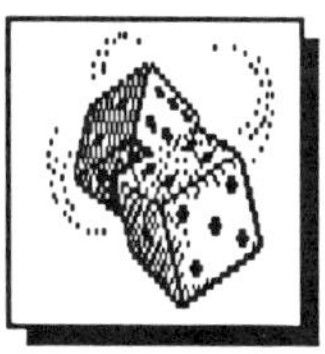

Emotional gratification. We are emotional beings. We thrive on positive emotions: excitement, elation, exhilaration, enthusiasm, love, joy, and a sense of accomplishment and well-being. Emotions are intense feelings involving physiological responses centered in the nervous and endocrine systems. Activation of the sympathetic nervous system provides a sense of excitement as it prepares for "fight or flight." The parasympathetic nervous system counters to keep the body in balance by providing a calming response. Adrenalin and norepinephrine intensify the feelings. Endorphins, sometimes called the natural morphine, provide relief from pain, produce euphoria, and suppress fatigue. We enjoy some of these feelings, and they are gratifying when they occur occasionally in life on special occasions. But some people seek to experience them on a frequent or constant basis. They become dependent on substances and behaviors that artificially induce these feelings. They become addicts.

Sensory gratification. We are also sensory demanding beings. We seek sensory stimulation. Like the fantasy robot character in the movie "Short Circuit," we call for ". . . input, input." We want to be entertained, to have our minds and senses occupied with faster, louder, more exciting sights and sounds. This may be a mindless type of entertainment that provides an

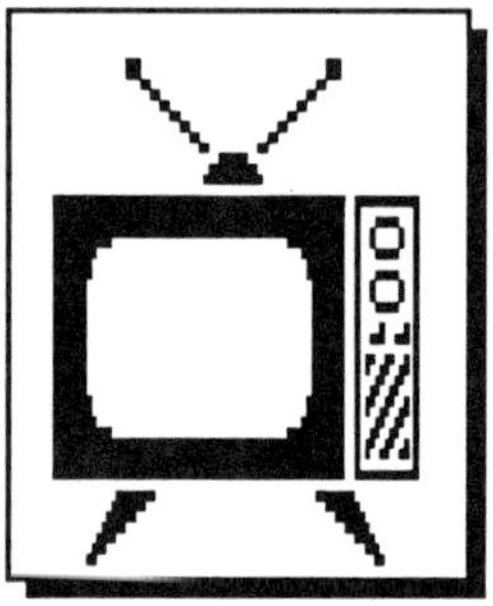

escape, but requires very little mental effort. The kinesthetic sense associated with rhythmic body movement may also fit in here. People do get hooked on physical activities such as jogging. An activity that provides an escape along with sensory gratification may become an addiction.

Reinforcement. Before addiction to a behavior or substance occurs, it must be reinforced. The reinforcement is the pleasure and relief the product or behavior provides. The power of the reinforcement should not be minimized. Even after the undesirable consequences become very apparent, the strength of the reinforcement makes it very difficult to stop.

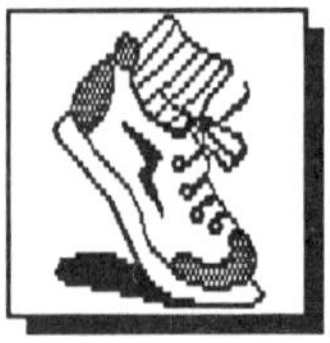

Positive addictions. Some addictions are called positive addictions because they are reinforced in the same ways negative addictions are. They are addictions because they are missed terribly when they have to stop. They are positive because they have some long-term health values, both physical and emotional. The benefits of a positive addiction may be very good, particularly for some people, but it can be carried to an extreme. Sometimes people lose perspective and become a slave to it. It is not easy to tell when normal behavior becomes an addiction. There is sometimes a fragile line between normal behavior and addiction. It is difficult for a person to recognize in themselves when they have crossed that line. To attempt self-analysis takes a lot of courage and time. It takes an honest and careful introspection merely to recognize a problem. Much more effort is required to overcome the problem, but identifying an addiction or something close to it is the place to start.

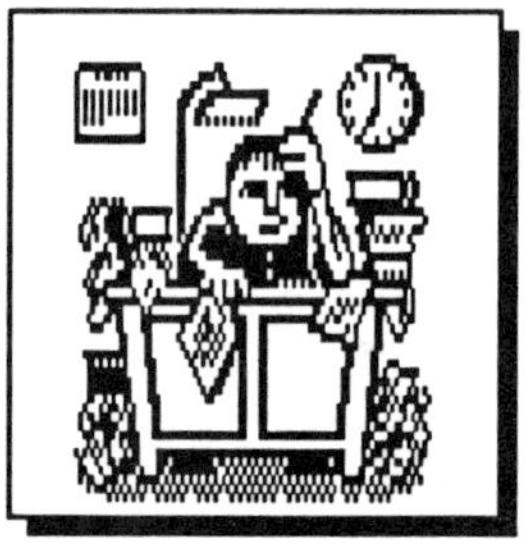

Normal behavior. It is not the behavior, but the way the behavior is incorporated into a person's life that makes the difference. If the behavior is normal, it tends to be spontaneous, rather than being predictable. The behavior is normal when it is integrated into the person's life, not a separate endeavor that detracts from the whole. The behavior is normal when it has an inherent value, not just because it has become a routine. The behavior is normal when it provides a level of satisfaction and when that is reached the person can go on to something else.

Addictive behavior. Addictive behavior, on the other hand, is quite the opposite. Addictive behavior is not spontaneous; it is compulsive and highly predictable. Addictive behavior is not integrated into one's life; it dominates life and causes the person to neglect other things of importance. Tolerance develops and no matter how much he does it, he can't get enough. The addict feels compelled to engage in the behavior even after its original appeal is lost.

He still continues his behavior in spite of the adverse consequence. He does it to avoid the withdrawal associated with stopping. Stopping will cause anxiety, jitters, disorientation, and the inability to function normally. Addictive behavior follows a spiral course of descent to destruction. An adverse consequence of addiction is the loss of self-respect, resulting in the person turning more and more to addictive behavior to hide this loss.

NOT PRONE TO ADDICTION		PRONE TO ADDICTION
	RESPONSIBILITY	
Accepts responsibility for his own behavior. Self-disciplined.		Blames others. Lacks basic skills. Lacks self-discipline.
	RIGHT vs. WRONG	
Sets standards. Chooses right from wrong.		Fails to recognize difference.
	REALITY	
Recognizes the ultimate good or bad consequences. Can defer gratification.		Denies the problem. Escapes through fantasy. Wants immediate gratification.
	REALISTIC	
Recognizes his own limitations and sets realistic goals.		Unable to set realistic goals.
	RELATIONSHIPS	
Has interest in others, can love and be loved. Respects others' rights.		Lack of interest in others, has poor social skills. Manipulates others.
	RESILIENT	
Optimistic, bounces back, from setbacks, withstands disappointment. Repentant.		Feels powerless, feels victimized, is pessimistic. Non-repentant.

EXAMPLES OF ADDICTION

Most people have some examples of addiction or behaviors approaching addiction, but they must first recognize them before they can overcome them. This and previous lessons have talked about some forms of addiction such as drug addiction, sex-related addictions, and various eating-related addictions. The following list of addictions includes those and some other examples of addiction:

- **Drugs** the depressant, stimulant, or hallucinogenic effect of drugs.
- **Eating** a sensual stimulation that relieves negative emotions.
- **Exercising** the neurological stimulation (endorphins) without dealing with life.
- **Sleeping** to avoid having to face life's problems.
- **Shopping** a reaction to disappointments.
- **T.V.** to escape life, a sensory stimulation.
- **Workaholic** to gain acclaim for success, to avoid dealing with other responsibilities.
- **Gambling** the excitement of taking a risk.
- **Risk Taking** the thrill of putting life in danger.
- **Sex** the sensual stimulation of pornography, fantasy, or promiscuity.
- **Violence** for the thrill of hurting others.
- **Traits** compulsive, almost unconscious nervous traits such as nail biting, etc.

ADDICTION PRONENESS

People with certain characteristics are more prone to addiction. The following list contrasts those characteristics which will help people to escape addiction to those characteristics which make a person more prone to addiction.

HELPING ADDICTED PEOPLE

An addict usually feels that as bad as his addiction is, it is better than life without it. To help him give up the addiction, we must help him find a better alternative. We must realize that the behavior is usually an attempt to meet unfulfilled needs. We should not attempt to change the behavior without finding better ways of meeting their needs. For example, if drugs are the problem, don't just suddenly take away the drugs. Find out what needs they are attempting to meet by taking drugs. Then help them find an alternative method for meeting the needs.

Basic physical needs. Start first with basic physical needs. It is hard to deal with emotional needs when the physical needs are a problem. Encourage them to follow good health practices--rest, exercise, proper nutrition, and personal cleanliness.

Basic emotional needs. Help them realize that someone cares about them and that they are a worthwhile individual. To do this, try to help her or him in the following ways:

- Get involved with things that bring success. Work on improving social skills and self-esteem.

- Confront the behavior, not the person. If they keep records, they might better recognize the problem.

- Avoid patterns that lead to the behavior. You don't gain strength by seeking tempting situations.

- Commit to realistic goals. People often want to do too much at once and become disappointed.

- Visualize the rewards for meeting their goals as well as the consequence of not meeting them.

Schools are not the only institution involved in minimizing those character traits that make people susceptible to addiction, but they are certainly one of them and they must do their part. The best way for schools to do their part is to help students develop healthy self-concepts and appropriate coping skills.

STUDY HELPS

1. What is the relationship between industrial and technological progress and the social upheaval that contributes to so many of our contemporary emotional and social problems?

2. Three social conditions are almost always found together: poor health, poverty, and inadequate education.

3. In regards to the behavior of young people, what are adults concerned about? What are young people concerned about?

4. Why are teachers in a unique position to do something about the contemporary emotional problems of youth?

5. While most adults are merely concerned about the problem, teachers are in a position to do something about it.

6. How has the commercial interests' (advertising) desires to exploit teenagers contributed to the emotional problems of our youth?

7. What is the danger of interpreting a person's motivation from observing his behavior?

8. How will a person with a positive self-concept generally differ from a person with a poor self-concept when something goes wrong?

9. Why is a negative self-concept almost universally associated with the contemporary emotional problems discussed in this lesson?

10. What is the most common emotional disorder in the United States?

11. What are the various kinds and degrees of depression? What are the characteristics of depression?

12. Among U.S. teenagers, where does suicide rank as a leading cause of death?

13. What are the leading risk factors for teenage suicide?

14. The Center for Disease Control lists several theories as to causes of suicide. What are they?

15. What percent of today's youth will live for at least a part of their school-age years in a single parent family?

16. What is the relationship between the risk of suicide and teenagers' drug abuse?

17. What are the comparative incidents of suicide and suicide attempts among males and females and what explains the differences?

18. What is probably the worst suicide myth? Why?

19. What makes the clues and warnings of suicide most significant?

20. The Center for Disease Control (CDC) has developed a list of recommendations to help communities develop a response plan for dealing with cluster suicides. What are the steps in this plan?

21. People with certain characteristics are more prone to addiction. What are those characteristics?

22. Why are educators sometimes afraid to talk to youth about suicide?

23. People usually respond to the news of a death by sequentially moving through a series of psychological stages. What are those stages? How long do they last?

24. People are often afraid of saying anything to the dying and the bereaved. What is probably the worst thing they could do?

25. It seems that adolescents get involved in cults for the same reason they become involved in other contemporary emotional problems. What is the reason?

26. There is a distinguishing difference between cults and traditional religious movements. What is it? What are the characteristics of cults?

27. Why are parents, educators, social workers, religious leaders, and community leaders concerned about young people's involvement with cults?

28. What are psychosomatic illnesses? What are some examples?

29. What is the relationship between the Latin word *addictus* and addictive behaviors today?

30. What are the components of the addiction scenario? How can one distinguish between normal behavior and addictive behavior?

Terms associated with contemporary social/emotional problems.

alienation
amoral society
automation
cultural lag
eroded values
job obsolescence
overcrowding
population displacement
social disruption
superfluous people
transient community
unemployment

Other terms of importance to this chapter.

acceptance
addiction proneness
addiction
addictus
anger
bargaining
chemical depression
cognitive
consequences
contemporary
cults
death and dying
denial
depression
developmental
distressing event
emotional gratification
emotional problems
intervention
motivation--popularity
needs
negative self-concept
positive addictions
postvention
prevention
problems
psychodynamic
psychological
reinforcement
sensory gratification
sociological theory
somatopsychic
stress
suicide clusters
suicide myths
workaholic

Chapter 8

EMOTIONAL PROBLEMS AND DRUG ABUSE

Substance abuse is one of the major problems in our society. Everyone needs to better understand this problem, but this knowledge is particularly important for school teachers. Within recent years, several states have added a drug education component to their teacher certification requirements. This chapter is designed to meet those needs.

DRUG USE, MISUSE, AND ABUSE

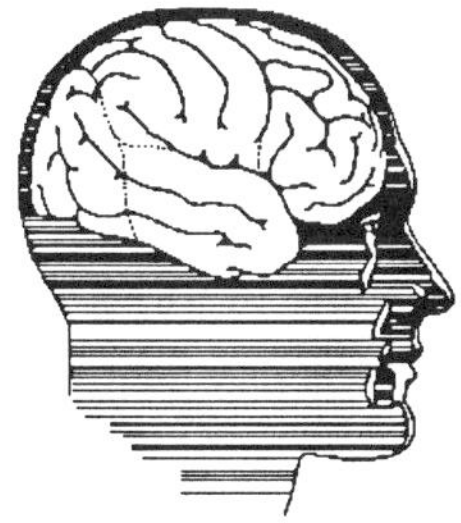

Central Nervous System

Throughout history in every culture, people have used substances which modify their moods, alter their perception, diminish their physical pains and emotional discomforts, and seem for awhile to make life bearable or pleasurable. These substances, whether found in nature or synthesized in the laboratory, are drugs of the central nervous system (CNS). A drug is any substance, other than food, that when taken internally alters the body functions. Specific types of drugs affect specific systems of the body, but the group of CNS drugs have a great potential for getting people into trouble. They affect a person's mood, alter perception, reduce physical and emotional discomfort, and provide a sense of pleasure. They also have the potential for developing strong dependence. They have been used in the natural state, brewed, and compounded. They have been inhaled, eaten, injected, and consumed in every imaginable way. They have been praised for their benefits and condemned for their destructive influences. Psychotropic drugs (drugs that act upon the psychic) have had a calamitous influence on the lives of individuals and the well-being of society. Some people feel that for every pain drugs have relieved, they have created a thousand miseries. But the perceptive recognize that drugs are not the problem; drug abuse is only a symptom of a problem that is seated in the emotions.

BENEFITS AND RISKS

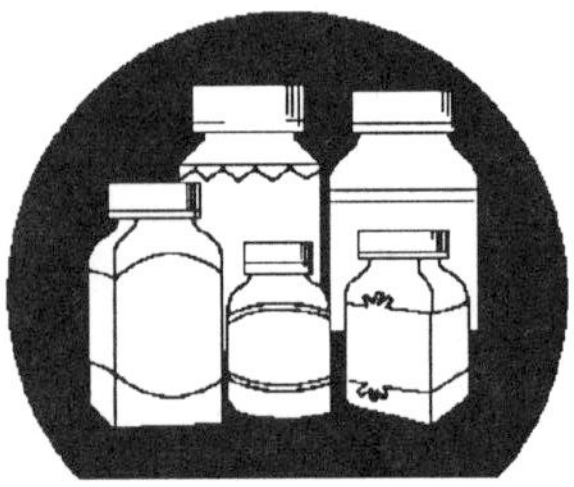

The human body is a chemical factory. It manufactures hormones, enzymes, and naturally occurring drugs which regulate body processes. The introduction of other drugs into the body is a risky business. Altering the chemical balance in the body can have serious consequences. In addition to their desired effect, drugs may also produce undesirable side effects, harmful interactions, and adverse reactions. Every drug has serious risks, at least for some people some of the time.

Drugs have both benefits and hazards. On the benefits side, drugs are used to reduce symptoms, diagnose, treat, and prevent disease. On the hazard side are side effects, adverse reactions, food and drug interactions, and dependence. Side effects are the minor irritations which a person might expect when using certain drugs. A person may continue to use the medication, but may have to limit some activities such as operating a vehicle or other machinery. Adverse reactions are unexpected, may present a major risk, and should signal the person to stop taking the medication and contact his or her physician. Interactions occur when a combination of drugs or food and drugs produce unexpected adverse conditions. Although interactions may range from mild to severe, a physician should be consulted. If comparatively safe medications can produce life-threatening adverse reactions or interactions, the abuse of unpredictable drugs is certainly dangerous.

In order to balance the benefits and risks, the federal government controls the distribution of drugs. The Food and Drug Administration (FDA) regulates the legal distribution of drugs for medical purposes. The Department of Justice enforces the laws pertaining to the illegal use and sale of controlled substances. New drugs must be proven safe and effective before the FDA can approve them for sale by prescription or over the counter.

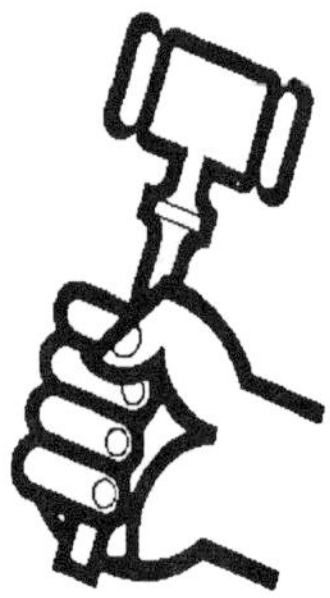

The Department of Justice, on the federal level, enforces the laws pertaining to the illegal possession and use of controlled substances--drug abuse. The Harrison Narcotic Act regulates the manufacture, distribution, use, and possession of morphine, heroin, marijuana, and cocaine. Penalties range from 2 to 40 years imprisonment and fines up to $20,000. The Drug Abuse Control Amendment (DACA) regulates amphetamines, methamphetamines, choral hydrate, barbiturates, LSD, and mescaline. Penalty for the first offense is a misdemeanor with fines up to $1,000 and/or imprisonment up to one year. A subsequent conviction is a felony with a fine up to

$10,000 and/or imprisonment up to three years. The distribution of alcohol and tobacco is controlled by the various states. Organic solvents are not a controlled substance.

The FDA's decision to approve or disapprove a new drug is based on a benefit-risk ratio. When the benefit versus risk factors are complex and when the directions for safe and effective use are complicated, the drugs are distributed by prescription. These drugs must be prescribed under medical supervision for a specific person in a specific situation. Some drugs must also be administered under medical supervision. Drugs designated as over the counter (OTC) are considered safe for distribution without prescription. The directions and warnings are relatively simple to understand and follow. Generally, they are not intended to be therapeutic, but are primarily for the relief of symptoms. However, there are still risks associated with their consumption, particularly when taken indiscriminately.

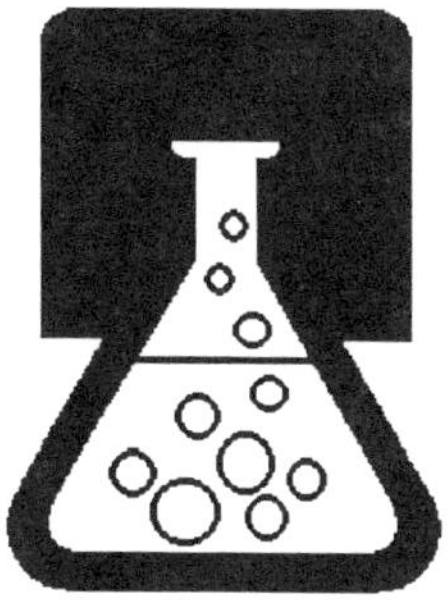

The benefits and risks associated with drugs have been analyzed on three drug consumption levels. Each level suggests some objectives for drug education programs in the secondary school. The three levels are use, misuse, and abuse.

Drug use. Drug consumption for a good medical reason and in a safe manner is considered drug use. Risks are minimal. School drug education programs should help students learn to appreciate the benefits of drugs on this level.

Drug misuse. Drug consumption for a good medical reason, but in an unsafe manner is drug misuse. Risks are considerable. School drug education programs should help students distinguish between drug use and misuse to avoid the dangers of misuse. Sharing prescriptions, not following directions, and combining drugs are frequent examples of drug misuse. This is a frequent problem in our society.

Drug abuse. The illegal consumption of drugs without a good reason and in an unsafe manner is drug abuse. The physical and psychological risks are among the greatest in our society. School drug education programs should help students recognize the risks associated with various drugs and help them avoid consumption. But more importantly, the whole school experience should help students develop a healthy self-concept, so they will be less apt to feel a need to get involved with drugs.

Drug abuse involves both the distribution of illegal substances and the illegal distribution of controlled substances. A number of federal agencies are involved in enforcing the laws against drug abuse. Prosecution of offenders comes under the jurisdiction of the

Bureau of Drug Abuse Control in the Justice Department. State and local agencies are also involved in combating drug abuse.

PRESCRIPTION DRUGS

℞ The Federal Food, Drug, and Cosmetic Act divides drugs into two main classes: prescription drugs and over-the-counter drugs. When a drug is so powerful that it should be used only under a physician's supervision, the law requires that it be sold only by prescription. A prescription is as personal as your name. It is designed for one individual alone and is based on his age, height, weight, condition of health, and other factors, as well as the illness being treated. It is a violation of federal law to sell a prescription drug without a prescription. A prescription must be written or telephoned in by a licensed physician who has had years of training and experience to enable him to know when a drug is necessary and when the calculated risk involved in its use is justified. Then only a registered pharmacist may fill the prescription. The physician will tell him how much, how often, and special instructions. The instructions should be followed exactly. The person taking the medicine should know when to check back with the physician on the effects of the drug. If he thinks the results are not what his doctor expected, he should check back with him promptly.

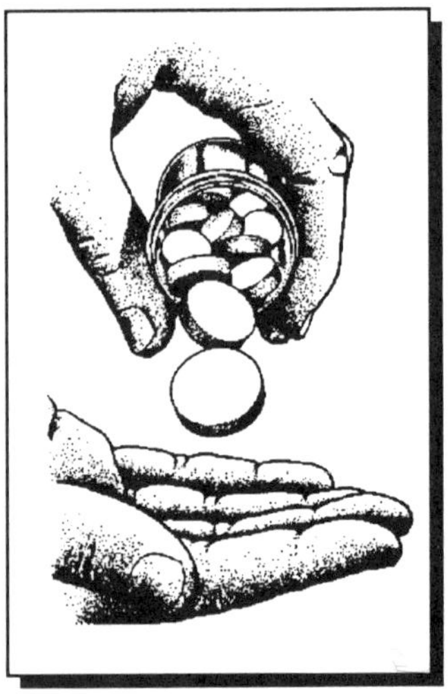

One should never take a prescription written for another person, even if he thinks he has the same disease. Prescriptions weren't meant to be traded over the back fence or passed around the family. A person should never take prescriptions written during a previous illness without first checking with the physician. The illness may not be the same or the drug may have lost strength. A pharmacist cannot refill a prescription unless the original prescription specifies refills are permitted. Special warnings in connection with the prescription, such as "do not drive if the medicine makes you sleepy or dizzy," should be followed. When some of the more powerful drugs are prescribed, thc doctor and pharmacist must report their use to the federal government. Some drugs require such tight restrictions that they are dispensed only through hospital pharmacies.

OVER-THE-COUNTER DRUGS

Drugs that are allowed by law to be sold over the counter, without a prescription, are safe and effective for most people if used according to directions on the label. The labels required by law give warnings, dosage, and ingredients. They tell how to use the drugs for specific conditions and give warnings on what to avoid. The package circular is considered part of the label, and it contains very important information. Warnings tell how to use the medication safely, when to stop taking it, and other important information such as when you should see a doctor.

OTC

Over-the-counter drugs are safe enough to use without a prescription, but this does not mean they should be bought and used indiscriminately. They should be used only for minor ailments that last a little while. The pill-taker who prescribes for himself for a continuing illness could be suffering from a serious disease. The over-the-counter drug he takes may relieve his symptoms, but that is all it does. He may think he is getting better while the disease is growing and spreading. One should never become a steady user of any drug except at a physician's order.

PRECAUTIONS

The combination of certain drugs may produce an undesirable effect. Drugs that produce the same general kind of effect, when taken together, may produce an exaggerated effect out of proportion to that of each drug taken separately. Such drugs are said to be synergistic. When two drugs are taken together, and one intensifies the action of the other, one drug is said to potentiate the other. When two or more drugs are given together and their effects represent the action of one plus the action of the other, their effects are said to be additive--half the dose of one drug plus half the dose of another drug produces the additive effect of one full dose. It would be unwise to take an over-the-counter drug while taking prescribed medications or to combine over-the-counter drugs.

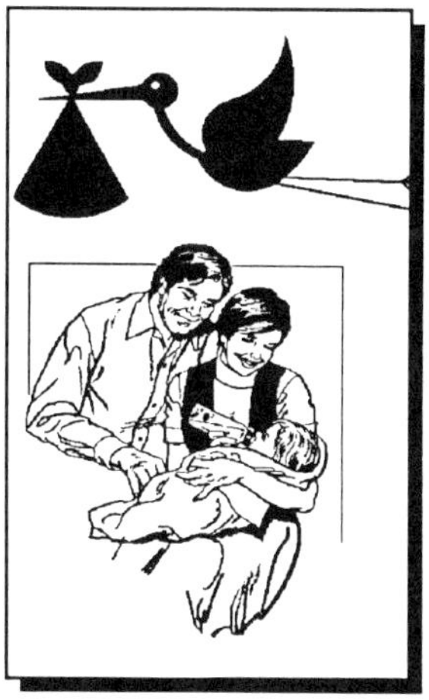

All drugs should be dated. Prescriptions are dated by the pharmacist. Old leftover drugs should be discarded by flushing them down the toilet, and the discarded container should be kept out of reach of children. Old drugs deteriorate and may become ineffective or even dangerous. Medicines should be bought in realistic quantities. Be sure to store all drugs out of the way of children. Safeguard drugs that may taste or look like candy. Never give or take medicine from an unmarked or falsely marked container. Never take medicine in the dark. Measure medicine carefully. Never buy drugs from a peddler, gas station, or other place not licensed to dispense drugs.

One of the most serious but very subtle risks associated with drug use is the effects on an unborn child. If a mother is taking or has been taking drugs, they may seriously effect the embryological development of the unborn child during the first trimester of pregnancy. Birth defects, reduced birth weight, and infant health problems are much higher when the mother has used alcohol, tobacco, or other drugs.

If a person is familiar with the safeguards that are necessary for the prudent use of drugs, he will understand why drug abuse is hazardous. If he is able to put drugs in their proper perspective while he is young, he will be less apt to have trouble when he is older.

DRUG TERMINOLOGY AND CLASSIFICATION

The vocabulary used to describe drugs and their effects is extensive and rapidly increasing. For a single drug, there is the trade name, the generic name, the chemical name, and a variety of street and slang names. The slang names are always changing from time to time and from locality to locality. It would be difficult for a teacher to keep up to date with the name changes as well as the names of the new drugs coming into popular use. This name change tends to separate those who are "in the drug scene" from those who are not. Yet a teacher should be familiar with some of the traditional names of drugs as well as their effects on the body.

The term "addiction" has been used as a general term to describe the compulsive use of drugs. It has also been used more specifically to describe both a physical and psychological compulsion to use drugs; whereas the term "habituation" was used to describe a compulsion that was psychological only. The term "addict" comes from the Latin word *addictus* which in Roman law meant "a debtor awarded as a slave to his creditor." It means the drug addict is a slave to a drug. More recently, the term "drug dependence" has replaced the terms "addiction" and "habituation." The type of dependence is specific to the type of drug. One of the most feared risks associated with drug use is dependence. There is a difference between physiological and psychological dependence. Dependence is a condition resulting from repeated use of a drug which causes the person to continue to use the drug.

PHYSICAL DEPENDENCE

Physical dependence is present when the individual must continue to take the drug to avoid *withdrawal* or *abstinence syndrome*. Physical dependence occurs when the cells of the body become so accustomed to the presence of the drug that they fail to operate properly without the drug. Physical dependence is overcome when a person successfully completes withdrawal. Withdrawal without medical assistance, "doing it cold turkey," may take several days of extreme agony. Some people on some drugs may not live through it; and others wish they could die. With medical assistance, withdrawal takes much longer, but

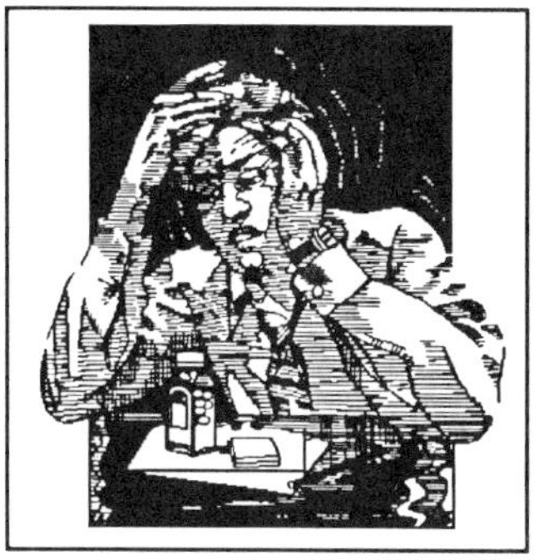

is less severe. Physical dependence may occur quickly or slowly depending on the drug and the individual. The severity of the withdrawal illness also varies, but when it is over the person is free from the physical dependence unless they start taking the drug again.

PSYCHOLOGICAL DEPENDENCE

Psychological dependence is when the individual must continue to take the drug to satisfy strong emotional need. People usually get involved with drugs to try to meet a psychological need; physical dependence may come later. Psychological dependence is overcome when the individual's personality is modified, when the individual learns to meet his emotional needs in a more positive manner. That takes months and years. Most people who have gone through drug rehabilitation and return to use drugs again do so because they are still psychologically dependent. All drugs that affect the central nervous system are capable of producing psychological dependence.

The opinions of experts regarding the potential for a certain drugs to produce dependence has also been changing. For example, for years physical dependence was not associated with cocaine, but more recent evidence indicates that cocaine, especially in the form of *crack,* has a high potential for producing physical dependence. All of the evidence is not in on the physical and psychological effects of drugs. It may take years to accurately compare the health risks of tobacco and marijuana.

DEFINITIONS OF TERMS

<u>Effects of Drugs</u>

Addiction condition resulting from repeated use of a drug in which physical dependence is established because of biochemical and physiological adaptations to the drug.

Analgesic a chemical or drug which has the ability to relieve pain.

Carcinogen chemical, substance, or agent that tends to produce a cancer in the body.

Depressant a drug which causes a reduction of the functional activity of a part of the body.

Dependence condition resulting from repeated use of a drug which causes the person to continue to use the drug. *Physical dependence* is present when the individual must continue to take the drug to avoid withdrawal or abstinence syndrome. *Psychological dependence* is when the individual must continue to take the drug to satisfy strong emotional need.

Euphoria feeling of well-being; in psychiatry, exhibiting abnormal or exaggerated sense of well-being.

Habituation condition resulting from repeated use of a drug in which a psychic, not physical, dependence is established.

Hallucination perception of objects or experience of sensations with no real external cause.

Hypnotic drug that acts to induce sleep.

Intoxication literally, state of being poisoned or drugged; condition produced by excessive use (abuse) of toxic drugs, alcohol, barbiturates, etc.

Narcotic having the power to produce a state of sleep or drowsiness and relief of pain.

Potentiation making a drug more effective or more powerful by the use of more than one drug.

Psychogenic originating in the mind.

Psychotoxic literally poisonous to the mind, having the ability to modify mood and change behavior.

Sedative depressant drug that allays excitement; quieting.

Stimulant chemical substance or other agent which has the ability to increase the functional activity of the body--uppers.

Synergism drugs which work together.

Tolerance increasing resistance to the usual effects of a drug, meaning that it gradually takes more and more of the drug to get the desired feeling. As tolerance builds, they may have to switch to a stronger drug or go through withdrawal to lower their tolerance. Reverse tolerance also occurs sometimes.

Tranquilizer drug that acts to relieve an overactive, anxious, or disturbed emotional state; a central nervous system depressant.

Withdrawal set of symptoms resulting when the consumption of certain drugs stops. It is also called abstinence syndrome.

<u>Depressant Drugs</u> * may cause physical dependence, + may develop tolerance.

Alcohol * + depressant of the central nervous system. Found in beer, wine, liquor.

Risks: intoxication, alcoholism, physical damage.

Opium * + a narcotic drug that comes from the opium poppy. Opiates are drugs derived from opium: heroin, morphine, and codeine act as analgesic, sedative, and hypnotic.

Barbiturate * + a drug group used in medicine as hypnotics or sedatives, includes luminal, veronal, nembutal, seconal, etc.

Risks: intoxication, severe withdrawal.

Chloral hydrate a sedative and hypnotic generally replaced in medical use by barbiturates. Combined with alcohol it is known as a "Mickey Finn" or knockout drops. It is not a street drug of choice.

Tranquilizers a group of drugs used in medicine to reduce anxiety and tension without causing sleep. Major tranquilizers such as Thorazine and Resperpine are used in a hospital for treating psychosis. Minor tranquilizers include librium and valium.

Nicotine * + acts as a depressant on some organs and as a stimulant on others. Nicotine is the drug in tobacco, but the carbon monoxide reduces oxygen transport and the tars contain cancer-producing substances.

<u>Stimulant Drugs</u>

Amphetamines + a drug group which acts as a stimulant to the central nervous system. Includes benzedrine, dexodrine, methedrine, speed, etc.

Caffeine an alkaloid chemical found in coffee, tea, and other substances; a stimulant to the central nervous system.

Cocaine * + a drug used in medicine as a local anesthetic; a stimulant to the central nervous system. May produce hallucinations.

Hallucinogens

LSD, DMT, PCP + a chemical substance or other agent capable of producing distortions of the senses which include hallucinations. Includes LSD, DMT, PCP, mescaline, peyote, and psilocybin.

Marijuana + the plant, *Cannabis sativa*, or parts of it. Hashish is the pure resin. Frequently classified as a hallucinogen and sometimes as a narcotic.

Psilocybin extract of a Mexican mushroom.

Mescaline alkaloid in peyote button of a cactus.

Volatile Solvent an easily vaporized substance capable of dissolving something; specifically, chemicals contained in lighter fluids, model airplane glue, and other common substances which produce a state of intoxication when inhaled.

THE SCOPE OF THE DRUG PROBLEM

There are many current misunderstandings about who the drug abusers are. They are not all young; neither are they all hippies. Drug abusers are physicians who recklessly prescribe amphetamines and tranquilizers rather than helping individuals learn to cope adequately with normal anxiety, frustration, depression, and fatigue. Drug abusers are pharmaceutical companies who advertise their products to deal with "the everyday problems of anxiety and tension."

Drug abusers are housewives who use amphetamines to give them the energy to complete everyday chores or allegedly to cut appetite and enable them to lose weight. Drug abusers are housewives and workers who live on tranquilizers and sleeping pills. Drug abusers are parents who give tranquilizers and diet pills to their children without a physician's prescription.

Drug abusers are businessmen who must have a martini with lunch; they are fathers who need a drink immediately upon returning home from the day's routine. Drug abusers are "the hidden alcoholic"--the housewives who drink several times each day.

National Adolescent Health Survey

	8th GRADE	10th GRADE
CIGARETTES	16%	26%
SMOKELESS TOBACCO	12% (boys)	1% (girls)
BEVERAGE ALCOHOL	34%	53%
MARIJUANA	6%	15%
COCAINE	2%	3%
GLUE	7%	5%

Drug abusers are persons who smoke one or more packs of cigarettes per day. They are persons who drink ten to sixteen cups of coffee or endlessly consume cola drinks each day. Drug abusers are persons who take twenty to forty aspirin tablets daily, strictly for a mood effect.

Drug abusers are children and adolescents who sniff glue, gasoline, thinners, and solvents. They are young people who try spices, their parents' medicines, nitrous oxide, or unknown tablets in search of a high.

Drug abusers are high school and college students who continue to smoke pot or take LSD, mescaline, or STP for alleged consciousness-expansion. They are businessmen, doctors, lawyers, etc. who daily take morphine or Demerol to avoid pain. This pain may be real, imagined, social, vocational, or psychological.

Statistically 25-35 percent of the adult population uses over-the-counter drugs frequently. These drugs are mainly barbiturates and non-barbiturate sedatives and tranquilizers. Seventy percent of the adult population uses alcohol, five percent of them are alcoholics. Nicotine from tobacco is another problem drug affecting around 30 percent of all youth and even a greater percent of the adult population. Drugs that are obtained and used legally constitute only about 30 percent of all drugs used. The other 70 percent come from the black market or illegal means.

The National Adolescent Health Survey released in 1988 asked 11,000 students if they had used the following drugs within the past month. The chart shows the percent of 8th and 10th grade students who said that they have used each drug within the past month.

A closer look at the problem reveals that among Utah high school students, as high as 30 percent use drugs. The students themselves estimated that up to 50 percent of the students use drugs. A few years ago society was alarmed about the drug problems among the youth, and the media made the most of it. Somehow the schools were blamed for the problem and for new shotgun educational approaches. Today the media has taken a quieter approach, the police have taken a low profile, and much of society feels the problem is over. But those who know, know differently. There is continuously a switch from one substance to another, but drug problems continue. Today a greater number of teenagers smoke cigarettes and drink alcohol than ever before, and illegal traffic of drugs into this country is at an all time high.

MOTIVATION FOR DRUG ABUSE

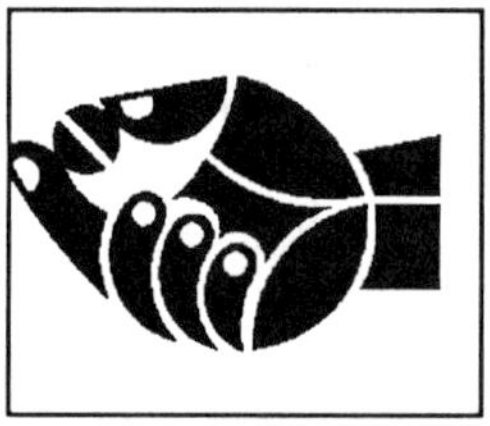

There are many motives for drug abuse but in general, some people take drugs merely to try to diminish their discomforts, while others seek to find excitement or a mind-altering sense of pleasure. There are many motives for starting to take drugs, and there are many motives for continuing to take them. Most of the drugs produce not only the effect for which they are taken, but also serious undesirable side effects. Although the undesirable physical and emotional side effects may be serious, the emotional condition that motivates a person to take drugs in the first place may be more serious. To truly understand the drug problem the investigation should start, not with the drugs, but with the personal motivation behind their use. The following is a list of emotional reasons why people take drugs.

Curiosity. The vast majority of young people who take drugs are experimenting. They desire an exciting risk-taking experience. Drugs offer a challenge. Young people are especially inclined to experiment when they are with a group and peer pressure is exerted. They often use drugs to overcome boredom. Unfortunately, this type of motivation often leads to a more intensified type of curiosity.

Pleasure. Some claim they take drugs because they enjoy the pleasure or taste as a form of recreation. The pleasure motivation includes the use of drugs to have fun. It also includes the use of drugs in a social setting as a refreshment or for the purpose of augmenting sociability. Social interaction is the main goal; the drug is the means to an end. However, it often ends up inhibiting that desired end. This social and pleasure motivation for drugs often introduces people to a more serious motivation in susceptible individuals.

Search for meaning. The search for self-transcendence--the meaning of life and the reason for existence--sometimes leads people to use drugs. Mind-altering chemicals are thought to assist in the communication with the ultimate power. While the use of drugs for spiritual and rehabilitative purposes may sometimes work with certain people, the drug experience may lead other, more vulnerable people into deeper psychological maladjustments which may become the motive for continuing to take drugs.

Rebellion. Many young people turn to drugs, because they feel anger and resentment against authority, e.g., parents, school, and the establishment. This defiant attitude is sometimes successful in getting attention and other desired results. But more often, it leads to poor and dangerous forms of communication. It can lead to more rejection and alienation. The drug pattern, once started, may continue in a more serious form.

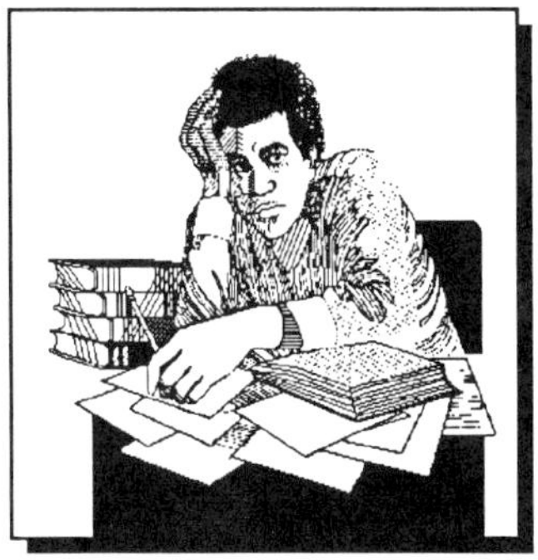

Alienation. People who have a feeling of estrangement and separation from the social and subcultural group may turn to drugs to fill that void or satisfy their other unmet needs. Individuals who share this lack of identity join together in a counterculture movement and assist each other in obtaining the drugs they desire.

Oblivion. In this instance, the drugged state of mind offers a pleasant respite from the stresses of the world around them. Some seek temporary oblivion only when the pressures get too big. Then, gradually the pressures get bigger and more frequent, so they desire to stay in a constant state of semi-oblivion. They feel incompetent and unable to live up to their own expectations or the expectations of others. With drugs they feel free from fears of failure.

Psychological. Many start on drugs because of psychological problems. Others may have started on drugs for some other reason, but psychological problems become the reason for staying on drugs. A major problem is the lack of identity. Those on drugs will do things they would not do otherwise, and this behavior may shatter previous identity.

One may use drugs for certain desired effects. He may gain them, but he may also gain some undesired effects. The thrills, the high, the trips, the euphoria, the relaxation, the sociability, and the pleasurable taste may all be desired. The mind may be bent, the mood may be modified, and all may appear well, but the risk that is involved with all drugs is that they can bring undesired consequences. The smoker enjoys the taste of his tobacco, but he hardly wants the lung cancer that comes twenty years later. The social drinker appreciates the fact that his beverage is a social lubricant, but he never expects it to become a crutch. The office worker drinks coffee to keep himself sharp and to settle his nerves, but when the coffee machine breaks down, he cannot pull his nerves together and get anything accomplished. The girl who drives while under the influence of marijuana is happy until the accident because of poor visual perception. At best, drugs produce a temporary maladjustment. Who knows how bad they are at their worst?

The major problem with drug abuse among adolescents is that they avoid the natural expression of emotions at a time when young people should be maturing by learning to deal with their emotions. Emotional growth and development comes through learning to control emotions, not by avoiding them.

RECOGNIZING DRUG ABUSE

Many teachers would like to be able to spot a student in class who is abusing drugs. This is often difficult and perhaps unwise. However, teachers should be aware and able to recognize some of the common signs often displayed by people using drugs, especially if they are teaching in the area of drugs. The effects of several types of drugs are described below. It is important to remember that these signs could be caused by something other than drug abuse, so if a student has one of the symptoms listed, jumping to conclusions is not wise. Your assumption may be inaccurate and could lead to inappropriate behavior. Careful observations and cautious judgment are important.

Depressants

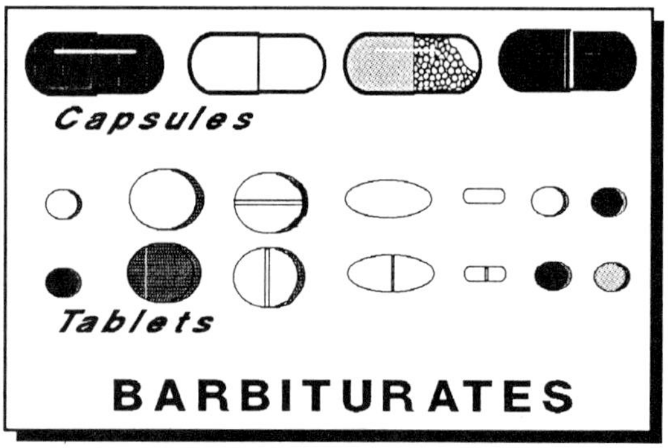

The depressants, such as narcotics, hypnotics, and tranquilizers initially tend to decrease activity, reduce alertness, and promote relaxation, sometimes to the point of drowsiness and sleep. A feeling of euphoria and a lack of ability to concentrate usually result. Larger doses cause lethargy, further reduction of activity and awareness, decreased breathing and pulse rate, constricted or pinpoint pupils, lowered temperature, and profuse sweating. An overdose may result in deep sleep or coma and respiratory failure. It may be necessary for someone to maintain an open airway, administer artificial respiration, treat for shock, and seek medical assistance.

Alcohol

Alcohol also acts as a depressant upon the body, but since it seems to be quite common for students to be involved with it, we will elaborate on it a little more. The frontal lobe of the brain containing the areas of judgment, values, conscience, and personal and social control is the first to be depressed. When this happens, normal inhibitions are released and more base, antisocial behavior may take place. Judgment, coordination, vision, hearing, balance,

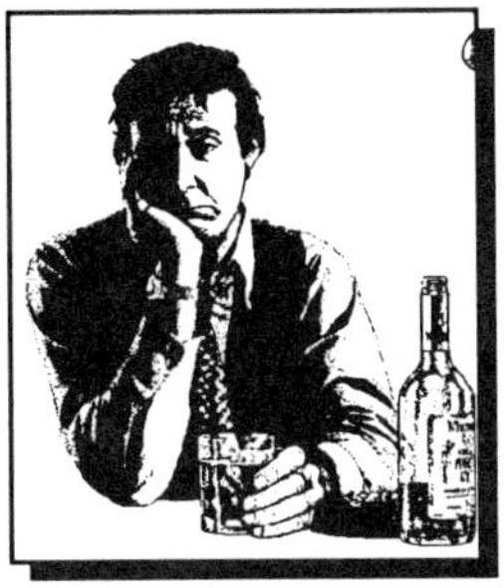

and reaction time are impaired. The student may say and do things he wouldn't normally do. It may be dangerous to operate machinery such as a car. He may become violent and require careful handling to keep him from harming himself and others. Large quantities of alcohol may depress the body's vital functions to the point that death results. The odor of alcohol on a person's breath does not mean he is intoxicated. He may have only consumed a little alcohol, or the odor may be from other substances, such as candy.

Stimulants

Normal doses produce wakefulness, alertness, talkativeness, confidence, and a feeling of initiative. Increased doses may cause confusion, compulsive repetitions of meaningless acts, suspicion, fear, hallucinations, delusions, and aggressive antisocial behavior. A "run" may last for several days without food or sleep, leaving the abuser exhausted, emotionally depressed, and lethargic. Psychiatric help may be necessary.

Hallucinogens

Psychological effects of hallucinogens are variable and unpredictable. A person may experience a feeling of euphoria or have mood shifts and be out of contact with reality. A bad trip may produce intense fear, terror, or panic and may induce a complete loss of emotional control. In other cases, hallucinations, profound depression, or extreme anxiety may occur. Sometimes the person needs to be protected from self-inflicted bodily harm, but those attempting to help should be careful they don't get harmed. Afterward, the person may need to be "talked down" from his disturbing experience in a quiet and non-threatening manner.

Marijuana

A marijuana user may have reddening of the eyes, throat irritation, occasional dizziness, uncoordination, increased appetite, and sleepiness. The effects may include feelings of exhilaration, hilarity, elation, and congeniality. There may be an exaggerated sense of ability, distortion of time and space, and disturbed psychomotor activity. Some users may experience psychotoxic effects similar to hallucinogens.

Volatile Intoxicants

The use of volatile substances as in glue sniffing often results in a sense of initial excitement and release of inhibitions. Auditory and visual hallucinations and illusions, mental confusion, light-headedness, headache, nausea, ringing in the ears, impaired vision, rapid eye movement, oral secretions, sneezing, coughing, chest pain, a dreamy, blank expression, staggering, loss of muscle control, stupor, blackout, or unconsciousness may result. Serious organic damage can occur. Sometimes an abuser will be found with a bag over his head. Artificial respiration and prompt intensive medical attention may be necessary.

Steroids

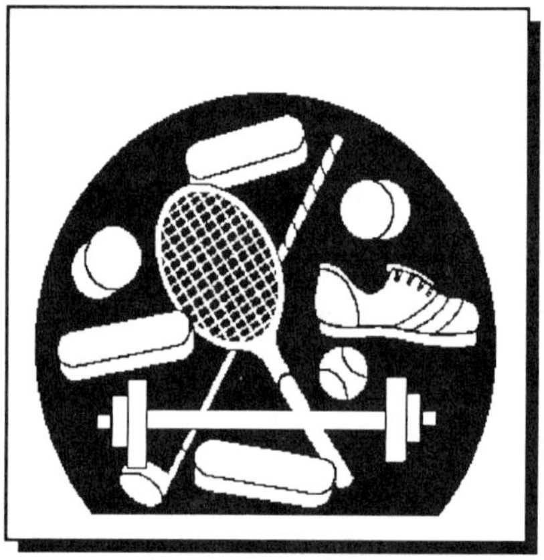

Anabolic steroids are a different type of problem. They are not CNS drugs and therefore do not fit in with the rest of the drugs discussed in this lesson. However, they do present a special threat, and this may be the best place to recognize it. Steroids are derived from the male hormone testosterone and can be ingested in pill form or injected as solution. They were given to German soldiers during World War II to increase aggressiveness. Soon after the war they were used by weight lifters and other athletes to build up their muscles. There has been widespread use of steriods by professional, collegiate, and high school athletes. There are serious health problems associated with their use, and most organized sports have banned their use. College, professional, and Olympic sports groups conduct tests to enforce the ban. The biggest problem now is among high school-age athletes. Most physicians have stopped using them, but black market sources are still available. It is estimated that the steroid black market is a 100 billion dollar business that sells to more than 250,000 high-school-age athletes. The 1988 amendments to the Food, Drug, and Cosmetic Act makes the distribution or steroids to minors punishable by a fine and up to six years in prison (*FDA Consumer*, 23 (2) p.3).

Steroids help the body utilize protein, and this builds muscles and adds weight. They also cause increased aggression, and this may be desirable in competition but detrimental in normal social relationships. There are other serious consequences of steroid use (*Health Education*, 18 (4) pp.32-34). They cause a chemical imbalance in the body, a retention of salt and water, and increased acne. They stop bone growth if taken by young people who have not reached their full physical maturity. They alter sexual development. Male users experience reduced natural testosterone production, testicular atrophy, decreased sperm production, enlarged breasts, and the development of male pattern baldness. Female users experience increased growth of body hair, deepening of the voice, general masculinization, and menstrual irregularities. Severe depression results from abrupt cessation of use. A number of suicides among outstanding student athletes have been linked with steroids.

In addition to these signs and symptoms, other clues may suggest drug use or abuse. There may be evidence of the drugs themselves, containers, or the apparatus used in taking the drugs. Hypodermic needles, eye droppers, teaspoons, constriction bands, and needle marks on the person's body are also significant.

WHAT THE SCHOOLS CAN DO

Much of what a teacher should do about the drug problem depends on the policies within the school and the general approach in the community. It also depends on the teacher's interest, time commitment, and ability to relate with the students. Some teachers would take one or more of the following approaches. What would you do?

1. Try to ignore the fact that students in class are using drugs.
2. Appreciate it when previously rowdy students, now taking drugs, sleep in class rather than disturbing others.
3. Be inclined to help the law catch the students.
4. Turn the information over to the school officials.
5. Try to work with the students and help them yourself.

The solution to the problem does not lie with any single individual, agency, or discipline. It is a multifaceted problem, and it will require a multi-faceted approach. A co-operative effort is essential, beginning in the home with the parents and extending to the medical profession, the pharmaceutical companies, government agencies, social agencies, and the schools.

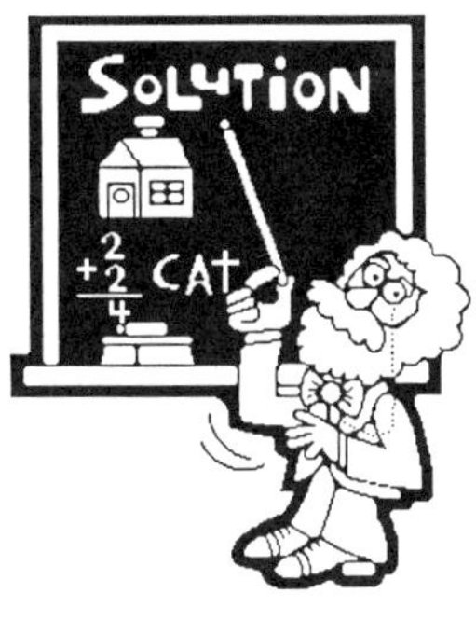

In most commun-ities, there are several agencies concerned with the drug problem, and frequently they include the police department, schools, churches, civic groups, rehabilitation centers, mental health centers, and crisis centers. A variety of rehabilitation approaches are used. Sometimes the individual voluntarily participates in a program, and other times the courts commit a person to a particular program. Some programs have more success than others, usually depending on how they are able to substitute something better than drugs into the person's life.

Prevention is the best approach and here is where the schools can make the greatest contribution. First, schools must make sure they are contributing to the solution of the problem rather than being part of the problem. Within the schools, drugs cannot be isolated as a separate course. Drug education must be incorporated into health education and family living courses. It should start in kindergarten and be interwoven continuously into the curriculum through the twelfth grade. It should be based on the "total person" concept rather than treated as an isolated subject. It should be based on humanistic behavior patterns rather than solely on content information.

In the *primary* grades, the emphasis should be on health development. Students should learn to respect drugs as both potentially dangerous and helpful. They should understand that drugs, when used under a doctor's prescription or under a parent's direction for a definite medical illness, are proper and beneficial. They should learn that unknown substances may produce adverse psychological and physical effects. The difference between candy and medicine that may resemble candy should be pointed out.

During the *intermediate* grades, they can learn generally how medicines affect the body. They can discuss how advertisements may be misleading. They can learn how various drugs, including alcohol and tobacco, have detrimental effects upon society. Also, they can learn why laws and agencies are needed to help protect people from improper use of drugs.

In *junior high*, the emphasis could be on moral, social, and legal aspects of personal behavior. Students need to learn about interpersonal relationships, communication, handling peer pressures, and developing personal awareness. Alternative highs should be suggested, and legal consequences of drug abuse should be understood.

Education in *senior high school* should review all that has been learned in the previous years. Students here are ready for a more in-depth study of the psychological, physiological, biochemical, and pharmacological aspects of drugs. They should also look at the social problems accompanying drugs and the responsibilities of government agencies and pharmaceutical companies for making sure drugs are safe and effective. Social and consumer issues such as drug safety, drug costs, rehabilitation problems, and problems of drug misuse should be explored.

Scare tactics or *conveyance of false information* should be avoided. Approaches to help students develop healthy self-concepts should be emphasized. Students should develop a sense of personal responsibility based upon the concept of total well-being.

This approach will deal with not only drug problems, but also with problems of sexual promiscuity and other forms of juvenile delinquency. When problems like these emerge, they are already deeply woven into a person's personality; they reflect attitudes that have been acquired over a long period of time. Therefore, to be effective in preventing them, a positive program must be developed on a long-term basis. Because of the many influences in the home and community, the schools will not be able to "save" everyone, but they must do the best job they can.

WHAT CAN SCHOOLS DO?

In 1986 the U.S.Department of Education published *Schools Without Drugs.* This 78 page booklet was distributed free of charge to anyone who would request it from the Consumer Information Center, Pueblo, Colorado 81009. William J. Bennett explains in the introduction that "the foremost responsibility of any society is to nourish and protect its children. In America today, the most serious threat to the health and well-being of our children is drug use."

Schools Without Drugs provides a practical synthesis of the most reliable and significant findings available on drug use by school-age youth. It provides detailed information on approaches that have worked in some schools and communities. The book calls for schools to unite with parents, students, and community resources to implement a plan for achieving schools without drugs. It emphasizes prevention, not treatment. The following information comes from that book.

EXTENT OF DRUG USE

Drug use is widespread among American schoolchildren. The rates were higher in 1985 than in 1975. The rates are higher than in any other industrialized nation. In 1985, 41 percent of the seniors reported using marijuana in the last year, and 26 percent said they had used it in the previous month. Thirteen percent had used cocaine within the last year (Martin et al., 1986).

Another source, the U.S. National Institute on Drug Abuse, reported a survey conducted in 1982 among 12- to 17-year-old youth. The survey showed that 26.9 percent had used alcohol within the previous month, 14.7 percent had used cigarettes, 11.5 percent had used marijuana, 2.6 percent had used stimulants, 1.6 percent had used cocaine, and 1.4 percent had used hallucinogens.

Another study reported in *Schools Without Drugs* indicated that 57 percent of the student drug users had bought most of their drugs at school. Among the seniors who used marijuana, one-third had smoked it at school and of those who had used amphetamines, two-thirds had used them at school. In 1985, fifty percent of the seniors in metropolitan areas reported illicit drug use. In non-metropolitan areas, the percentage was slightly lower, forty-five percent. More male students report using drugs than do females, but the gap between the sexes is lessening. Comparing blacks and whites, except for marijuana, the use is slightly higher among whites. Initial drug use is occurring at an earlier age; in the 1960s marijuana use was virtually nonexistent among 13-year-olds, now 16 percent of the 13-year-olds have used marijuana.

HOW DRUG USE DEVELOPS

The first temptation to use drugs may come in social situations in the form of pressure to "act grown up" and "have a good time." As children get older, peer pressure to use cigarettes, alcohol, or marijuana increases. Initial attempts may not produce much of a high, but with continued use, children learn that drugs can alter their feelings. When they get involved with the feelings, they seek other drugs or ways of using drugs to intensify the feelings. Drug use usually progresses in stages, from occasional or recreational use, to regular use, to multiple drug use, and then to total dependency.

DRUGS AND DEPENDENCY

Drugs cause physical and emotional dependency. Users may develop an overwhelming craving for specific drugs, and their bodies may respond to the presence of drugs in ways that lead to increased drug use.

Tolerance. Regular users of some drugs develop tolerance, a need to take larger doses to get the same initial effect. They may react by taking larger doses of the drug, switching to a more potent drug, or by combining drugs.

Physical dependence. Certain drugs create physical dependence. With prolonged use, these drugs become part of their body chemistry. When the regular user stops taking the drug, the body experiences the physical trauma known as *withdrawal.*

Psychological dependence. All drugs are capable of producing psychological dependence. Drug taking becomes the center of the user's life. This will erode school performance and can destroy ties with family and friends. Interests, values, and goals are lost. The child goes from taking drugs to feel good to taking drugs to keep from feeling bad. But the bad feelings gradually get worse and the person resorts to other approaches, including suicide to get rid of the bad feelings. More than half of all adolescent suicides are drug-related.

Side effects. The harmful side effects of drugs can remain in the body long after the drug use has stopped. The fat soluble drugs such as marijuana hallucinogens settle and build up in the fatty tissues such as the brain. Months later they may experience *flashbacks.*

DRUGS AND LEARNING

Drugs erode the self-discipline and motivation necessary for learning. Drug use among students creates a climate in the schools that is destructive to learning. Drug use can cause a decline in academic performance, grades go down. The decline in grades often reverses when drug use is stopped. Drug use is closely tied to truancy and dropping out of school. Drugs are also associated with crime and misconduct. Drugs transform schools into a marketplace for dope deals. They lead to classroom disorder and to the destruction of property. A drug-ridden environment is a strong deterrent to learning, not only for drug users, but for other students as well.

WHAT CAN WE DO?

Schools Without Drugs indicates that the most effective way to combat drug abuse is to involve the entire community: parents, schools, students, law enforcement authorities, religious groups, social service agencies, and the media. They all must transmit a single consistent message that drug use is wrong, dangerous, and will not be tolerated. This message must be reinforced through strong, consistent law enforcement and disciplinary measures. The following recommendations are examples of what can be done to stop drug use:

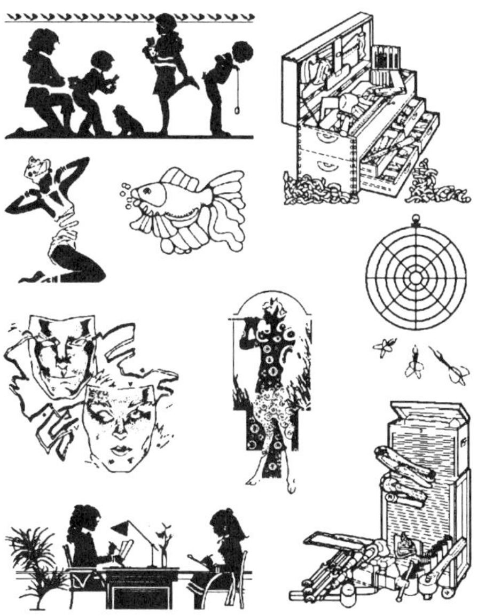

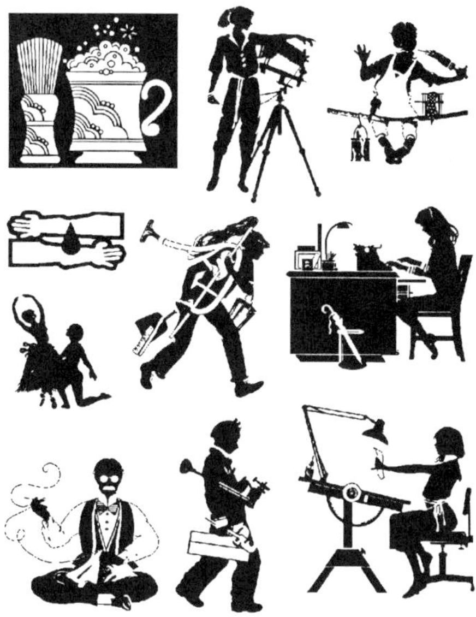

Parents

1. Instilling responsibility. Teach standards of right and wrong and demonstrate these standards thorough personal example.

2. Providing supervision. Help children to resist peer pressure to use drugs by supervising their activities, knowing who their friends are, and talking to them about their interests and problems.

3. Recognizing drug use. Be knowledgeable about drugs and signs of drug use so that if signs are observed there can be prompt response.

Schools

4. Assessing the problem. Determine the extent and character of drug use and establish a means of monitoring that use regularly.

5. Setting policy. Establish clear and specific rules regarding drug use that includes strong corrective action.

6. Enforcing policy. Enforce established policies against drug use fairly and consistently. Implement security measures to eliminate drugs on school premises and at school functions.

7. Teaching about drug prevention. Implement a comprehensive drug prevention curriculum from kindergarten through grade 12, teaching that drugs are wrong and harmful and supporting and strengthening resistance to drugs.

8. Enlisting the community. Reach out to the community for support and assistance in making the school's anti-drug policy work. Develop collaborative arrangements in which school personnel, parents, school boards, law enforcement officers, treatment organizations, and private groups can work together to provide necessary resources.

Students

9. Learning the facts. Learn about the effects of drugs, the reason why drugs are harmful, and ways to resist pressure to try drugs.

10. Helping fight drug use. Use an understanding of the danger posed by drugs to help other students avoid them. Encourage other students to resist drugs, persuade those using drugs to seek help, and report those selling drugs to parents and the school principal.

Community

11. **Providing support.** Help schools fight drugs by providing them with the expertise and financial resources of community groups and agencies.

12. **Providing tough law enforcement.** Involve local law enforcement agencies in all aspects of drug prevention: assessment, enforcement, and education. The police and courts should have well-established and mutually supportive relationships with schools.

TEACHING ABOUT DRUG PREVENTION

An effective drug prevention curriculum covers a broad set of educational objectives. *Schools Without Drugs* contains a model program that might help local schools design a drug education program. The four objectives in this model are as follows:

1. **To value and maintain sound personal health; to understand how drugs affect health.** At the early elementary school level, children learn how to care for their bodies. They learn how medicine can help the body and how poisons can harm the body. Older students learn how to tell when a substance is safe, how to read labels, and how to follow the doctor's directions. On the secondary level, students learn the effects of specific drugs on the body, how drugs increase stress, and the effect of drugs on adolescent development.

2. **To respect laws and rules prohibiting drugs.** In the early grades, students should learn to identify rules and understand their importance. Schools should teach children to respect rules and laws, because they maintain social values and protect individuals and society. Older students learn about the school's drug code and the laws regulating drugs in the society.

3. **To recognize and resist pressures to use drugs.** Students learn to identify the social and internal pressures that encourage them to use drugs. They learn responsible decision making, how to counteract persuasive messages, and how to say no to drugs.

4. **To promote activities that reinforce the positive drug-free elements of student life.** School activities that provide opportunities to have fun without drugs builds momentum for peer pressure not to use drugs. Make participation in school activities dependent on not using drugs. Make sure that drugs are not available at school-sponsored activities. Train students to exercise leadership in peer drug prevention programs.

SIGNS OF DRUG USE

For parents and schools to do their part in preventing drug use, they must know how to recognize the signs of drug use. The book, *Schools Without Drugs,* lists the following signs of drug use.

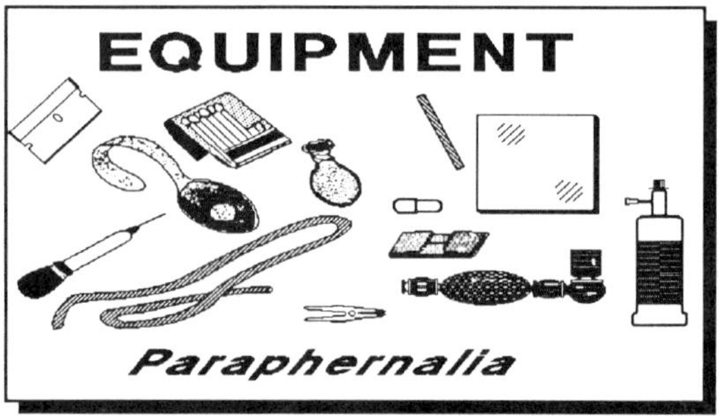

Drugs and drug paraphernalia. There may be drugs or evidence of drugs such as odors of drugs or the smell of incense to cover up the odor of drugs. There may be peculiar plants, butts, seeds, leaves, etc. Drug paraphernalia includes pipes, rolling papers, small bottles, or small butane torches.

Identification with drug culture. Hostility in discussing drugs, jokes and conversations that are preoccupied with drugs, or the presence of drug-related magazines, slogans, and clothing may indicate an association with the drug culture.

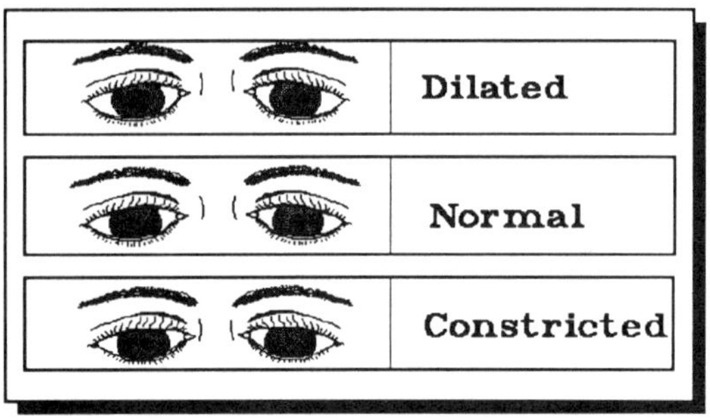

Signs of physical deterioration. Blood shot eyes, dilated pupils, memory lapses, short attention span, difficulty in concentration, slurred or incoherent speech, poor physical conditioning, unhealthy appearance, and indifference to hygiene and grooming are signs of drug use.

Changes in school performance. Drug use is frequently associated with distinct downward turns in students' grades, assignments not completed, and increased absenteeism or tardiness.

Changes in behavior. Changes in behavior may signal use of drugs. There may be a change in friends or evasiveness in talking about new friends, secretiveness, diminished interest in usual activities and hobbies, reduced energy motivation, poor self-esteem, lack of self-discipline, increasing anger and hostility, irritability, dishonesty (lying, stealing, cheating), and possession of large amounts of money. Changes that together form a total pattern may be associated with drug use.

SEARCHING FOR DRUGS

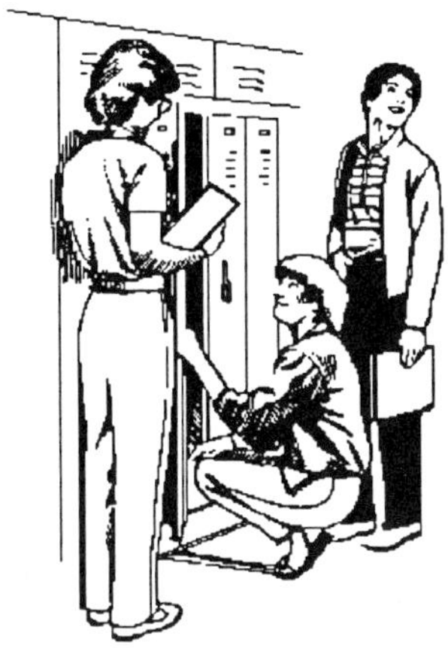

Schools committed to fighting drugs should do everything they can to prevent the use of the school grounds to facilitate the possession, use, or distribution of drugs. An effective program of drug searches is an important tool, but it has its problems. First, administrators should identify specific areas in the school where drugs are likely to be found or used, such as lockers and rest rooms. Second, administrators should clearly announce in writing at the beginning of the year that those areas will be subject to unannounced searches. The students should know that those areas are considered *public* rather than *private.* Searches may be subject to litigation, but the courts have usually upheld locker searches where schools have established prior written policies under which the school retains joint control of student lockers.

If students know that their lockers may be searched, drug users will be less likely to store drugs there. The effectiveness of locker and building searches may be improved with the use of specially trained dogs.

In some circumstances, teachers or other school personnel will wish to search a student whom they believe to be in possession of drugs. The courts have recognized that the need of school authorities to maintain order justifies searches that might otherwise be unreasonable if undertaken by police officers in the larger community. School officers, unlike the police, do not need "probable cause" or a search warrant to conduct the search. School officials may institute a personal search if there are reasonable grounds to believe that the search will reveal evidence that the student has violated or is violating either the law or the rules of the school. However, the searches must employ only measures that are reasonably related to the purpose of the search. The search must not be excessively intrusive.

It is important to remember that any illicit drug and drug-related items discovered at school are evidence that may be used in a criminal trial. Care must be take to not compromise the integrity of the evidence. Schools must keep up-to-date with local policies and procedures in conducting searches, in handling evidence, and in administering penalties.

PENALTIES

A school policy may lawfully provide for penalties of varying severity, including suspension and expulsion, to respond to drug-related offenses. It is helpful if school policies are explicit about the type of offenses that will be punished and about the penalties that may be imposed for each. Students facing suspension or expulsion from school are entitled under the law to common sense due process protection of notice and an opportunity to be heard. The more severe the penalties, the more formal the notice and hearings must be. A student may be subject to school discipline, regardless of the outcome of criminal proceedings.

School officials need to report drug-related crimes to the police and assist local law enforcement authorities in detecting and prosecuting drug offenders, but the schools need to take steps to ensure compliance with federal and state laws governing confidentiality of student records. Under the Family Educational Rights and Privacy Act (FERPA), disclosure of information on education records to individuals or entities other than students, parents, and school officials is only permissible in specified situations. Such disclosure is permitted if requested by a court order or subpoena or if warranted by a health or safety emergency. FERPA does not apply to information school officials become aware of through personal observation or to evidence secured during a search.

Suits may be brought against a school district or its employee or both on the basis that the student's constitutional or statutory rights have been violated. The courts have generally tried to discourage such litigation unless the actions are clearly unlawful, unreasonable, arbitrary, or discriminatory. However, schools should exercise care. Since the area of law is complicated, it is important that an attorney be involved in formulating school policy.

CLASSIFICATION OF COMMONLY ABUSED DRUGS

The charts on the next several pages answer the following questions about drugs. The illustrations show where the drugs come from, what form they may be in, and what they look like.

LEGEND

DRUG:

Name:	What are the names for the drug?
Slang:	What is it commonly called?

DESCRIPTION:

Form:	What does it look like?
Source:	Where does it come from?
Mode:	How is it taken?

EFFECTS:

Medical:	What are its medical uses?
Abuse:	What are the desired effects in abuse?
Reactions:	What are the bad effects of abuse?
Dependence:	Does it cause physical dependence? Does it cause psychological dependence? Does it cause tolerance?
Signs:	What are the signs of abuse?

CANNABIS (MARIJUANA)

DRUG:	
Name:	Marijuana, Hashish, *tetrahydrocannabinol*, THC.
Slang:	Pot, Grass, Weed, Tea, Reefer, Dope, Mary Jane, Acapulco Gold, Roach, Thai Sticks, Hash, Hash Oil.
DESCRIPTION:	
Form:	Dry parsley, mixed with stems/seeds.
Source:	Indian hemp plant, *cannabis sativa*.
Mode:	Smoked or mixed with food.
EFFECTS:	HALLUCINOGEN.
Medical:	None, under investigation.
Abuse:	Euphoria, relaxed inhibitions, reduced appetite, exaggerated sense.
Reactions:	Fatigue, paranoia, altered sense of time and space, poor coordination.
Dependence:	Psychological, moderate physiological.
Signs:	Materials and paraphernalia, mild intoxication, blood shot eyes.

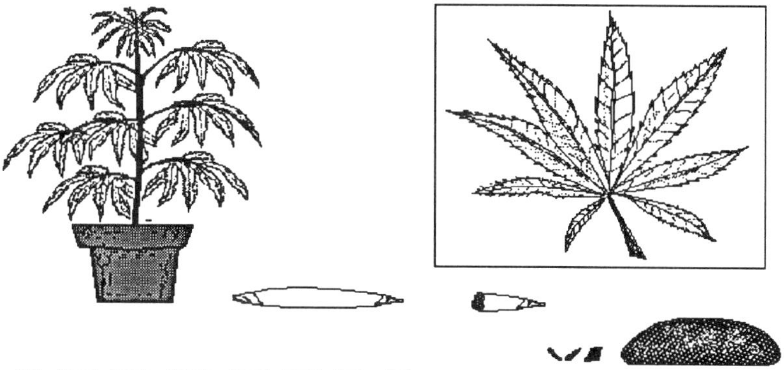

CANNABIS

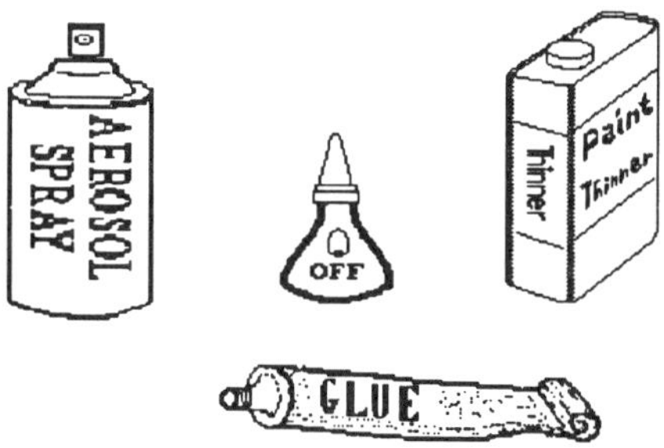

Inhalants

INHALANTS

DRUG:	
Name:	Solvents (hydrocarbons), aerosol sprays (chlorohydrocarbons), laughing gas (nitrous oxide), amyl nitrite, butyl nitrite.
Slang:	Whippets, Poppers, Snappers, Rush, Bolt, Bullet, Climax, Locker Room.
DESCRIPTION:	
Form:	Solvents, sprays.
Source:	Glue, paint thinner, gasoline, aerosol spray cans, ampules, cylinders, small bottles.
Mode:	Inhaled.
EFFECTS:	
Medical:	Clinical and laboratory reagents.
Abuse:	Euphoria, auditory and visual hallucinations and illusions, unconsciousness.
Reactions:	Sneezing, coughing, nausea, nosebleed, fatigue, lack of coordination and judgement, loss of appetite, incontinence, headaches, irregular pulse and respiration, and suffocation (due to displacement of oxygen depression of nervous system). Long term use may cause permanent nerve damage, and hepatitis.
Dependence:	Psychological.
Signs:	Similar to alcohol intoxication, substance and paraphernalia, see reactions above.

COCAINE

DRUG:	
Name:	Cocaine, Crack.
Slang:	Coke, C, Snow, Flake, White, Blow, Bog C, Lady, Snowbird, Crack, Nose Candy, Rock, Freebase Rock.
DESCRIPTION:	
Form:	Cocaine: White crystalline powder; Crack: Light brown or beige pellets or crystalline rocks.
Source:	Cocaine: alkaloid from coca leaf; Crack: Cocaine is mixed with baking soda and water to form a paste which when dry is cut into chips, slivers or pellets.
Mode:	Cocaine: snorted (3 min.), injected (15 sec.); Crack: smoked (5 sec.), freebasing--heated to form vapors and inhaled.
EFFECTS:	STIMULANT.
Medical:	Local or topical anesthesia, stimulant.
Abuse:	Excitation, exhilaration, invigoration, rush, reduces hunger and fatigue, quick pickup.
Reactions:	Depression after effects wear off (1 hour). Delusions, hallucinations, paranoia. Inflammation and permanent damage to nasal passages and septum. Increased heart rate and blood pressure, respiratory failure, convulsions, and instant death.
Dependence:	Cocaine: psychological; Crack: Strong psychological, physical (most addicting drug today).
Signs:	Insomnia, anxiety, irritability, paraphernalia: a vial, folded paper, or aluminum foil.

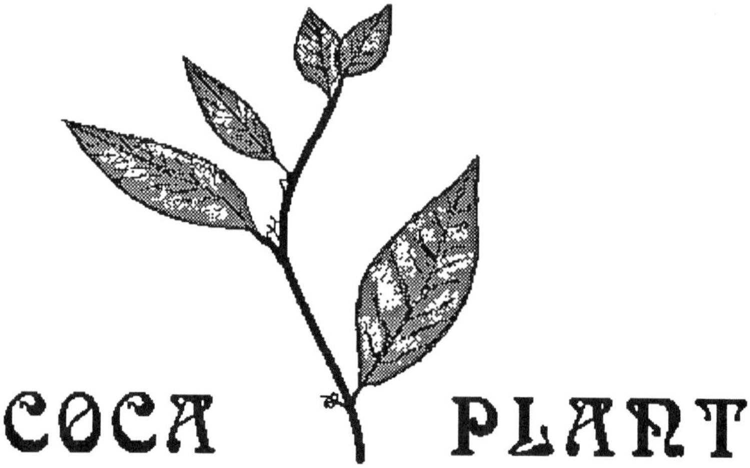
COCA
PLANT

STUMULANTS

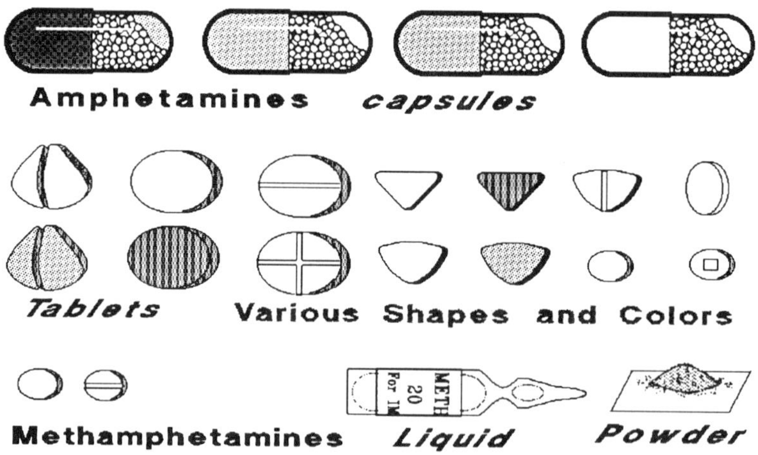
Amphetamines
capsules
Tablets
Various Shapes and Colors
METH 20 For IM
Methamphetamines
Liquid
Powder

AMPHETAMINES

DRUG:	
Name:	Benzedrine, Dexedrine, Methedrine, Dextroamphetamine, Methylphenidate.
Slang:	A, Uppers, Bennies, Dexies, Copilots, Hearts, Bumblebees, Pep-Pills, Wake-ups, Black Beauties, Footballs.
DESCRIPTION:	CNS stimulant.
Form:	Tablets, capsules, liquid, or powder.
Source:	Synthesized.
Mode:	Swallowed or injected.
EFFECTS:	STIMULANT.
Medical:	For overweight and fatigue (largely useless). For narcolepsy and some childhood behavioral disorders.
Abuse:	Euphoria, increased energy, improved performance, and alertness. To get up after taking depressant drugs.
Reactions:	Headaches, irritability, dizziness, insomnia, loss of appetite, delusions, toxic psychosis, probable organic damage, tolerance.
Dependence:	Psychological dependence, tolerance.
Signs:	Dilated pupils, dry nose and mouth, excessive perspiration, mood swings, abnormally cheerful, exaggerated emotions, extreme restlessness, paranoid tendencies.

METHAMPHETAMINE

DRUG:	
Name:	Methamphetamine, methedrine.
Slang:	Speed, Meth, Crystal, Crank, Splash, Crystal Meth.
DESCRIPTION:	CNS stimulant.
Form:	White powder, pills, or a rock which resembles a block of paraffin.
Source:	Synthesized in undercover illegal laboratories.
Mode:	Orally, injected, inhaled.
EFFECTS:	STIMULANT.
Medical:	None.
Abuse:	Feeling of extreme pleasure, a tingling or buzzing sensation. Runs or episodes lasting for several hours or days of continued injections without food or sleep. As the run continues the mood changes from euphoria to hyperactive aggression.
Reactions:	Weight loss, nervousness, psychotic states. May require de-pressants to come down. Depression, hallucinations, dizziness, psychosis, death from overdose.
Dependence:	Strong psychological dependence, tolerance.
Signs:	Excitation and hyperactivity, anxiety, confusion, sweating, dilated pupils.

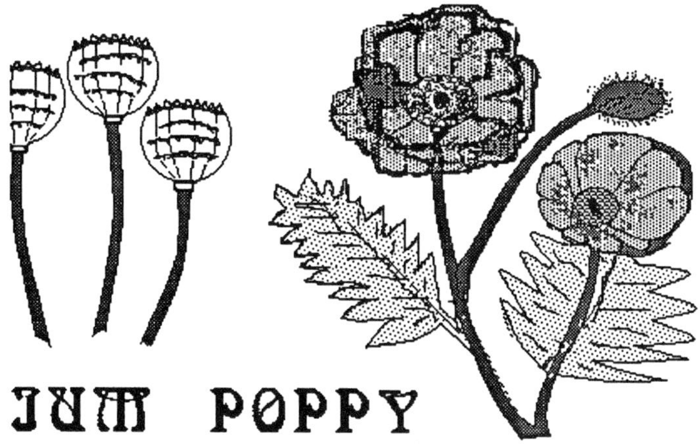
JUM POPPY

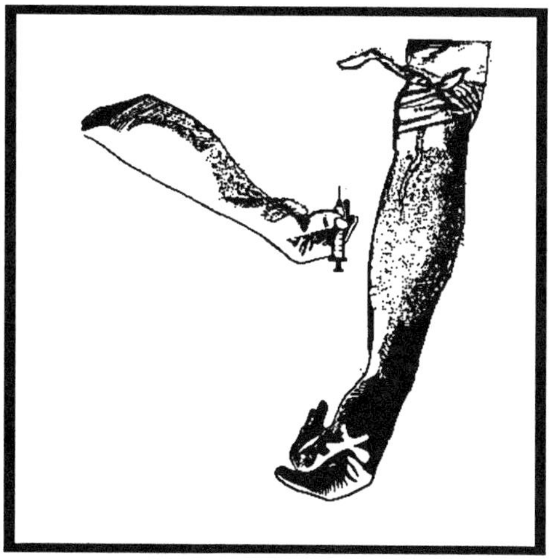

NARCOTICS--OPIUM AND OPIUM DERIVATIVES

DRUG:	OPIUM, MORPHINE, HEROIN, CODEINE, PAREGORIC.
Name and Slang:	OPIUM: O, Dope; MORPHINE: M, Emma, Monkey, Caps, White; HEROIN: H, Horse, Scat, Junk, Smack, Stuff; CODEINE: Schoolboy; PAREGORIC: Pg, Po, Gee.
DESCRIPTION:	
Form and Source:	OPIUM: dried milky juice from poppy pod; MORPHINE: white crystalline powder, cubes, or tablets processed from raw opium; HEROIN: white crystalline powder processed from morphine base; CODEINE: tablets or liquid derivative of opium or morphine; PAREGORIC: liquid tincture of opium and camphor.
Mode:	OPIUM: smoked, snuffed, eaten. DERIVATIVES: swallowed or injected.
EFFECTS:	CNS DEPRESSANT.
Medical:	OPIUM and HEROIN: none; MORPHINE: for pain; CODEINE: for pain and coughing; PAREGORIC: for sedation and diarrhea.
Abuse:	For euphoria and to avoid withdrawal.
Reactions:	Drowsiness, nausea, vomiting, constipation, loss of appetite, indirect organic damage. Overdose results in clammy skin, convulsions, coma and death due to respiratory failure. Infection from contaminated needles. Criminal activities to support addiction.
Dependence:	Physical and psychological, rapid tolerance.
Signs:	Constricted pupils, watery eyes, itching, symptoms of intoxication, slow (on the nod), needle marks (tracks), blood stains on cloths, burns, and paraphernalia.

SYNTHETIC NARCOTICS

DRUG:	METHADONE, MERPERIDINE, DILAUDID.
Name:	METHADONE: *methadone hydrochloride*, Dolopine, Meth-adone, Amidone, Dolly (slang); MEPERIDINE: *meperidine hydrochloride,* Pethidine, Demoral, Mepergan; DILAUDID: *hydromorphine*.
DESCRIPTION:	CNS depressant.
Form:	White powder, tablet, or solution.
Source:	Synthesized.
Mode:	Orally or injected.
EFFECTS:	DEPRESSANT.
Medical:	Pain relief (substitute for morphine), used to treat narcotic dependency.
Abuse:	Euphoria and to prevent withdrawal illness. Abusers turn to synthetic narcotics when they can't get natural narcotics. The effect is shorter and addiction follows a slightly different pattern, but is still addiction. Withdrawal patterns appear more slowly and are of less intensity.
Reactions:	Addiction, constipation, loss of appetite, indirect potential for organic damage.
Dependence:	Physical, psychological, tolerance.
Signs:	Constricted pupils, watery eyes, symptoms of intoxication, same as natural narcotics.

DEPRESSANTS

DRUG: Name and Slang:	BARBITURATES: Nembutal, Seconal, Amytal, Tuinals, Luminal; METHAQUALONE. METHAQUALONE: Quaaludes, Ludes, Sopors; BARBITURATES: Downers, Barbs, Goofballs, Yellows, Yellow Jackets, Blues, Blue Devils, Blue Heavens, Blue Birds, Reds, Red Devils, Red Birds, Seggy, Rainbows, Double Trouble, Christmas Trees, Purple Hearts, Candy.
DESCRIPTION: Form: Source: Mode:	CNS depressants, hypnotic. BARBITURATES: yellow, red, blue, red and blue, or purple capsules or tablets; METHAQUALONE: tablets. Synthesized from barbituric acid. Orally and injected.
EFFECTS: Medical: Abuse: Reactions: Dependence: Signs:	DEPRESSANT. BARBITURATES: Sedative hypnotic to relieve anxieties and tension by inducing sleep, for high blood pressure and epilepsy. Anxiety reduction and euphoria, to induce sleep, to come down from a stimulants high. Small doses may calm and relax, but larger doses can cause intoxication. Very large doses can cause coma and death due to respiratory depression. When combined with alcohol, the effect is multiplied. Physical, psychological, tolerance. Withdrawal is mild or fatal. Appearance of drunkenness with alcohol odor, kit including needles, syringe, needle marks, blood spots, dilated pupils.

DRUG:	
Name:	MAJOR TRANQUILIZERS: Reserpine, Thorazine; MINOR TRANQUILIZERS: *meprobamate*--Equanil, Miltown, Kesso-bramate; *benzodiazepine*--Valium, Librium.
Slang:	T's.
DESCRIPTION:	CNS depressants, hypnotic.
Form:	Tablets or capsules.
Source:	Synthesized.
Mode:	Orally.
EFFECTS:	DEPRESSANT.
Medical:	MAJOR TRANQUILIZERS: Used in mental hospitals for treating psychosis; MINOR TRANQUILIZERS: Used as mild sedative to relieve anxiety, tension, and muscle spasms, but do not produce sleep.
Abuse:	Anxiety reduction, prescribed excessively, used as street drug.
Reactions:	May cause clumsiness, drowsiness, and dizziness. Decrease memory and motor functions. Persistent use may produce side effects such as lethargy, rashes, menstrual irregularity, constipation, hypertension. Dangerous during pregnancy or when combined with alcohol. Withdrawal characterized by violent shaking and possible seizures.
Dependence:	Habit forming, physical dependence.
Signs:	Pills or container, reactions as listed above.

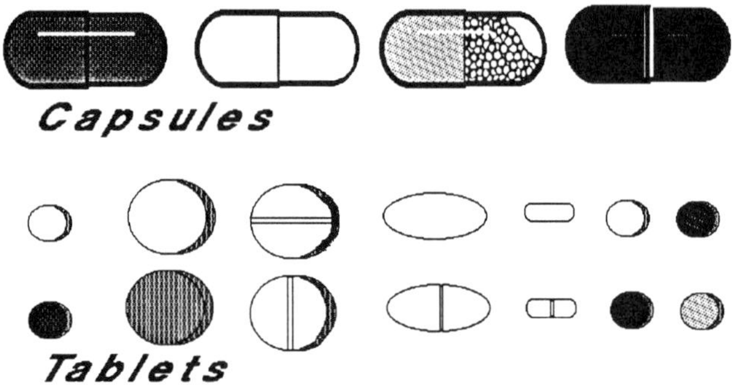

BARBITURATES

HALLUCINOGENS

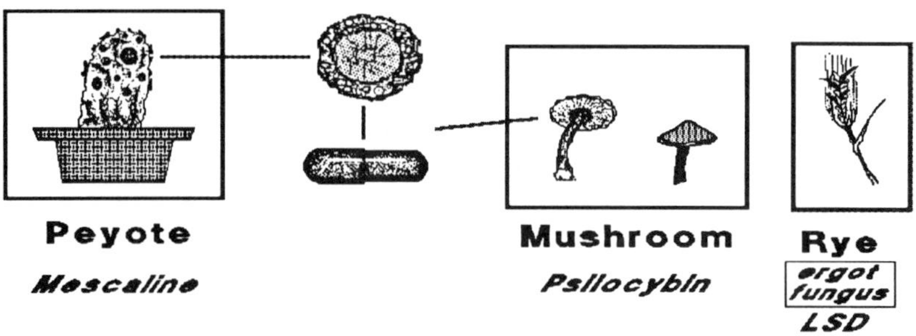

HALLUCINOGENS

DRUG:	LSD, PCP, MESCALINE, PSILOCYBIN.
Name and Slang:	LSD *Lysergic Acid Diethylamide*: Acid; PCP *Phencyclidine*: Angel Dust, Loveboat; MESCALINE: Mesc, Buttons, Cactus; PSILOCYBIN: Magic Mushrooms.
DESCRIPTION:	
Form and Source:	LSD: clear liquid, colored tablets, thin gelatin squares, or on blotter paper. Made from ergot fungus on rye or from chemicals in morning glory seeds. PCP: synthetic liquid, capsules, white powder, or pill. MESCALINE: active ingredient in peyote cactus, hard brown cactus discs, tablets, capsules. PSILOCYBIN: fresh or dried mushrooms.
Mode:	Swallowed, inhaled, injected.
EFFECTS:	HALLUCINOGEN.
Medical:	None.
Abuse:	Euphoria, exhilaration, altered mood, psychedelic perception, good trip or hallucinations--altered color, sight, sound, and taste.
Reactions:	Difficulty in concentration, bad trips or hallucinations (bum-mers), unpredictable behavior, panic, violence, depression, "flashbacks," self-destruction, chromosome aberrations, in-creased temperature, heart rate, and blood pressure, convul-sions, coma.
Dependence:	Psychological dependence.
Signs:	Emotional, out of contact with reality, mood swings, dilation of pupils (dark glasses at night).

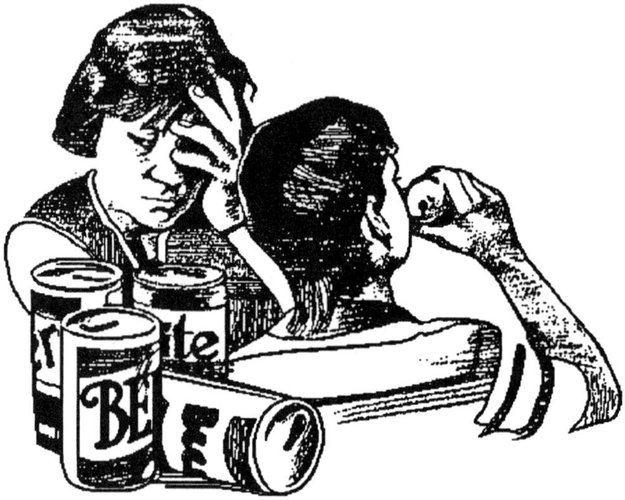

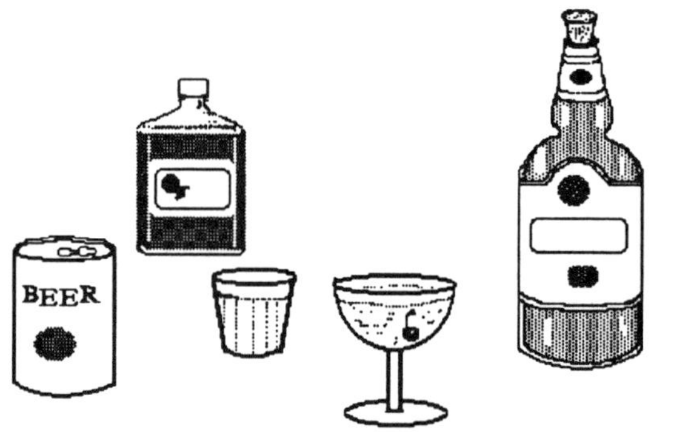

ALCOHOL

ETHYL ALCOHOL

DRUG:	BEER, WINE, LIQUORS.
Name:	Ethanol, ethyl alcohol.
Slang:	Booze, Juice, Sauce.
DESCRIPTION:	CNS depressant.
Form, Source, and Mode:	BEER: Fermented grains, malt, hops, water. 2-8%. WINE: Fermented fruit juices. 8-16%, (fortified 18-21%). LIQUOR: Distilled beverages. 40-50% or 80-100 proof. Whiskey--grains, Brandy--fruit, Rum--molasses, Vodka-- potatoes. COMPOUND LIQUORS: Gin, Cordial, Cocktail, Martini, Highball. Percentage depends on mix.
EFFECTS:	DEPRESSANT.
Medical:	Some physicians suggest alcohol for a variety of minor ailments, but most prefer more effective drugs.
Abuse:	For relaxation, euphoria, escape, a sense of confidence, to reduce anxiety and inhibitions, a social practice, etc.
Reactions:	Intoxication (depends on concentration of alcohol in blood), loss of inhibitions, reduced reaction time, loss of coordination, loss of consciousness, loss of life. Reduced safety, altered personality, exaggerated emotions. Damage to liver, brain, etc.
Dependence:	Physical, psychological, tolerance.
Signs:	ALCOHOLISM: preoccupation with drinking, gulps, alone, morning drinks, tolerance, hidden bottle, blackouts, tremens.

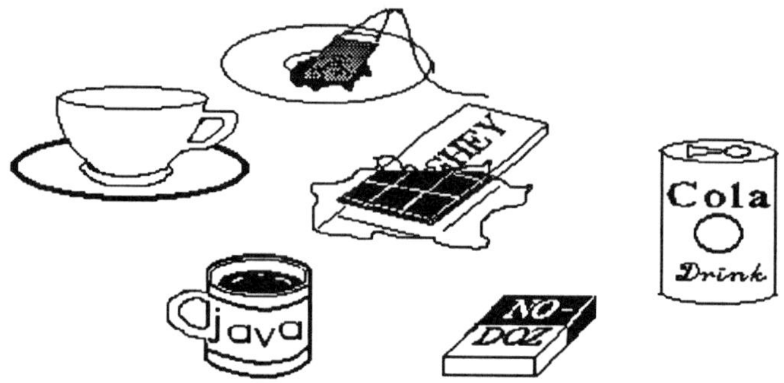

Caffeine

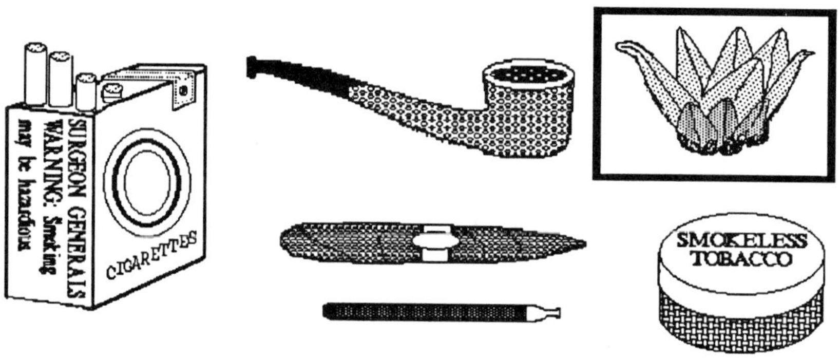

Tobacco

CAFFEINE

DRUG:	
Name:	Caffeine, *theophylline, theobromine.*
Slang:	Java, Coke.
DESCRIPTION:	CNS stimulant.
Form:	Liquid beverage, coffee, tea, cola, chocolate.
Source:	Natural.
Mode:	Swallowed or eaten.
EFFECTS:	STIMULANT.
Medical:	Mild stimulant.
Abuse:	Alertness.
Reactions:	Stimulation is followed by depression. Occasional use stim-ulates mental alertness, habitual use reduces effect. Heavy use produces undesirable side effects: headaches, interocular eyeball pressure, reduced visual accommodation, ringing in ears, skin irritation, elevated blood pressure, irregular heart beat, digestive disturbances, feelings of irritation, and insomnia. It masks fatigue, uses reserves, and delays rest and recuperation.
Dependence:	Psychological dependence.
Signs:	Irritability when caffeine is not available.

NICOTINE

DRUG:	
Name:	Nicotine, *nicotinic tobacum.*
Slang:	Fag.
DESCRIPTION:	CNS toxin, stimulant to some parts of the body, depressant to other parts.
Form:	Tobacco, cigarette.
Source:	Dried tobacco leaf.
Mode:	Smoked, chewed, sniffed.
EFFECTS:	STIMULANT, DEPRESSANT.
Medical:	An emetic, a topical poultice.
Abuse:	Relaxation.
Reactions:	Loss of appetite. Nicotine constricts arteries in skin and in heart, paralyzes cilia hair in lungs. Other harmful ingredients in tobacco are carcinogens and co-carcinogens which cause cancer, carbon-monoxide which reduces the body's oxygen-carrying capacity, and other toxic substances. High probability of organic damage depending on tobacco consumption patterns. Smoking contributes directly to cancer, coronary artery disease, burgers disease, chronic bronchitis, and emphysema. Smoke-less tobacco contributes directly to oral cancer.
Dependence:	Psychological, and possible physical.
Signs:	Nicotine dependency is manifest by irritability when smokes are not available.

DESIGNER DRUGS

Controlled substances are classified according to a schedule starting with Schedule I which includes drugs with the highest potential for abuse and addiction and no accepted medical use. Heroin, LSD, and marijuana are schedule I drugs. Schedule II drugs have high potential for abuse and addiction and restricted medical use. Schedule V drugs have the lowest potential for abuse and are accepted for over-the-counter (OTC) distribution.

Drugs are defined by law according to their chemical formulas. Underground chemists have tried to circumvent the laws by modifying the chemical structure of certain illegal drugs. These drugs are referred to as designer drugs. They can be many times stronger than the drugs they are designed to imitate.

One synthetic heroin drug is called China White. Others are called MPTP (New Heroin), MPPP, and PEPAR.

Synthetic amphetamines and methamphetamines designed to act as hallucinogens are called MDMA (Ecstasy), XTC (Adam Essence), MDM, STP, PMA, DMA, TMA, DOM, and DOB. Synthetic Phencyclidine PCP are PCPy, PCE, and TCP. They are all available in white powder form. The amphetamines are also available in tablet or capsule form. Some of them are inhaled, some injected, some are taken orally, and some are smoked.

The designer drugs have a strong potential for causing very severe health problems even as a result of the first use.

STUDY HELPS

Answer the following questions:

1. Distinguish among drug use, drug misuse, and drug abuse.
2. Distinguish between prescription drugs and over-the-counter drugs.
3. Distinguish between physical dependence and psychological dependence.
4. Distinguish among the various motivations for drug use.
5. Discuss the motivation and consequence of steroid abuse.
6. Discuss the value of scare tactics and false information in drug education.
7. What are the main points to remember when conducting a drug search at school?
8. What should the teacher do with incriminating information about drug use?
9. Discuss the extent of the substance abuse problem among youth in this country.
10. Identify the symptoms of drug abuse that a teacher might become aware of.
11. Explain how you might persuade a young person not to smoke or abuse drugs.
12. Indicate what schools and teachers might do to reduce the substance abuse.

Match the drugs with the effects they are likely to produce.

DRUGS		EFFECTS
1. alcohol	___ ___ ___	A. addiction
2. amphetamines	___ ___ ___	B. analgesic
3. barbiturate	___ ___ ___	C. carcinogen
4. caffeine	___ ___ ___	D. depressant
5. chloral hydrate	___ ___ ___	E. euphoria
6. cocaine	___ ___ ___	F. habituation
7. crack	___ ___ ___	G. hallucination
8. heroin	___ ___ ___	H. hypnotic
9. marijuana	___ ___ ___	I. intoxication
10. methamphetamine	___ ___ ___	J. narcotic
11. morphine	___ ___ ___	K. physical dependence
12. nicotine	___ ___ ___	L. psychic dependence
13. opium	___ ___ ___	M. potentiation
14. peyote	___ ___ ___	N. psychogenic
15. psilocybin	___ ___ ___	O. sedative
16. tranquilizers	___ ___ ___	P. stimulant
17. volatile solvent	___ ___ ___	Q. synergism
18. LSD	___ ___ ___	R. tranquilizer
19. DMT	___ ___ ___	S. tolerance
20. PCP	___ ___ ___	T. withdrawal

Chapter 9

POSITIVE MENTAL HEALTH

Much of what has been written under the heading of mental health is really about mental illness. This chapter however, is about positive mental health in the classroom. There are several ways in which schools and teachers can take affirmative steps to modify emotional health problems and contribute to positive mental health.

CONTRIBUTING TO POSITIVE MENTAL HEALTH

Most of what we read about mental health is really about mental illness. Those who are emotionally disturbed certainly need help, but a more positive approach in the past may have helped prevent their problems. Positive steps today may help modify the behavior of students who have emotional conflicts. People who are normal and above average in intellectual and emotional health can also profit from some special attention. That is a positive approach to mental health.

After reading the previous chapters, a prospective teacher may be overwhelmed. But all youth are not depressed, likely to commit suicide, using drugs, promiscuous, involved in cults, or suffering from eating disorders. Most of your students will be normal well-adjusted teenagers.

Some of your students will have serious personality problems that will only respond to extensive professional help, if at all. It take years to form a personality, and it may take years to change a personality. A teacher cannot be expected to be a miracle worker, but what a teacher can do, he or she must do. If they can't be a part of the solution, at least they can avoid being part of the problem. It is the small things that count.

DEALING WITH STUDENT PRESSURES

There are two major ways in which schools and teachers can modify emotional health problems. First, they can help prevent emotional problems by reducing unnecessary pressures within the school setting. Second, they should try to deal with the problems when they arise.

STUDENT PRESSURES

Pressures are placed on students from a variety of sources. One at a time, most students are able to handle them, but when the pressures pile up, the student may lose his effectiveness or even experience emotional problems. When the pressures become too great, the student may turn to some maladjustment measure to relieve the tension and anxiety. Frequently, the teachers, schools, parents, students, and community organizations need to evaluate the situation so that unnecessary pressures can be reduced. It should be remembered that not all students respond to pressure the same, and one student may be more affected by the same pressure at one time than another. Individual differences should be considered. The following outline indicates the sources of pressure and how they can be minimized.

Pressures From Teachers

1. Some teachers frequently seem to consider their own assignments as having precedence over other school activities. As a result, they create situations which make it difficult for the student to complete all of the assignments for a given day, particularly if two or three other teachers are making similar demands.

   A teacher can help minimize this pressure by:

   a. giving appropriate rather than excessive amounts of homework.
   b. coordinating due dates with other faculty members so that they will not overlap.
   c. giving enough time for assignments.
   d. refusing to give homework over school and national holidays when the student is not likely to complete it.

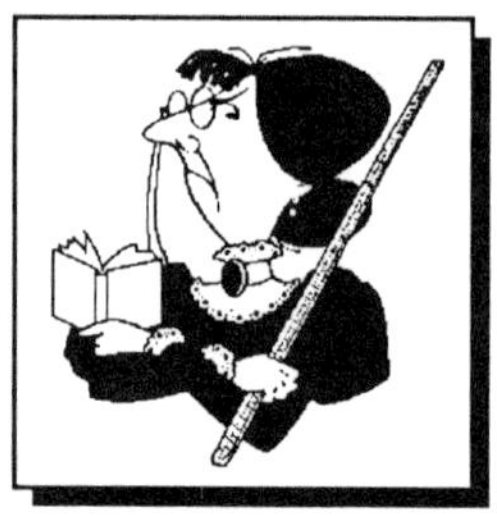

2. Some teachers seem to be unduly preoccupied with grades rather than learning. Unfortunately, teachers who emphasize grades to the exclusion of all else foster an atmosphere of excessive competition which can lead to cheating. If the teacher uses of a lot rules and procedures to prevent cheating, it shows that the teacher distrusts the students and expects them to try to cheat. The students will respond by finding more elaborate ways of cheating. The best prevention for cheating occurs when cheating is made taboo by a student's own peer group.

   A teacher can minimize this pressure by:

   a. de-emphasizing grades as the ultimate goal of education.
   b. scrutinizing testing devices and techniques.

c. establishing a grading system which does not call for the student to compete excessively.

3. The harmful effects of pressures can be minimized if the teachers show genuine interest in their students. Some teachers seem to take little interest in the student.

Teachers can minimize the apparent lack of interest by:

a. showing love and concern for each individual student.
b. demonstrating concern by word and deed.
c. being democratic rather than autocratic in the classroom.
d. teaching the students to understand their own and others' feelings.
e. establishing communication lines in the classroom.
f. being consistent and fair with all students.
g. becoming aware of individual student needs.
h. demonstrating flexibility.

4. A teacher is in an unusually good position to detect the first signs of a developing problem. To be able to recognize these signs, he must have a close and continuous relationship so that when there is a change, it can be noticed. But an adult who is going to help needs to do more than recognize a possible problem. His response to an upset adolescent is very important. A teacher should not act defensively when a student is emotionally upset. An adult should not regress to adopt the adolescent's point of view. The adolescent needs someone to talk to and someone who will listen. What he doesn't need is to have someone order him around or to criticize him. Just listening can do more than people realize. It is one of the most important steps in establishing a positive relationship. It may result in a transfer of the teacher's positive attitude to the listener. Occasionally, all that is needed is a flash of insight that could change the whole emotional balance.

Pressures From Parents

1. Parents occasionally exert pressures upon their child which can cause certain emotional difficulties. Some of these pressures are related to grades, athletic success, social acceptance, and recognition for other talents. While many parents maintain that such pressure is exerted for the child's benefit, it is often an expression of the parents' need to feed their own ego. Parents who expect their child to perform beyond his abilities create an impossible situation; this is particularly true in the case of a child who desperately wishes to please his parents but is not able to do so. If this pressure is not offset by some other source of success, it may have disastrous effects.

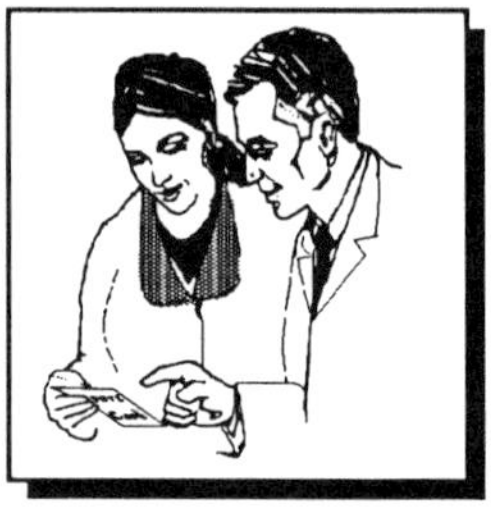

2. Pressures are created when parents try to impose their value systems upon their children at a time when they are dealing with the value systems of the outside world. A teacher is in a unique position to help provide some balance between the apparent contradictions and also to help the child discover his own values.

3. Most home situations are beyond the school's scope and teachers must use discretion when dealing with such problems. There are ways in which schools and teachers can help. Parents need to be made aware of the pressures which they create for their children.

Teachers can make parents aware of the pressures they are causing by:

a. Parents can be invited to attend a meeting where teachers, counselors, students, and parents can alert others to the importance of eliminating parental pressures.
b. Parents can be alerted to the pressures they may be causing by attending a parent/teacher conference.

<u>Pressures From Students</u>

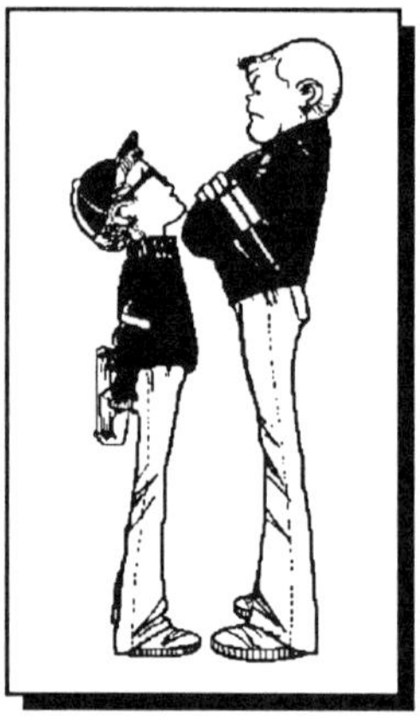

1. Students can frequently exert tremendous pressure upon themselves. Some students take upon themselves an unbearable work load without realizing it. They get involved in many activities such as music lessons, team sports, church activities, jobs at home and outside the home. This leaves the student who tries to excel in all of these activities little time to rest.

2. There is also considerable pressure placed upon students by one another. Social pressure among young people is an extremely potent force and may influence their feelings about such things as clothing, dating partners, drugs, drinking, sexual relations, and school. There is a great deal of pressure to be popular and to conform to crowd norms. During adolescence, peer pressure is usually at its strongest.

3. Although it is unrealistic to assume that these pressures can be eliminated entirely, the school can exert some influence in this area.

Pressure can be eliminated by:

a. Teachers can work with peer groups to reduce peer pressure.

b. The school can set guidelines which will help a student to refrain from overloading himself.

Pressures From School

1. School policies and procedures can create pressure for the student:

Pressure results from the following ways:

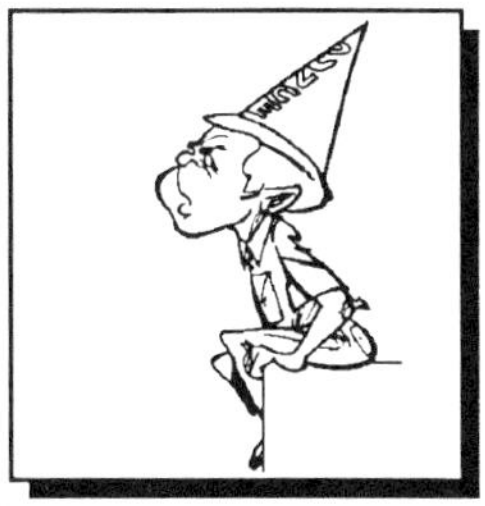

a. Some school personnel think that students exist to serve the school staff rather than vice versa.

b. Many rules and regulations are adopted to meet the needs of the school staff rather than those of the students. Regulations are necessary, of course, but when they are overdone, they create unnecessary pressure and cause many students to drop out either physically or mentally.

c. Policies which dictate what type of equipment a student must buy for certain classes such as P.E., shop, or home economics can create pressures for the student who cannot afford to purchase such materials.

d. School scheduling may also create some problems for the student. For instance, what should a student do if he needs a pencil for his first period class but the bookstore does not open until after school starts?

e. Some students feel pressured by dress and grooming standards.

2. It is easy to see that some school policies and procedures can indeed cause pressure for students; many feel hopelessly trapped within a system that is unresponsive to their individual needs, which leads to frustration and rebellion. A wise school board will try to alleviate the unnecessary pressures it may be placing upon its students by frequently reviewing its policies and modifying them when necessary.

DEALING WITH EMOTIONAL DISTURBANCES

In a lifetime of teaching, you will face many emotional disturbances. Most of the time the person who is emotionally disturbed will be someone else; occasionally, you may be the person who is emotionally disturbed. In either case, you should know how to deal with the problem.

BE A GOOD LISTENER

When a teacher is faced with an emotionally disturbed person (a student, a parent, or a colleague), the main approach at that time is simply to be a good listener. To do this one should follow these guidelines:

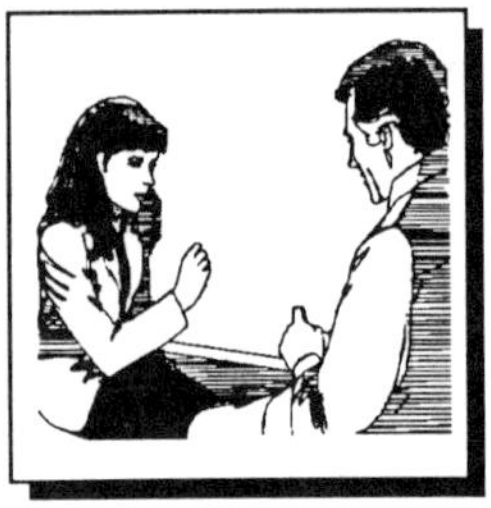

- **Don't talk, listen.** This listening process is disrupted when the listener blames, criticizes, pities, or offers logic. To explain to someone why he is upset is unwise. Allow the person to ventilate his feelings and ideas without interruptions of your opinions or actions. However, an occasional short comment to let him know you are listening, caring, and thinking about what he is saying may be necessary.

- **Don't belittle the problem.** Sometimes the problem may seem trivial to you but to the person with the problem, it is serious. Also, there may be more than meets the eye, as often the problem a person speaks about may be leading up to a bigger one which the person will only disclose if properly listened to.

- **Don't be impatient.** Realizing the potential difficulty in self-expression, the listener must be willing to tolerate considerable repetition or vagueness.

- **Don't provide the answer.** The person must come to his own decisions. The role of the listener is either to serve as a sounding board for the expression of feelings or to bring into view possible alternative actions. However, the more serious the emotional distress and the less control the troubled person has, the greater control someone else must assume.

If the above techniques don't seem to solve the problem, do not overestimate your ability and continue on as counselor, but refer the troubled person to a more professional source of help such as a psychologist or counselor.

DEALING WITH HYSTERIA

If the teacher is faced with an acute psychiatric emergency, specific do's and don'ts should be followed until professional help can be obtained.

- **Don't try to treat the problem yourself.** Call a family doctor, a mental clinic or hospital, the mental health association, the student health center, or the counseling center for competent advice on what action to take.

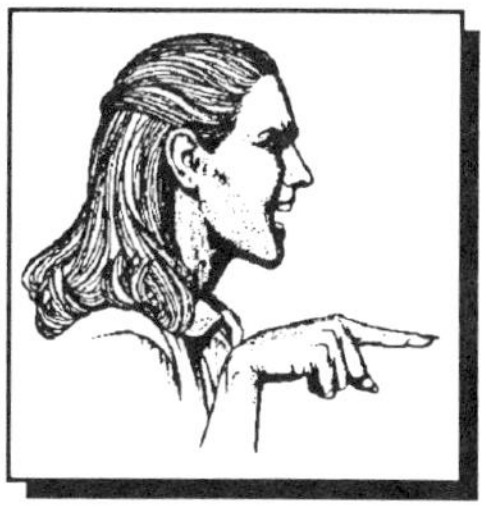

- **Don't become anxious yourself, even if the attack does not subside immediately.** You should be forewarned of the fact that outbursts of emotion can be contagious. Those in the immediate vicinity tend to become overanxious as they feel unable to cope with the outbursts. Most people's nervous attempts to calm the hysterical person only serve to intensify the attack.

- **Don't shout at the hysterical person.** Shouting only conveys anxiety and loss of control on your part and puts the situation under less control.

- **Don't use physical methods such as slapping the face or throwing water on the person.** These time-honored customs may bring success, but it is more likely to be viewed as an act of desperation and make the situation worse.

- **Don't scold the person, argue with him, or criticize him.** Do not tell him it is his own fault and that all he needs to do is just snap out of it.

- **Show sympathy and really listen.** Do not talk too much. Listening implies your willingness to help. When speaking, do so quietly but firmly. Reassure him that everything is in hand or that the danger is past. If there are several people trying to help, leave it to the person who seems most able to take command of the situation.

- **Don't restrain a person who is throwing himself about unless there is a danger present.** It is often better to pay no attention until his movement ceases. Then give reassurance and support.

For violent or self-destructive behavior, do not leave the person unattended. You may not have time to get the help you need. However, unless the person is coming in or out of a state of depression, he is not likely to be dangerous.

DEALING WITH A PERSONAL CRISIS

In your lifetime, you will come face to face with many little and probably at least one big crisis. It may be when your marriage is threatened or a close loved one dies. These are times that are very trying and when decisions have to be made. The unknown seems threatening, and we fear that we may make the wrong choices. Whether we can successfully handle the crisis or not depends largely on our basic psychological strength. In order to do this and be properly prepared to handle future crises, some practical steps are suggested.

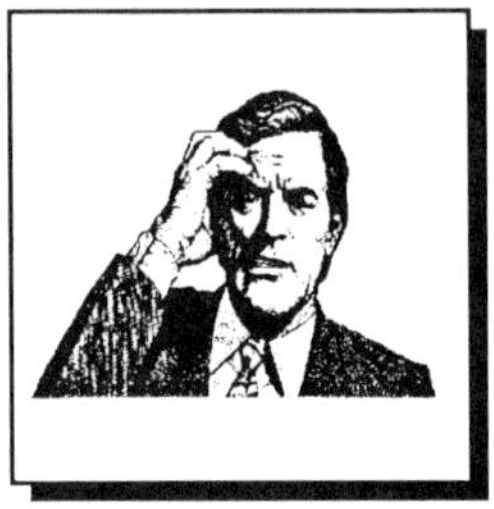

- <u>Take a breather</u>. It is always hazardous to make a decision during an emotional turmoil--a cooling-off period is wise. Turn your attention to something else for a little while--a hobby, a movie, a book, or a long walk. Then give your decision some thought and it will be easier.

- <u>Talk it out</u>. A crisis is a time when "a fella needs a friend." Talking it out, or even writing it out, usually gives a new slant on the situation. You can't expect your listener to solve your problems, but talking about them will make you feel better.

- <u>Understand yourself</u>. Your success in handling a crisis depends to a large extent on how you picture and value yourself. If you have an accurate idea of your intelligence and capabilities, you will have greater courage. If you know your true capacity, you will be able to work within those bounds.

- <u>Attack one point at a time</u>. Break the problem down into components. The big dilemma consists of a number of small, not too difficult problems. Taking them one at a time, they are less frightening and easier to handle.

- <u>Stay healthy</u>. A time of crisis is, above all others, a time to guard your health. Make sure you eat sensibly, have some exercise, and get enough sleep. Even a slight illness now will make your problems more difficult. A healthy, rested body gives psychological strength.

THE EMOTIONAL HEALTH OF TEACHERS

The emotional health of teachers can have a direct influence on the emotions of the students. Students are very perceptive of a teacher's mood. Negative emotions displayed by a teacher will make a big difference in the lives of the students. Teachers, like other human beings, develop emotional conflicts and are susceptible to emotional illness. But when teachers are helping mold the lives of young people entrusted to their care, the impact of emotional problems may be more significant. An emotionally unstable teacher may be able to get by with most well-adjusted students, but the results of interactions between an emotionally ill teacher and an emotionally immature student may be drastic in the lives of one or both.

Emotionally disturbed teachers frequently exhibit impulsive hostility, irritability, and negativism. In handling interpersonal relations with students, they tend to reflect a mirror image of the student's negative emotions. They tend to exhibit excessive concern and unnecessarily strict discipline for minor infractions. Grades are over-emphasized as a

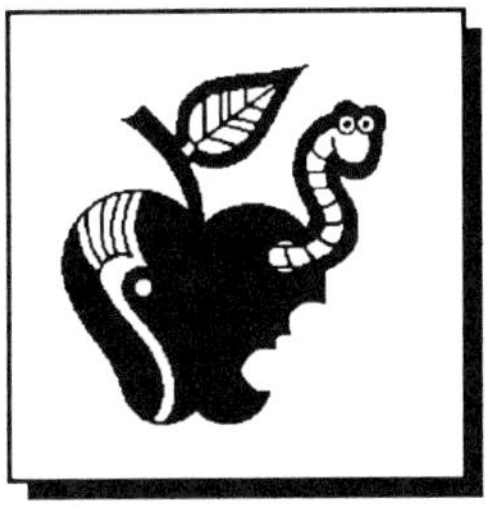

reflection of the students' performance to the point of producing a failing complex in the minds of low achievers.

School districts can and should do much to help improve the emotional health of its teachers. Providing job security and economic stability is one important need. This includes appropriate benefits and retirement programs. A teacher who is forced to moonlight in order to support his family will not do his best job or feel good about what he is doing. Teachers need to have the facilities and materials required to do a good job in their teaching. A good type of health insurance that provides for routine medical and psychological evaluations for the teachers with good coverage for their dependents should be provided. Teachers need to have a place to escape for a few minutes each day from the pressures of teaching. This place may be a faculty room lounge that is restful and relaxing, a separate dining facility, or a private office area. Opportunities for personal growth and achievement such as in-service education programs in their subject area, in teaching procedures, and in areas of personal interest should be offered. The gym and shop areas may be made available to faculty so that they maintain physical fitness, have an opportunity to relax and create, and interact socially with other teachers and staff members. They should have the opportunity for advancement and to have their achievements recognized.

Probably most important, they should feel that the administration is fully behind them. They need to feel that they are part of a team. Proper rapport and communication between members of the team are important. Teachers should be able to work closely with school counselors concerning students.

MODIFYING STUDENT BEHAVIOR

William Glasser is well known as a practicing psychiatrist and consultant in the educational and correctional fields. His first book, *Mental Health or Mental Illness?* presented a sound and sensible approach to psychiatry for practical action. It helped laymen and professionals better understand how normal and abnormal people function. Some of the concepts presented in lesson seven were based on that book.

While working with juvenile delinquents, Dr. Glasser developed an approach he called reality therapy. To share and explain that approach, Dr. Glasser wrote his second book with the title of *Reality Therapy.* That book was so well received by educators that he was asked to conduct training seminars for school administrators, counselors, and teachers around the country. He later established the Institute for Reality Therapy in Los Angeles to further refine his philosophies of behavior.

The next several pages will summarize Reality Therapy's approach. We will also explore some ideas presented in two other books by Dr. Glasser. His third book, *Schools Without Failure*, challenged some of the traditional practices in education. But of his seven books, William Glasser says his most recent, *Control Theory,* has given him the greatest sense of personal satisfaction. It explains how people can better control their emotions and actions to live healthier and more productive lives.

REALITY THERAPY

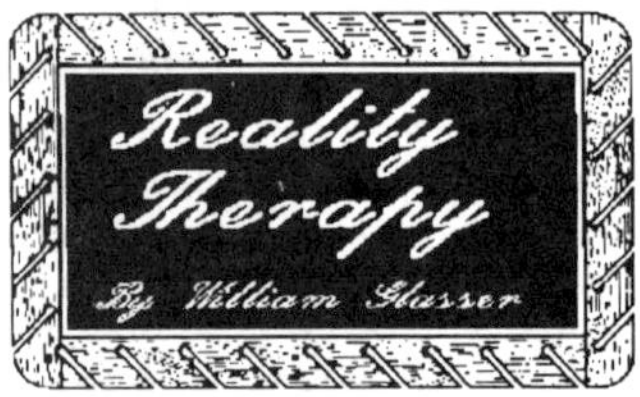

For years teachers have been using an approach called reality therapy adapted from Doctor Glasser's book, *Reality Therapy--a New Approach to Psychiatry.* Doctor Glasser has also conducted many seminars and workshops to help teachers learn to use this approach successfully in the classroom. This approach can be used on a day-to-day basis to help students whose inappropriate behavior has been due to emotional problems.

In the following eight pages the author has outlined and summarized the major points of reality therapy. Teachers can use this approach to make a valuable contribution to their student's positive mental health. The principles that may apply in a patient-therapist relationship in a clinical setting may also apply in a student-teacher relationship in an educational setting, except that in school the behavioral problems may be much less severe. When problems become too severe, professional counseling may be necessary; however, if teachers apply these principles early, the problems may never become severe. This summary starts out by asking and answering several questions.

WHAT IS WRONG WITH THOSE WHO NEED PSYCHIATRIC TREATMENT?

All psychiatric patients have a common characteristic. Regardless of how a problem is expressed, everyone who needs psychiatric treatment suffers from one basic inadequacy: they are unable to fulfill their essential needs. Unable to fulfill their needs in the normal ways, they begin to deny the realities of the world around them and try alternative ways of meeting their needs. No matter how irrational, inappropriate, or bizarre their behavior seems to us, it has meaning and validity to them. The harder it is to satisfy their needs, the stranger their behavior.

Therapy will be successful when they are able to give up denying the world and recognize that reality not only exists, but that they must fulfill their needs within its framework. Therapy will be a process of helping them strengthen their mental function so that they can satisfy their needs more normally. Interestingly enough, the process of strengthening the mental function of a mature person with a mental or emotional problem is much the same as the process of developing the mental function of a child in the first place. It is a process of helping the person learn how to satisfy his basic needs through reality. A therapy that leads a patient toward reality might actually be called a therapy toward reality or simply Reality Therapy.

WHAT ARE THE BASIC NEEDS?

The basic needs do not vary with age, sex, or race. It is generally accepted that all humans have the same psychological and physiological needs. Fulfillment of the physiological needs for food, water, oxygen, warmth, and rest are rarely the concerns of psychiatry. Psychiatry is concerned with the psychological needs which are: the need to love and be loved, and the need to feel that we are worthwhile to ourselves and to others. We all have the same needs, but we vary in our ability to fulfill them.

HOW DO WE FULFILL OUR NEEDS?

These psychological needs are only fulfilled through involvement with other people, one at the very minimum and hopefully more than one. At all times in our lives, we must have at least one person who cares about us and whom we care for ourselves. If we do not have this essential person, we will be unable to fulfill our basic needs. This person is usually a parent in the case of a child, or the therapist in the case of a mental patient.

One characteristic of the other person is essential; he must be able to fulfill his own needs. Parents who are unable to satisfy their needs usually rear children who are also unable to satisfy their needs. And these children never fully mature psychologically until they develop a close, caring relationship with a capable individual, perhaps a teacher, another relative, someone from church, a coach, a friend, a spouse, a parole officer, a social worker, or a therapist. Although the other person may change at times throughout our lives, if at any time we are not involved, we will very quickly become unable to satisfy our needs.

First is the need to love and be loved. In all of its forms ranging from friendship to conjugal love, this need drives us to continuous activity in search of satisfaction. To either love or allow others to love us is not enough; we must do both.

Second, and equally important, is the need to feel that we are worthwhile, both to 3ourselves and to others. To be loved is not enough; we need to feel of worth. Although these two needs usually are satisfied together, this is not always the case. For example, although an overindulged child may receive an abundance of love, the parents do not make the critical distinction between loving him and accepting his behavior, good or bad. Receiving love for behavior he knows is wrong does not allow him to feel worthwhile. For another example, a beautiful and capable woman often finds herself in a position of being recognized only for her beauty. Being the object of someone's love does not in itself give us worth.

To be worthwhile, we must maintain a satisfactory standard of behavior. To do so, we must learn what is right and wrong and then correct ourselves when we do wrong and credit ourselves when we do right. Morals, values, and standards of right and wrong behavior are essential to the fulfillment of our needs. The worth of behavior cannot be valued without standards. Thus, when we are unable to fulfill one or both of our needs, we feel pain or discomfort in some form.

HOW DO WE LEARN TO FULFILL OUR NEEDS?

Learning to fulfill our needs must begin in infancy and continue all our lives. If we fail to learn, we will suffer, and suffering drives us to unrealistic means to fulfill our needs. A person who does not learn as a little child to give and receive love may spend the rest of his life unsuccessfully trying to love. The younger and more thoroughly we learn to fulfill our needs, the more satisfactory our lives will be. However, from time to time in everyone's life the world and situations change, requiring one to learn and relearn to fulfill one's needs under different conditions and stresses. Whether we learn young or later in life, we must stay involved with people to continue to fulfill our needs.

Responsibility

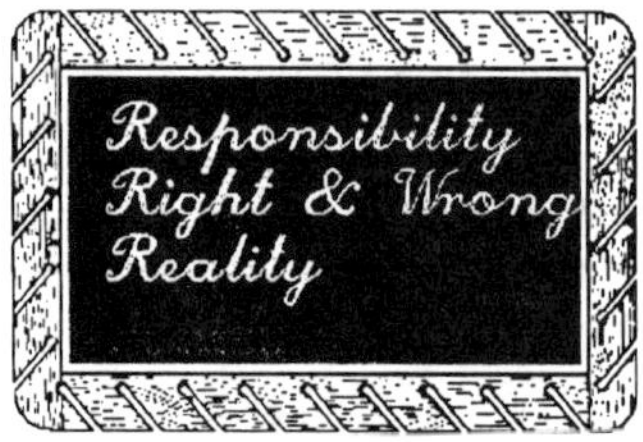

A responsible parent maintains the necessary involvement with his child. He teaches him responsibility through the proper combination of love and discipline. Responsibility can be learned at any age, but it is easier to learn correctly at the first than to have to overcome previous bad learning. For some children, the learning of responsibility does not come easy. Children do not know that what seems easy to them will not fulfill their needs. From infancy, they struggle against the reality that they must learn from their parents how to fulfill their needs. When they are older and can recognize reality, they test their parents with irresponsible behavior to see if what they have been taught is valid. Through discipline tempered with love, parents must teach their children to behave better. The child learns from this that the parents care.

Parents who are willing to suffer the pains of the child's intense anger by firmly holding him to the responsible course are teaching a lesson that will help him all of his life. Parents must understand that taking the responsible course will never permanently alienate the child. Parents must not only hold the child to the correct course of action, they must also show by example that they are capable of taking the responsible course. Parents who have no self-discipline cannot successfully discipline a child. When discipline is responsible and has with it the element of love, and when the parents' own behavior is consistent with their demands on the child, he will love and respect them even though on the surface he might not show it. He will understand the action of his parents to say, "I care enough about you to force you to act in a better way" and "I love you because you are a worthwhile person, because I respect you and feel you respect me as well as yourself."

When a person learns responsibility through involvement with other responsible persons, he will be given freedom to try out his newly acquired skills as soon as he is ready to do so. Reality Therapy defines responsibility as the ability to fulfill our needs and to do so in a way that does not deprive others of the ability to fulfill their needs. Acquiring responsibility is a complicated lifelong problem. Those who fill our mental hospitals, prisons, and psychiatric clinics testify that it is not an easy task. They are described as irresponsible.

Right and Wrong

All society is based on morality and if the important people in a person's life do not discuss whether his behavior is right or wrong, there will be no basis for feeling worth. Also, if a disparity exists between the values a person recognizes as the acceptable norm and the life he leads, there will be an absence of the feeling of worth.

"Right and wrong" is a concept basic to Reality Therapy. The therapist poses the question, "Are you doing right or wrong?" Patients are confronted with their behavior and are asked to judge what they are doing. Unless they judge their own behavior, they will not change.

Getting a person to acknowledge the values he really believes in is part of the art of therapy. Once acknowledged, the major task is to help him live by those standards. When standards and values are not stressed, the most therapy can accomplish is to help the patients become more comfortable in their irresponsibility. For the purposes of therapy, almost all behavior which leads to the fulfillment of our needs within the bounds of reality is right, good, or moral. In other words, when a man acts in such a way that he gives and receives love and feels worthwhile to himself and others, his behavior is right or moral. All of the implications of the decisions one makes about what is right or wrong must be examined in terms of reality and responsibility.

Reality

Like responsibility and right or wrong, reality is also a concept basic to Reality Therapy. It is concerned with the question, "What is realistic?" An action can be called realistic or unrealistic only when its remote as well as immediate consequences are taken into consideration. If the ultimate consequence of an action produces evil, pain, or suffering, that action may be termed unrealistic. If the ultimate satisfaction resulting from an action is greater than the immediate effort or sacrifice, the action can be called realistic. Reality Therapy is concerned with the person's ability to reason and properly appraise the consequence of his action.

When a person is suffering from irresponsible behavior, it would be incorrect to assume that the patient is fully conscious of his present behavior. In a sense he is aware, but it is only a meager awareness. The practice of Reality Therapy is only concerned with present behavior, the behavior closely preceding the session, and the therapist insists that the patient face his present behavior. They go over and over what he is doing to make him understand that his present behavior does not fulfill his needs. No outsider can solve the problem; he must do that alone.

If reality therapy stopped when it succeeded in getting the patient to face reality, the job would only be partially done. As important as confronting reality is, the patient must also learn to fulfill his needs in the real world.

REALITY THERAPY INCLUDES INVOLVEMENT

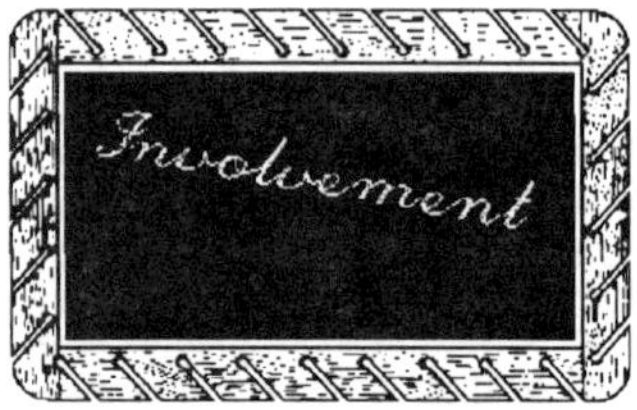

When the patient is suffering from irresponsibility, it indicates undersocialization. In ordinary socialization, parental love serves as a compensation for the immediate satisfactions the child is asked to give up. In Reality Therapy, the involvement the patient experiences with the therapist also serves this function.

Usually, the most difficult phase of Reality Therapy is gaining the involvement that the patient so desperately needs but which he has been unsuccessful in attaining or maintaining. Unless this requisite involvement exists between the therapist and the patient, there can be no therapy. The therapist needs to achieve a proper involvement, a completely honest, human relationship in which the patient, perhaps for the first time in his life, realizes that someone cares enough about him to not only accept him, but also to help him fulfill his needs in the real world.

The ability of the therapist to get involved is the major skill of doing Reality Therapy. It is a difficult task to quickly build a firm emotional relationship with a patient who has failed to establish such relationships in the past. The patient is desperately looking for a person with whom he can have the necessary involvement to satisfy his needs, but his past failures have created a wall against pseudoinvolvement that is difficult to penetrate. The patient is looking for a person with whom he can become emotionally involved, someone he can care about and who he can be convinced cares about him; someone who can convince the patient that he will stay with him until he can better fulfill his needs.

The therapist must be a very responsible person, able to satisfy his own needs. He must be interested, human and sensitive, and be willing to discuss some of his own struggles so that the patient can see that acting responsible is possible, though difficult. He must have the strength to become involved, to have his values tested by the patient, and to withstand intense criticism by the person he is trying to help. He must always be strong, never expedient. He must withstand the patient's request for sympathy. Never condoning an irresponsible action on the patient's part, he must be willing to watch the patient suffer if that helps him toward responsibility. To some extent, he must be affected by the patient and his problems and even suffer with him. Through all of this, the therapist must remain personal, subjective, and supportive. The patient must be able to see that the therapist really does care about him, considers him of worth, and sincerely wants to help.

Once involvement is gained and reality is faced, therapy becomes a special kind of education, learning to live more effectively. Reality Therapy takes every opportunity to teach patients better ways of fulfilling their needs. Much time is spent painstakingly examining the patient's daily activities and suggesting better ways for him to behave. Patients' questions are answered, and possible ways of solving problems are suggested. Patients who have not been able to solve their needs learn how to approach people so that they can become involved with more people. They learn how to accomplish things so that they can gain an increased feeling of self-worth.

REALITY THERAPY VERSUS CONVENTIONAL THERAPY

Often people wonder what goes on between the patient and the therapist. As part of becoming involved, the therapist must become interested in and discuss all aspects of the patient's present life--his interests, hopes, fears, opinions, values, and ideas of right and wrong. The therapist is interested in him as a person with a wide potential, not just as a patient with a problem. They always focus on the present. They are not interested in the patient's history. Without denying that the patient had an unsatisfactory past and that it certainly contributed to what he is now, we cannot change the past, only the future. Reality therapists rarely ask "why?" They ask "what?" They want to know what is going on now in all aspects of a patient's life that makes him act irresponsibly. This is a radical departure from conventional psychiatry where the patient's past history is as essential to psychiatry as the scalpel is to surgery.

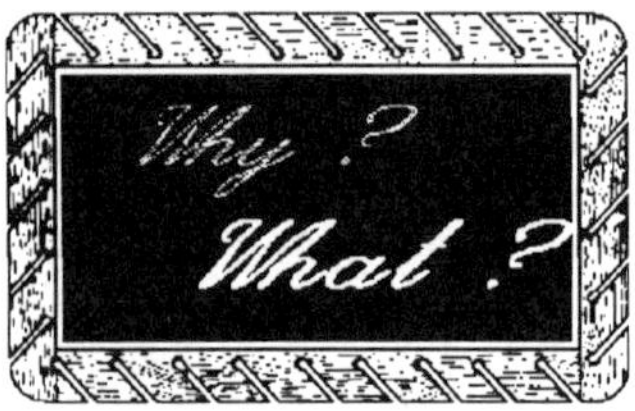

Conventional therapy also contends that unconscious motivation is highly important and that for successful therapy the patient must become aware of previously unconscious reasons for why he behaves as he does. The conventional psychiatrist uses projective tests, free association, dream analysis, and slips of the tongue to gain insight into the patient's unconscious mind. Reality Therapy acknowledges that talking in one's sleep, slips of the tongue, phobias, and compulsions are examples of behavior obviously based upon unconscious mental processes, but knowledge of it does not help therapy. Emphasis upon the unconscious sidetracks the main issue of the patient's irresponsibility and gives another excuse to avoid facing reality. Patients treated with conventional psychiatry may know the unconscious reasons for every move they make, but they still do not change, because knowing the reason does not lead to fulfilling needs. Delving into a person's unconscious mind is detrimental to therapy.

Another difference between Reality Therapy and conventional therapy has to do with the concept of mental illness. Reality Therapy contends that if there is a medical analogy which applies to psychiatric problems it is not illness, but weakness. While illness can be cured by removing the causative agent, weakness can be cured only by strengthening the person to cope with the stress of the world. Psychiatrists discovered long ago that as much as they would like to follow medical parallels and cure the patient of his brain disease, they were unable to do so with functional and personality disorders because no brain pathology exists. Of course organic disorder is another thing entirely. Instead of giving up on the illness concept, psychiatrists seized on the discovery of unconscious conflict as the cause of mental illness. Also misleading, but an important part of the mental illness concept, is the use of psychiatric diagnosis to label a wide variety of mental illnesses. The purpose of diagnosis is to select proper treatment. Where there is a variety of conditions, each with a specific treatment, diagnosis is vital. In Reality Therapy, all that needs to be diagnosed is whether the patient is suffering from irresponsibility or from organic illness. With irresponsibility, there is no essential difference in the treatment. Reality Therapy substitutes irresponsibility due to mental weakness for mental illness.

REALITY THERAPY IN PRACTICE

After one understands the concepts of Reality Therapy, qualifies as a person who satisfies his own needs, and gains involvement with a person, he may be able to use the four steps in a Reality Therapy dialogue.

1. **Get the person to identify his behavior**. The therapist and the person must be sure they are talking about the same behavior. The therapist never asks *why.* The preferred question is *what.* When you ask why, it looks like you are asking for excuses to justify the inappropriate behavior. Asking what identifies the behavior that

needs changing. The answer to why may interfere with behavioral change. If excuses are volunteered, don't accept them as justification for unacceptable behavior. The person is responsible for his behavior no matter how good the reasons are. Similarly showing too much *sympathy* can also get rid of needed change. *Empathy* is preferred because it shows you understand how they feel, but you also understand their need for change.

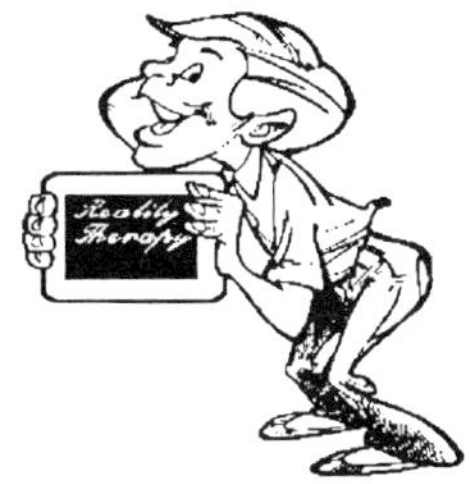

2. **<u>Get the person to identify the consequences of his or her actions</u>.** The reality of life is that if a person performs an act, he or she will experience the consequences of that act.

3. **<u>Get the person to make value judgments, either of the action or the consequence of the action</u>.** This is where standards of right and wrong come in. They should not be the therapist's values, but the values of the person. Is that action right? Is the ultimate consequences of the act desirable? Will it satisfy your greater needs?

4. **<u>Get the person to make plans for changing his behavior</u>.** He should change his behavior to that which he judges to be good and to that which results in the consequence he desires. Before deciding on a specific plan for change, the person should suggest and consider the possible alternatives.

After the person has decided on a plan of action, the therapist can help him follow through. He may help the person decide when he is going to do it. He may give some assistance, but the major responsibility rests with the person. It is essential that the therapist be subjective and personal throughout.

Although Reality Therapy was originally conceived as a process taking place between the psychiatrist and the patient, its principles have application to the teacher-student situation, the parent-child relationship, or any counseling situation. The concepts of Reality Therapy are also of value to the individual as he reasons with himself and makes decisions about his own behavior and involvement with others. The application of Reality Therapy requires:

- intense personal involvement
- facing reality
- rejecting irresponsible behavior
- learning better ways to behave

Compared to conventional therapy, reality therapy may appear harsh, but it can produce noticeably different results; it can change behavior. The principles involved in Reality Therapy can help teachers to help their students make better decisions.

SCHOOLS WITHOUT FAILURE

While *Reality Therapy* focuses on student behavior, *Schools Without Failure*, another book by Doctor Glasser, focuses on school practices that may be detrimental to the emotional health of the students. Dr. Glasser said,

> Too much of our present educational system emphasizes failure and too many children who attend school are failing. Unless we can provide schools where children, through a reasonable use of their capacities, can succeed, we will do little to solve the problems of our country. We will have more social disturbances, more people who need to be kept in jails, prisons, and mental hospitals, more people who need social workers to take care of their lives because they feel they cannot succeed in this society and are no longer willing to try.

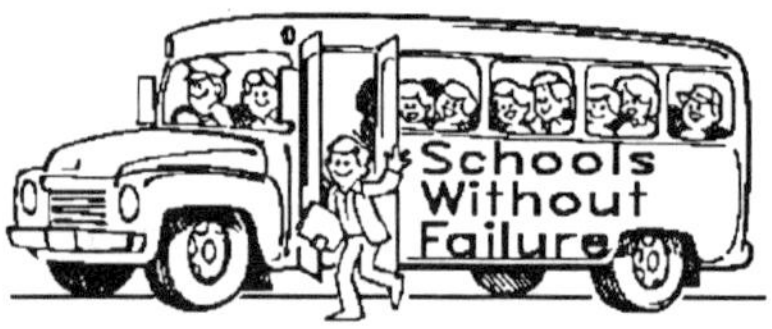

Hopefully, the schools will be able to provide experiences which will help break a child's failure cycle started at home, but some practices traditionally followed in education may accentuate the failure cycle. In the next three pages, the authors summarizes Doctor Glasser's suggestions.

Labels

Failing children will continue to fail if their teachers continue to remind them of their failures. Sometimes the records and anecdotal information passed from teacher to teacher interferes with a child's chance for success. Glasser maintains that the only information worth gleaning from the past is concerned with the child's successes. Very few children come to school as failures; they are optimistic, but the schools begin to hang labels of failure on them. The shattering of student optimism is the most serious problem in education, and the first few years are most critical.

Emphasis on Memorizing

Children learn to use their brain to explore their interests and solve problems, but sometimes in school they just use their brains to memorize facts. It is unfortunate when schools make memorizing more important than thinking. It is even more unfortunate if what is memorized is irrelevant. Some students tend to give up when they realize that what is important in school may not be important in life. Nothing should be taught in school that is not relevant to life. Failure to help students learn how to think and how to discover for themselves what is relevant is one of the major failures of education. Although it feels good to be right, if being right is based on memory alone, there is little lasting satisfaction. But there is more lasting satisfaction when being right is based on thinking, judgment, and decision making.

Most examinations depend on memory. The closed-book examination is based on the fallacy that knowledge remembered is better than knowledge looked up. The world says look it up, use a reference book, check the tables, make sure, and don't rely on your memory. Schools say memorize it until the exam. A rational basis for examinations is to test how well students can use the tools of education.

Irrelevance of Education

Because memorization without relevance leads to boredom, schools are turning more and more to grades and the threat of punishment as external motivations. Students lose interest and refuse to learn. Their bodies may remain in school, but their minds leave. To correct this problem, the schools should relate every subject taught to something that children now do or will do later in their own lives outside of school. Because children will not necessarily see this relevance, teaching relevance is a part of effective education.

Homework is often excessive, tedious, and irrelevant. Homework that students are not prepared for is frustrating. Homework that the students already understand is redundant. Poor students don't do homework. Good students don't need to do it. Homework tends to widen the gap between the successful and failing students.

Education Without Emotion

To a large extent, emotions have been eliminated from education. This is a problem, because emotions help students see relevance in what they are studying. Most materials have little reference to the rich emotional aspects of the students' cultures. A totally quiet, orderly, unemotional classroom rarely provides a good learning experience.

Grading

Probably the school practice that produces the most student failure is grading. Grades are supposed to stimulate the student to work harder, but they do not work that way. Grades are frequently substituted for learning. Grades are primarily a measure of the student's ability to remember facts rather than to think. Several studies have shown almost no relationship between the grades a student gets in college and his competence and success in a profession. Often in college, a student has to select between concentrating on grades and giving up learning and thinking or concentrating on learning and giving up grades. Although grading systems may state that a "C" grade is passing or average, most people recognize that the only real passing grades are A's and B's. Grades are also bad, because they encourage students to cheat. As long as grades remain so important, few students will study anything that will not be covered on a test.

The normal curve used in grading reduces motivation and encourages mediocre performance. Although the normal curve is used to provide accuracy and objectivity in grading, it actually shows that education is ineffective because only a minority of the students earn the A's and B's. More effective teaching would produce a skewed grade distribution. Grades provide incentives and a sense of satisfaction for students who get A's and B's, but for the rest of the students, grades are a sign of failure and a signal to give up.

Instead of concentrating on failure, the schools should concentrate on success. The grading system should not be used to label any student a failure. Almost everyone succeeds to some degree. Positive mental health emphasizes those successes. That does not mean lowering standards or de-emphasizing learning skills. Progress must be measured to determine where students need help, but a student's progress should be assessed by a standard, not against other students. Working at their own pace, children are less aware of their relative competencies, less discouraged, and more apt to be part of a school without failure.

CONTROL THEORY

In the next four pages the author summarizes the key points in a more recent book by Doctor Glasser. In *Control Theory*, he points out that we all have the same basic needs; however, we may only become aware of them when they are not satisfied. One immediate need is to breathe. We may not be aware of it until we get short of breath, but then everything else becomes unimportant. Then as soon as one need is satisfied, other needs begins to push for satisfaction. First, there are basic biological needs for survival; then the psychological need to belong, to have power, and to be free. Dr. Glasser adds the need to have fun.

The purpose of Control Theory is to help people take effective control of their lives. We feel good when the important things in our lives are under our control. We feel bad when we iose control. Many of our emotional problems arise, because others are competing with us for control of our lives. The key to our success as an individual is to learn to take effective control of ourselves. The key to helping others is to help them learn to take control of their lives.

PICTURE ALBUM

To help us visualize the Control Theory concept, Dr. Glasser relates our behavior to a set of pictures in our mind. Through our experiences, we acquire a set of pictures of how we might act to satisfy our needs. Early in life, we start to assemble what may be described as a picture album in our minds. Throughout our lives, we fill the album with pictures of what will satisfy our needs and wants. As we gain experience, we add and delete pictures from this album. An extraordinary camera in our mind takes pictures of everything we perceive through our senses.

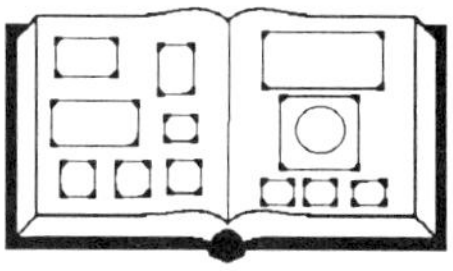

At times, our needs and wants are rather vague, but when we want something we sort through our album and try to match our wants with our pictures of how to get it. If we come up with several similar pictures, we will try to find the best picture of how to get what we want. If we do not have a picture of what will satisfy our wants, we try to make new contacts with the world through our senses so that the camera in our minds can take additional pictures to add to the album.

It is the pictures we have in our mind that cause us to do what we do. It is hard for us to change our pictures, but is even more difficult to get someone else to change their pictures. It may take a lot of time. The only way to get an old picture out of our minds is to replace it with a new picture.

Because of the need to belong, most of the pictures we store in our album come from our perception of the people we care for and respect. They become our teachers. They are the ones from whom we learn how to control our lives.

CONTROL

In Control Theory, the motivation comes from within. We see many examples of competition for control all around us. Parents attempt to control children, husbands try to control wives, wives try to control husbands, doctors try to control patients, teachers try to control students, and principals try to control teachers. Much of the time it looks like one person is allowing himself or herself to be controlled by another and this seems to fit in with the Stimulus-Response Theory. But we do not realize that when people seem to be controlled, they acquiesce only so long as following satisfies their needs. When following no longer satisfies their needs, they stop following and begin struggling to try to gain or regain control over their own life. Much of the time this struggle is manifest in a variety of emotional problems, self-destructive behaviors, and psychosomatic illnesses. Many of our social and emotional problems result because people are struggling not only to gain control of their lives, but also to gain control over other people.

Often the pictures in our album are competitive. We can choose from among the pictures associated with satisfying a particular need. There are four competitive components of our total behavior. What we are *feeling*, what we are *thinking*, and what we are *doing* are all accompanied by complex *physiological* voluntary and involuntary mechanisms. When we encounter a displeasing situation, we tend to be aware of just one component, usually our feelings. When we are able to recognize each component as a part of our total behavior, we will be in better control of our lives.

When we are in control of our lives, we will recognize our feelings, not as something that happens to us, but as something we choose to do. If I am feeling depressed after failing an exam, it would be more accurate to use the verb "depressing" to describe what I am doing. The difference between the noun and verb forms of the word is important. According to Control Theory, being depressed is not something that happened to me, it is what I choose to do.

Out of the several things I might choose to do when I receive bad news, choosing to feel miserable may for a time make the most sense. But when or if I want to change my total behavior, I cannot do it by changing how I feel directly, I must do it by changing what I do or think. We have almost complete control over what we do, some control over what we think, but almost no control over how we feel. If we markedly change what we do, we cannot avoid changing what we think and what we feel. The physiological components will change as well.

It is not accurate to say, "Because of what you did, you made me feel angry." It is more accurate to say, "In response to what you did, I choose to feel angry." The reason a person may choose to feel angry may be to exercise inappropriate control over another person. Sometimes it works, particularly for children, but as people get older they will more likely make another choice.

Depression is chosen as a way to get others to help. People might simply ask for help, but they don't because they are afraid of being turned down, or they do not want to admit to a weakness. Depression allows a person to plead for help, but at the same time maintain some self-esteem by denying that they need it. Some people become almost professional at being depressed. They are always able to steer a discussion around to their miseries, and no matter what others do for them, it is not enough. They will suffer much in order to maintain control. Dr. Glasser emphasizes, however, that not all aches and pains are chosen by the person who suffers from them. If there is a medical reason for the suffering, medical care should be provided. A person might be suspected of choosing painful behaviors to gain or maintain control only when there is no definite cause and when medical treatment remains ineffective.

Sometimes people turn to criticism to exercise control, though it may be disguised as "constructive criticism." What may be regarded as constructive criticism by the giver is almost always perceived as a "put-down" by the recipient. The one being criticized loses power and tends to resent it. Children, students, and newly hired workers may accept criticism in the proper spirit, but soon may resent it if too much unsolicited criticism is offered. Dr. Glasser says, "nothing that we encounter leads to greater and quicker loss of control than to be criticized." People are more apt to accept criticism if it comes from an outside source where there is no reason for a power struggle. In elementary school, there may not be a power struggle between a teacher and students, but teenagers are prone to construe even mild correction as criticism. It is best not to use even constructive criticism until the student has had a chance to find the problem himself. One should try to center on the idea that you are trying to build the student up, not tear him or her down.

WHAT A TEACHER CAN DO

A teacher should never do anything to a student or for a student that would cause the student to lose control. A teacher may be able to help a student gain effective control of his or her life. During a conference with a student, the teacher may briefly explain the "picture album" concept to help the student to focus more precisely on his behavior and alternatives. When there is a need for the student to modify his behavior, the teacher may do the following:

- **Conference**. If a student needs discipline, try to wait until you both have calmed down, then have a conference.

- **Recognize**. In the conference, try to find out if the student is satisfied with his or her behavior, or if he or she recognizes the need for a change.

- **Negotiate**. If the student is not satisfied with his or her behavior, try to negotiate a better way. Try to find agreement between what you want for the student and what is reasonably satisfying to the student.

- **Sanctions**. If the student continues to be satisfied with his behavior and doesn't want to change, you may have to evoke sanctions. Be sure that any sanctions will cause little or no loss of control. The loss of freedom or privileges should not last too long.

Students tend to be on either a failure cycle or success cycle, but the teacher is in a position to help break a failure cycle by helping students get on a success cycle. A successful experience may start a sequence of events that will lead to more success.

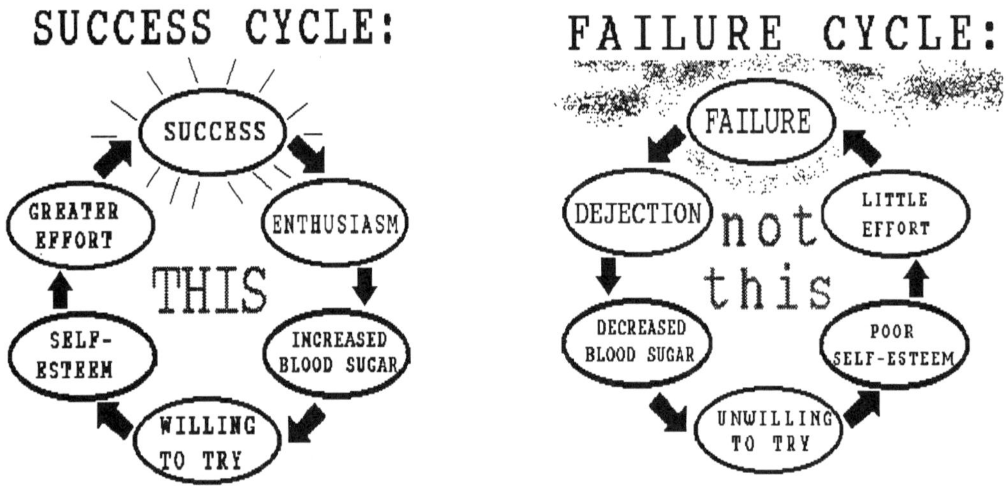

BEHAVIOR CHANGE PLANNING

If a person wants to become what he or she is capable of becoming, it is best to have a plan. People are much more likely to change their behavior if they follow a plan. Teachers may be able to help their students plan and follow through on a self-directed behavior change project that involves the following skills:

- **Positive self-analysis.** The first skill of behavior change planning is self-analysis, and the most important part of self-analysis is recognizing your own strengths. This helps you take courage from your strength before you target a weakness that needs changing. This includes recognizing the changes you have previously made and realizing that with an organized effort you can make greater changes. Appreciate your potential.

- **Goal setting.** The second skill in behavior change planning is identifying a health-related barrier that, unless changed, will limit your realization of your potential. List several behaviors you may consider changing. Consider the advantages of changing and the advantages of NOT changing. The first time you try this approach to behavior change it is best to select a goal that:

  1. you are likely to be successful at keeping.
  2. you have strong commitment to keep.

3. you think will make a difference in your life.
4. you have support from others to help you keep it.
5. you can measure, it is observable and specific.

- **Monitoring.** The third skill, monitoring, is the key to self-directed behavior change planning. The goal must be measurable. Planning includes working out a system for observing and recording. You should record:

    1. **Baseline data.** Monitor your behavior for a week to obtain you baseline data before you start to implement the change. The baseline data helps you understand the magnitude of the problem and allows you to measure your success with the project.
    2. **Progress chart.** Keep a simple daily record of your success or failure. Be accurate and strict in your counting.

- **Strategies.** The fourth skill is to plan one or more support techniques or strategies that will help you reach your goal. The more strategies that can be employed, the greater the chance of success. Some strategies are:

    1. **Shaping.** Divide your new behavior into small, but steady and compatible parts or steps.
    2. **Modeling.** Identify some individuals whose behavior you can imitate to serve as your model.
    3. **Rehearsals.** Practice the behavior in an actual situation or use imaged rehearsals.
    4. **Alternatives.** Recognize behaviors and situations incompatible with your goal and plan alternatives.
    5. **Witnesses.** Identify someone who can help monitor and motivate your behavior change.
    6. **Rewards.** Recognize some intrinsic rewards or provide some extrinsic rewards for desired behavior.

- **Do it!** Put your plan to work. If you come up short, revise your plan if necessary and try again. After succeeding on one behavior change planning project, identify another goal and start on it.

POSITIVE MENTAL HEALTH IN THE CLASSROOM

Positive mental health is not merely being able to satisfy one's needs and defend against the stresses of life; it is also expanding one's identity. It is not merely being able to get along without undue tension and anxiety, but it is also being productive, creative, and more closely reaching one's potential. It means developing one's value system, improving one's personality, and increasing one's performance to better enable a person to love others and be loved in return, to feel a sense of worth to himself and to others, and to experience excitement from a variety of activities in life.

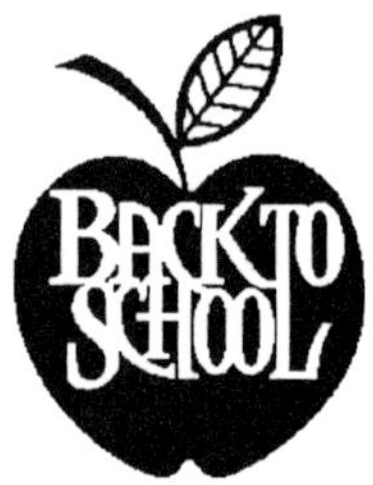

If one of the goals of education is to improve the mental health of students, schools should maintain an atmosphere in the classroom that is conducive to mental health. The proper social-emotional climate in the classroom is necessary to contribute to this positive mental health. Some classrooms have a negative tone which produces psychological tension and prohibits this type of positive emotional growth, even though the required academic objectives are achieved. Teachers who create an atmosphere of trust, friendliness, and fairness will be able to foster the interest and enthusiasm necessary for positive emotional and intellectual growth.

Effective teachers exhibit characteristics which contribute to positive mental health. Likewise, a positive atmosphere in the classroom can benefit the students' mental health.

The teacher should be:

- Friendly, warm, and supportive.
- Well organized and communicative.
- Able to catch the students' interest.

The classroom should be:

- Furnished to be provide a pleasant atmosphere.
- A place where friendliness is encouraged.
- A place where individual differences are honored.

The school should be:

- A place that tries to catch the students doing good.

The teacher is friendly and tries to encourage friendliness among the students. The teacher takes time to chat with students about their special interests. The teacher recognizes students' achievements and helps them to feel personally significant. The teacher is sensitive to students' feelings and lets them know they are still accepted as an individual even when their behavior is out of bounds and their schoolwork is below par. Teachers who are most effective in helping their students reach their potential take the positive approach. They do a lot of complimenting and very little criticizing.

TEACHING VALUES AND MENTAL HEALTH

If one of the goals of education is to improve the mental health of students, schools should incorporate activities that will best achieve that goal. Somewhere in the school curricula there should be an opportunity for students to be exposed to teaching strategies that concentrate on positive approaches to mental health such as value clarification, overcoming self-destructive behaviors, improving study habits, and developing life skills. This goal can and should also be an incidental part of every class. This is more likely to be achieved in an interactive classroom than in a traditional academic environment. The teaching strategies might appear more like games than lectures and discussions. Activities will focus on preventing illness and maintaining health. It should prevent feelings of alienation and tendencies toward self-deception. It will explore perceptions, values, and feelings. Such an approach will result in a much closer-knit group, better rapport between students and teachers, and a more effective group of learners.

SELF-ESTEEM

Self-esteem is at the center of positive mental health. Teachers can and do affect the students' self-esteem. The self-concept is composed of all the internal beliefs and attitudes an individual holds about the self. These attitudes and beliefs determine who we are, what we think we are, and what we become. Students respond favorably to learning when a teacher understands their feelings. Students must feel reasonably comfortable in their learning environment before they can focus their attention on learning. Teachers play a significant role in helping students perceive themselves more positively.

- **Belonging**. One of the conditions of self-esteem is a sense of *connectivity*. This means belonging to and being needed by groups such as family, church groups, clubs, teams, professions, and other affiliations. Students need to develop skills related to forming and maintaining a *network* of satisfactory group relationships. Teachers can provide opportunities for students to contribute to the class.

- **Confidence**. Another condition of self-esteem is a sense of power over self. This comes when they are successful at setting and reaching specific goals. Teachers can help students experience the sense of pride at completing a meaningful task. The more frequently this occurs, the more self-confidence people develop. There is a positive correlation between confidence and self-esteem.

- **Distinctive**. Another characteristic of self-esteem is the sense of being unique, special, distinctive. Everyone should be very good, perhaps the best, at something. Although differences are sometimes difficult to accommodate in a classroom, teachers should help students satisfy these needs constructively. Teachers can help students succeed in their own unique area, even if they have to find an area of limited competition.

- <u>Modeling</u>. A positive role model can aid the development of self-esteem. Teachers can encourage students to consider key people as role models in their lives, but to distinguish between the positive and negative characteristics of the models. Teachers may become mentors and enhance their students self-esteem by providing unconditional acceptance.

- <u>Decisions</u>. A person's self-esteem may be negatively affected by poor decision-making skills. Teachers can help students recognize, analyze, and evaluate alternatives in terms of their benefits and consequences.

- <u>Communication</u>. Communication skills are important goals of education. Self-esteem is influenced by one's ability to communicate with others. This includes listening skills. It includes both verbal and nonverbal communication. Communication skills include the ability to express one's true feelings (self-disclosure), to affirmatively respond to other's comments (confirmation), to speak to others on the appropriate level (transaction management), and to be versatile (adaptable).

Some educators avoid the introduction of values and emotions into the classroom and, in doing so, eliminate the most powerful assets to learning, and also the most important objectives of learning. What would life be without emotions and values? It is through our positive emotions that we get our rewards for living. It is through our values that we recognize worth.

It is because of values and emotions that we seek for improvement. Man is a multi-dimensional being who learns intellectually (cognitively), emotionally (affectively), and physically (empirically). These three types of learning can take place together or independently. When two or three types of learning take place together, resultant knowledge is more readily transferred to practical life situations. When a person learns physical skills in an atmosphere that is emotionally enjoyable, he is more apt to continue those skills after he leaves the class. The same is generally true when learning facts. The emotional atmosphere is often remembered longer than the facts. The student can intellectually understand a principle but fail to put it into practice in his daily life, because his emotions are more influential than his logic.

As the teacher responds to the needs and goals of students in a multidimensional setting and atmosphere, students will be more capable of utilizing these learned experiences in real life situations. As the learning processes that take place in the classroom situation more closely resemble those that take place in the real world, students will begin to identify classroom learning as meaningful experiences which will be beneficial in attaining their goals and purposes.

Much of what schools teach is about a non-loving world. History and many of the ways of man as depicted in the newspaper emphasize wars and crimes of violence. Often the teacher's relationships with his students are based on class rules and school regulations creating an atmosphere for learning. But enlightened educators who possess a sincere love for their students can teach love and other positive emotions and traditional values in the following ways:

- Start first with your own example, which is the highest form of influence. What a teacher is becomes his most powerful lesson.

- Use teaching methods and techniques that will result in student success. Praise a student for his or her success, and he or she will develop a healthy self-concept. Self-love is necessary before students can have a concern for family, regard for fellowmen, devotion to country, or reverence for God.

- School subjects such as music, art, and literature provide opportunities to help students understand the role of various types and levels of love. Students can be helped to distinguish between selfish infatuation and the serving and caring forms of love.

The school has a tremendous influence upon the mental health of the students, and that effect may be either beneficial or detrimental or both. The schools should do the following:

- Work to alleviate unnecessary pressures on the students.

- Provide a stimulating and meaningful curriculum.

- See that every student has a successful experience.

- Provide an atmosphere that is conducive to intellectual, emotional, social, moral, and physical growth.

This requires teachers who are prepared in their academic field and who have a high level of mental health so that they can interact well with students and other teachers. It also requires that the schools make deliberate efforts in the areas of personality improvement and value clarification. Much can be done to develop healthy self-concepts, emotional maturity, and value awareness as an incidental byproduct of the traditional curriculum and extracurricular activities.

Adolescence is a time of trying to find out how to think, what to believe, and what to do. Adolescents face decisions every day and have to make choices about how to live. Their choices will be based on their values; but in this confusing world, they frequently are not clear about their values. They are surrounded by a bewildering array of alternatives. Youth are confused by the many sets of standards and inconsistencies. Parents say to do one thing, but frequently do another. The church, the school, the peer group, and the public media all offer different values. Young people bombarded with all of these influences are ultimately left to make their own choices about whose advice to follow. Their choices should not be made on the basis of peer pressure, unthinking submission to authority, or the power of propaganda. Frequently, a dichotomy exists between theory and practice. Lip service may be paid to certain standards, but behavior contradicts those values.

Young people need to learn the process of valuing. They need to learn how to develop their own sense of identity. They need to learn how to determine their own moral and ethical standards. They need to learn how to relate to people whose values differ from their own. Most young people do not want or need adults to do this for them, but they do want and need help.

Frequently adults, motivated by a sincere desire to have the younger generation lead happy and productive lives, have attempted to guide them by moralizing. The assumption behind moralizing is that adults can pass on to the youth the values the adults have learned and thus save the youth the problems of having to learn them on their own. The direct transfer of values works best when there is complete agreement upon the source or basis of values. The problem here is that people often say one thing and do another. On the other hand, some adults maintain a laissez-faire attitude toward the transmission of values. The assumption is that no value system is right for everyone, and each has to make his own values. They let their students do and think what they want without intervening. The problem with that is that young people, left completely on their own, experience conflict and confusion. Other adults take the approach of transferring values by example. They try to be an attractive model, so the young people will be impressed and adopt their values. It is important for young people to have teachers who set a good example, but the young people are exposed to so many models it is difficult to sort out which values to emulate. Neither does it work for secondary students to simply be told what to believe and do; nor to be left entirely alone to resolve the confusion and conflict. They need the organized help that can be provided by the schools. The teachers have the responsibility of providing this help in a professional manner.

The teacher will have to determine how much time to spend on value clarification and plan activities accordingly. The teacher has the responsibility to create and maintain a classroom climate that is conducive to value clarification. He should develop an atmosphere of freedom so that the students will feel free to express themselves openly and honestly, but still have the right to pass if he does not want to respond. He should develop a sense of trust within the class, so they will know what they say will not be rejected or ridiculed, but will be listened to and respected. People need to learn to listen to each other. Verbal and nonverbal expressions should indicate interest and serious consideration for the ideas expressed. The teacher should develop a sense of responsibility among the students, so they will not divulge confidential information either in or out of the class. The teacher will have to establish a structure of role relationships and bounds so that the process will take a positive approach and not degenerate into destructive sensitivity sessions or encroach into areas that are inappropriate. The teacher has to be careful to select the appropriate value education activities for the maturity level of his students. A variety of material relating to value education is available to teachers and youth leaders. A teacher who is serious about teaching values should turn to one of these sources for specific value clarification activities.

Some schools have a separate course emphasizing value clarification, while others integrate it into specific courses. A teacher who decides to use value clarification can either set aside a specific block of time or tie it into the regular subject matter so that students learn both at the same time. The valuing process will motivate students to more interest in a class.

Value education has four goals:

- to help students develop a concept of what values are.
- to help students become aware of their own goals.
- to help students develop the ability to discover their values on their own.
- to help students respect other people's values.

Valuing involves the following processes:

- choosing--one must be free to choose, select from alternatives, and be ready to accept the consequences of his own choice.
- prizing--one must cherish his choice and be ready to affirm his choice in public.
- acting--one must be willing to do something on a repeated basis to attain his value.

IMPROVING STUDY HABITS

Most of the material discussed here has dealt with improving emotional health, but some attention should be applied to improving intellectual health through more effective study techniques. Of course, emotional stability is important to effective study, and conversely, ability to reason and solve problems helps a person avoid situations that otherwise may cause emotional problems. Certainly, students who follow effective study programs will avoid many of the emotional problems that accompany poor preparation and poor grades. Teachers should have some good suggestions in mind to give to their students who need help in organizing an effective study program. Perhaps a teacher could suggest the following points to his or her students:

1. Try to recognize that learning takes place only through the effort of the learner. The school can invite you to learn, and your teachers can try to make the invitation attractive, but the student must be actively involved in the learning process--and that means study.

2. Try to find an acceptable time and place to study. The time should be regularly scheduled every day and at a time when the student is alert. The place should be free from noise and other distractions.

3. Try to get the big picture of the entire course, including the course objectives, techniques, assignments, and deadlines.

4. Try to get involved in what you are studying. Find a reason to want to learn it besides just getting a grade for the course. Ask yourself questions, and try to find the answers while you are studying. Ask the teacher questions and make comments in class. Discuss what you are studying with other people.

5. Try to focus on three class periods at a time--the previous class period, the next class period, and the class period after that. Between class periods, you should have a post-class review, a pre-class study, and a preview for the class after next. In the review and preview, relate the material to the whole course. In the review, restate in your own words the ideas learned. In the preview, scan the material you expect to cover in the class after next. In the pre-class study, first scan the whole reading assignment. Then read it in detail, think about it, and summarize the important points in a notebook, in the margin, or in the text by underlining.

Students should be exposed to the intellectual problem-solving technique. Not only is it a good method of learning the subject matter, but it also has application in helping students learn how to solve problems. The scientific or experimental technique of surveying the situation, defining the problem, developing a theory, gathering the data, drawing conclusions, and retesting has application in making decisions throughout life. It will help a person make decisions based on proven cause-and-effect relationships rather than on chance or coincidence. The ability to solve problems logically and objectively is a component of mental health.

CONCLUSION

Most people face about the same problems in life, the difference is how they deal with the problems. One person can be overwhelmed by a problem that another person takes in stride. The difference is not the problem, but how they view themselves in relationship to the problem. William James, the most widely read American philosopher of the 1900s, said:

"The greatest discovery of this generation is that man can change his whole life just by altering his attitude of mind."

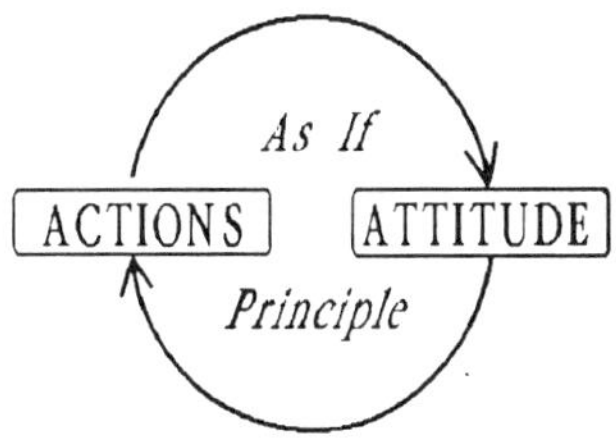

James was a pragmatist, and he believed that attitude could make a difference. He introduced the *"As If" Principle.* If you would like to have a certain characteristic, act as if you already had that characteristic, and you will develop that desired characteristic. It will become a natural part of your personality. For example, if you want to be happy, first ask yourself, "What do happy people do?" Then do it. At first it may seem unnatural, but if you keep at it, soon it will become automatic and you will be happy. The accompanying illustration shows the relationship between action and attitudes. Attitudes influence behavior and behaviors influence attitudes. By changing one, you can change the other. Except in cases where there may be a biological basis, people can replace negative emotions with positive emotions by applying the *"As If" Principle.* It would be well for teachers to help their students discover this principle.

Happiness is linked to mental health. Dr. Murray Banks, a popular psychiatrist and entertainer, taught a valuable lesson. If you want to find out about a person's mental health, ask them this simple question, "Are you happy?" He said "Happiness is not a station you arrive at, it is a byproduct of effective living."

"I have discovered that people are just about as happy as they make their mind up to be." *Abraham Lincoln*

It is the little things in life that make a difference. We should try to live a little more effectively day by day. We should also be prepared to accept the setbacks. The prayer of Alcoholics Anonymous has application for all.

Lord, grant me the strength to change the things that I can change, the serenity to accept the things I cannot change, and the wisdom to know the difference.

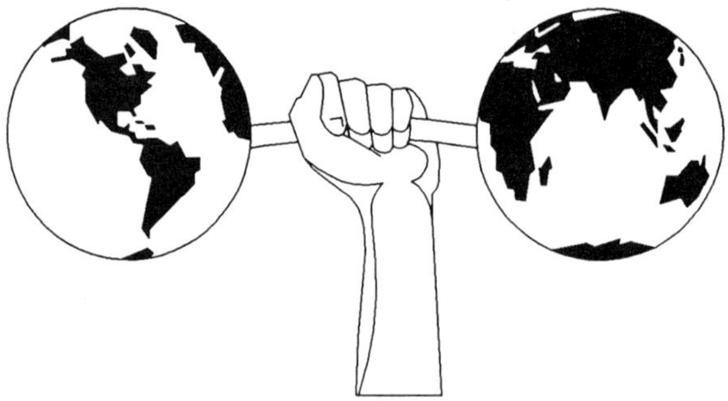

TEN LITTLE BIG THINGS THAT TEACHERS CAN DO TO ENHANCE THE DEVELOPMENT OF POSITIVE SELF-CONCEPTS IN STUDENTS*

*By George L. McMahon, with some revisions

1. **Speak to each student by name in your class each day**. Collectively, or better yet, individually, people like to be acknowledged.

2. **Make positive statements as often as possible**. No human being can survive a steady barrage of no's and don'ts.

3. **Dispute only inaccurate facts, accept opinions as opinions even though they may differ from yours**. Opinions need to be accepted with the understanding that they may be based upon different values.

4. **Reach out and physically touch students when needed and where appropriate**. A handshake or hand on a shoulder communicates much better than words, "I like you," "I care about you." A refusal to touch communicates the opposite.

5. **Smile often**. It is contagious.

6. **Address students as responsible human beings**. In order to be responsible, people must have responsibility.

7. **Be honest with students--their trust in you is tied to your trust in them**. They will learn that you trust them.

8. **Express anger toward misbehavior rather than toward the student or a group of students**. Better for a student to think, "I did something bad," than, "I am bad."

9. **Try to stay in the present time--learn to forgive and forget**. Recalling past behavior merely causes hurt in the present. Dealing with present behavior can be a learning experience.

10. **Work to develop your own positive self-concept**. Happy, well-adjusted, self-aware human beings who genuinely care for other people make good teachers.

STUDY HELPS

1. What can teachers do to help minimize the pressures homework might put on students?

2. What can teachers do to help minimize the pressures that the grading system might put on students?

3. In what ways can schools and teachers help parents become aware of the pressures which they create for their children?

4. In what ways can teachers help students reduce the pressures they impose on themselves and on each other?

5. Explain the significance of the following "don'ts" in regard to being a good listener.
   a. Don't talk, listen.
   b. Don't belittle the problem.
   c. Don't be impatient.
   d. Don't provide the answer.

6. Which of the following are considered effective ways of dealing with another person with hysteria? What are some better ways?
   a. Most teachers should be able to treat the problem.
   b. If you shout, it tends to calm the hysterical person.
   c. Show physical force, slap them or throw water on their face.
   d. Scold, argue, or criticize the person and point out it's his or her own fault, so just snap out of it.

7. What are some good points to remember in dealing with a personal crisis?

8. What are the characteristics of a teacher who consistently contributes to the positive mental health of his or her students?

9. What is the relationship between the expression of emotions and the teaching of values in the classroom?

10. Is there a place for teaching love and other positive emotions and values in the classroom? How is it done? Can it go too far?

11. What can a teacher do to help his or her students to improve their study habits?

12. What can a teacher do to help his or her students to improve their personality and eliminate self-defeating behaviors?

13. What is the meaning of the following terms as they relate to *Reality Therapy, Control Theory*, and *Schools Withnout Failure* ?

responsibility	right and wrong	reality	involvement
labels	memorizing	irrelevance	grading
emotion	picture album	control	needs
conference	recognize	negotiate	sanctions

14. How does Reality Therapy differ from conventional therapy on the following points?
    a. The questions "why?" and "what?"
    b. The role of unconscious motivation
    c. The concept of mental illness

15. What is the significance of the following steps in the practice of Reality Therapy?
    a. Identify the behavior
    b. Identify the consequences
    c. Make value judgments
    d. Make plans for changing

16. What is the significance of the following questions in Reality Therapy?
    a. What is wrong with those who need psychiatric treatment?
    b. What are the basic needs?
    c. How do we fulfill our needs?
    d. How do we learn to fulfill our needs?

17. What is the significance of the following parts of behavior change planning?
    a. Positive self-analysis
    b. Goal setting
    c. Monitoring
    d. Baseline data
    e. Progress chart
    f. Strategies
    g. Modeling
    h. Rehearsals
    i. Alternatives
    j. Witnesses
    k. Rewards
    l. Do It!

18. What is the difference between a teacher showing *sympathy* and *empathy*?

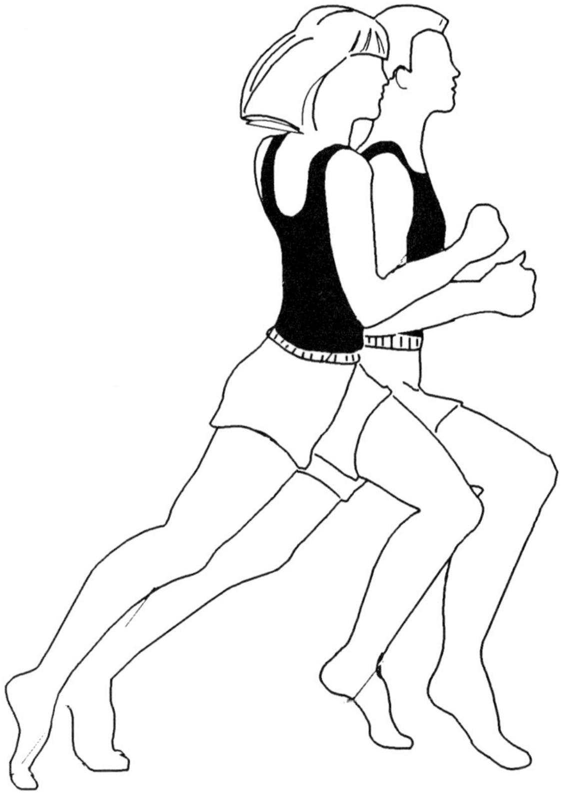

UNIT 3

PROBLEMS OF GROWTH AND DEVELOPMENT

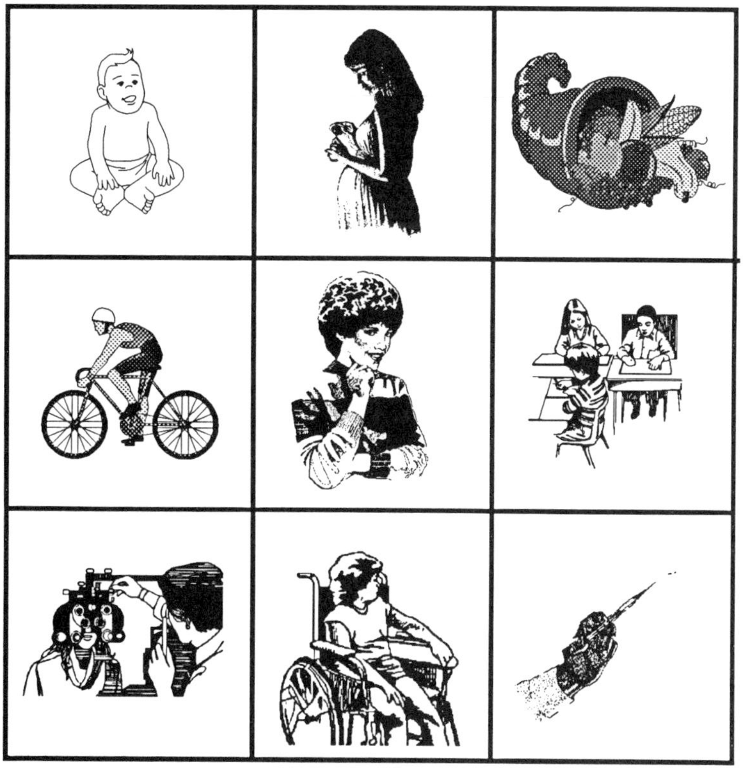

An effective teacher is a positive role model for students.

GROWTH AND DEVELOPMENT

Adolescence is a time of rapid physical growth and development, and young people are sometimes preoccupied with this phenomenon. This concern also has a strong influence on other dimensions of their lives. To better understand the students and to be able to give them appropriate council if the opportunities arise, teachers must understand not only the normal patterns of growth and development, but also the departures from normal.

Departures include various learning disorders, chronic health problems, and acute diseases. Competent teachers will observe their students for possible departures from normal and make appropriate referrals. A teacher is also responsible for following school policies for excluding students from class if they exhibit possible signs and symptoms of a communicable diseases.

An important ramification of adolescent growth and development is the effect of sexual maturation. This is tied to the student's emotional, moral, and social health. Prospective teachers should become familiar with the various community views regarding sexuality and sex education.

In all respects, a teacher should be prepared to exert a positive influence on the values of their students. A teacher should be a good example to the students. A teacher should practice the principles of physical fitness not only to be a role model, but also as a means of maintaining the health vigor necessary to be an effective teacher.

OBJECTIVES

At the conclusion of this unit, you should be able to meet the following objectives.

1. GROWTH AND DEVELOPMENT

UNDERSTAND THE STRUCTURE AND FUNCTION OF THE BODY SYSTEMS AS THEY RELATE TO GROWTH, DEVELOPMENT, AND MATURATION.

- Explain the various maturation patterns of teenagers.
- Identify the internal and external factors influencing growth and development.
- Describe the basic process for providing structure, maintenance, and regulation for the various body systems.
- List growth and posture problems that may be identified by a teacher.

2. MAINTAINING PHYSICAL FITNESS

KNOW AND PRACTICE THE PRINCIPLES RELATING TO THE MAINTENANCE OF GOOD HEALTH AND PHYSICAL FITNESS.

- Explain why good health is important to effective learning.
- Explain how physical fitness contributes to effective teaching.
- Identify the principles of good nutrition.
- Identify the principles of maintaining physical fitness.
- List the prevalent myths related to nutrition and fitness.

3. MATURATION AND ADOLESCENT SEXUALITY

DESCRIBE THE SEX-RELATED VALUE CONFLICTS EXPERIENCED BY ADOLESCENTS AND EXPLAIN A TEACHER CAN BE A POSITIVE INFLUENCE.

- List value conflicts related to sexual adjustment.
- Evaluate various approaches to sex education.

- Describe problems associated with teenage pregnancy.
- Explain the problems associated with deviant sexual behavior and promiscuous sexual relationships.

4. TEACHER OBSERVATION

OUTLINE THE TEACHER'S RESPONSIBILITIES FOR STUDENT OBSERVATION AS PART OF THE SCHOOL HEALTH SERVICES PROGRAM.

- Explain how teacher observations relate to other components of school health appraisal.
- Explain how to conduct teacher observations and screening procedures.
- Describe the nature of common learning disabilities and indicate how a teacher can help a student with such problems.

5. DEALING WITH CHRONIC HEALTH PROBLEMS

UNDERSTAND THE NATURE OF COMMON CHRONIC HEALTH PROBLEMS THAT MAY AFFECT STUDENTS AND BE ABLE TO MAKE APPROPRIATE ACCOMMODATIONS.

- Identify the major chronic health problems among adolescents.
- Suggest ways a teacher should deal with chronic health problems among his students.

6. CONTROLLING COMMUNICABLE DISEASE

OUTLINE THE TEACHER'S RESPONSIBILITIES IN THE PREVENTION AND CONTROL OF COMMUNICABLE DISEASES THAT MAY AFFECT STUDENTS IN HIS CLASSES.

- Explain the control measures to break the chain of infection.
- Describe the normal course of a communicable disease.
- Identify the communicable diseases found among school children, youth, and school personnel.
- Suggest steps a school should use to stop the spread of infection.

Chapter 10

GROWTH AND DEVELOPMENT

Adolescence is a time of rapid growth, change, and adjustment, and many of these changes are related to physical growth and development. While maturation is a very interesting process, it brings its share of problems to teenagers and to the adults who are closely involved with them. This lesson is intended to provide prospective teachers with a basic understanding of patterns of growth and development.

PATTERNS OF GROWTH AND DEVELOPMENT

Although physical growth and development usually occur almost simultaneously, they should be regarded as independent phenomena. Growth has to do with size, development has to do with function. Growth is the addition of additional or larger cells to the various parts of the body. Development is the maturation of the complexity and effectiveness of the body's functions. One child may have experienced a more rapid growth rate in size than another child of the same age, but has not developed in physiological functions as rapidly as the other child.

During infancy, growth can be measured easily by weight and length, but assessing development requires careful observation. Pediatrics and experts in child development are trained to observe subtle neurological reflexes that indicate the physiological maturation of infants. Eye movements, response to stimuli, muscular-skeletal movements, and the functions of internal organs are indicative of development. The functioning of the nervous system and its coordination with other parts of the body determine the stage of development.

Certain characteristics of growth and development take place during each of the stages of life: infancy, childhood, adolescence, adulthood, and aging. The study of each of these phases of life is interesting, but at this point our interest is in adolescence. Adolescence, the period of transition from childhood to adulthood, is generally considered to last roughly from *puberty* to age 18 or 20. Puberty is the period of life when hormonal changes take place, preparing the body for sexual reproduction. The terms puberty, adolescence, and teenager are generally interchangeable.

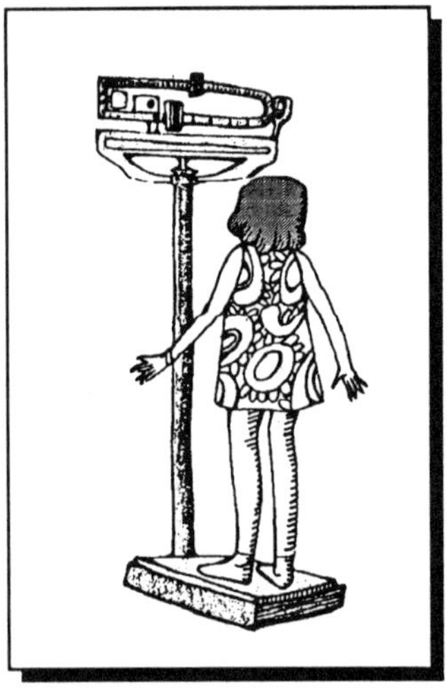

During adolescence, growth and development takes place at various rates. While puberty brings some difficulties to most youth, it brings greater problems to a few, particularly those whose growth and development patterns vary considerably from the norm. Since a typical school population will have students in all stages, a teacher needs to be aware of both the physical and psychological effects of growth and development. Teachers need to understand the impact that extreme patterns in growth and development can have on students. Teachers should not only perceive the problems, but also aid their students in understanding and accepting themselves.

Adolescents who mature much earlier than others are *precocious* developers. Those who mature much later are *latent* developers. But nearly all teenagers experience rapid growth spurts at times and growth plateaus at other time. At times, growth is emphasized in certain body parts, and it seems the body becomes "gangly" and disproportionate. During this period of rapid growth, the body becomes less coordinated and clumsiness is noted. The arms and legs grow faster than the head and trunk, resulting in the gangling, gawky appearance. The chin and nose seem to be more prominent than other facial features, adding to the picture of disproportion. Add to this the changes in internal functions such as the endocrine glands which affect emotions. It is no wonder that teenagers begin to question their own identity.

Although these changes may appear to be rapid to the adults, to the teenager these changes are agonizingly slow. The boy may fondle the fuzz on his lip wondering when it will be ready to shave. The girl may measure her bust weekly wondering if she will ever reach the size she considers ideal. Early development presents some special problems. An early-maturing girl may feel out of place and strange with her classmates. She may be embarrassed by her height and developing bust, and to hide it she may slouch. Her classmates may tease her or shun her. On the other hand, she may receive too much attention from older boys. Late development presents other problems. The late-maturing boy may feel inadequate, and he may be made the object of jokes and ridicule. The late-maturing girl may feel pangs due to lack of attractiveness and social success. Adults have a tendency to forget what it was like to be a teenager. Adults who work with teenagers should try to understand.

PRENATAL DEVELOPMENT

A variety of factors may influence growth and development. These factors have been separated into two groups, internal and external. The internal factors include heredity and the functions of the endocrine system. The external factors include the influence of institutions such as the home, church, and school.

CONCEPTION

Conception is one of the marvels of nature. At that moment, a series of hereditary features coming from the parents are combined to produce a unique individual. Those hereditary characteristics will affect the life of an individual and perhaps the lives of others he or she will be closely associated with. Approximately halfway through a menstrual cycle, a mature female reproductive cell called an egg or ovum is released from one of the mother's two ovaries. Conception occurs if, as the egg travels along the fallopian tube toward the uterus, it is fertilized by a male reproductive cell called a sperm.

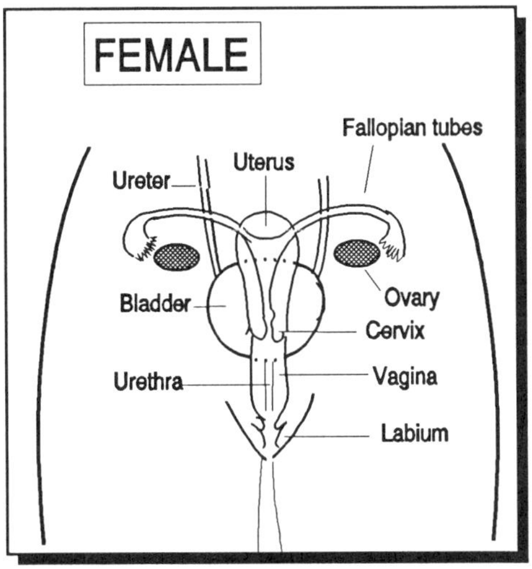

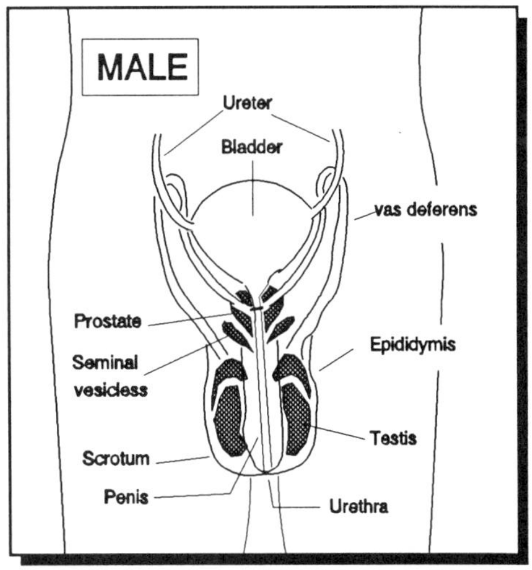

A female has two ovaries which contain thousands of immature eggs. After puberty, it is normal for a single egg to mature each month. About midway through the menstrual cycle (see the section of this lesson on the endocrine system), a mature egg is expelled from a follicle on the ovary in a process called ovulation. The egg is then drawn into the fallopian tube and begins to descend toward the uterus. An egg is large enough that if it could be isolated outside of the body, it could be seen without the aid of a microscope. In comparison, sperm are minute in size. Sperm are formed in the many coiled seminiferous tubules in the two male testes. The sperm pass from the testes into the epididymis where they are stored until ejaculation. Sperm are tadpole-shaped cells with a tail which provides mobility. During intercourse, millions of sperm and other fluids which make up the semen are deposited near the cervix of the uterus. The sperm migrate through the uterus and up the fallopian tube. If one sperm cell penetrates the membrane of an egg, fertilization occurs.

HEREDITY

Chromosomes are strands of material within a cell which contain the codes that regulate the functions of that cell. The codes in the chromosomes come in the form of DNA molecules called genes which are the body's internal directions. Normal human cells contains 23 pair of chromosomes (46 total). Half of each pair of chromosomes comes from the mother through the egg, and the other half comes from the father through the sperm. The combination of inherited recessive and dominant traits will determine most of the body's features and may influence some of the individual's personality characteristics. Heredity is important in the child's growth and development.

Unlike other body cells which contain 23 pairs of chromosomes, egg and sperm reproductive cells contain only 23 single chromosomes. When fertilization occurs, the 23 single chromosomes from the mother unite with the 23 single chromosomes from the father to form 23 pairs of chromosomes. With the normal number of chromosomes, the fertilized egg is able to undergo cell division. As the fertilized egg continues its descent through the fallopian tube, it divides to form two cells. Each of these divide into two which again divide, and so on until birth and on throughout the life of the individual.

Sexual reproduction is a process of sharing genetic characteristics, and it is interesting to see which features the child will inherit. There are thousands of characteristics carried by the genes on the chromosomes and how they will match up is difficult to predict because some genes are *DOMINANT* and others are *recessive*. A gene for a particular characteristic is located at a certain point on each chromosome in a certain pair of chromosomes. If both genes are *DOMINANT*, the person will not only exhibit that characteristic, but will also pass it on to all of his or her children. If one gene is *DOMINANT* and the other is *recessive*, the person will exhibit the dominant trait, but may pass on either trait to his or her children. Only when both genes are *recessive* will a person exhibit and pass on the recessive trait.

Some of the physical features that may give a teenager some concern may be due to heredity. The combination of inherited features can cause genetic disorders ranging from minor to serious. A person can also inherit a predisposition to some health problems which may or may not show up later in life depending on other factors. The combination of inherited physical features may not be compatible and may result in some abnormalities. For example, a girl may require some special dental work if she inherits her mother's dainty jaw and her father's big buck teeth. Fortunately, many of the patterns that appear to be abnormal during adolescence may disappear as the person matures.

SEX DETERMINATION

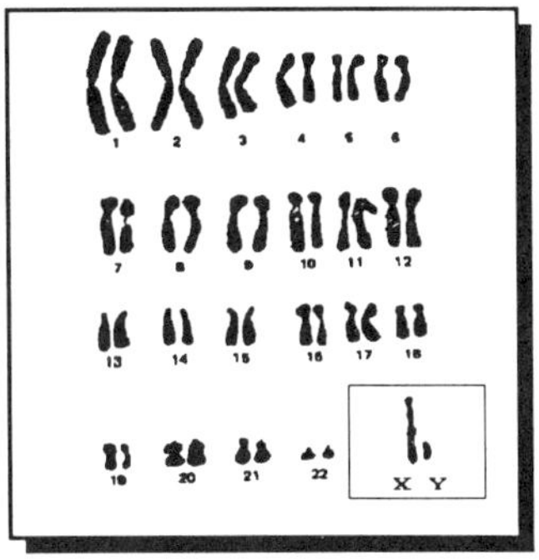

One pair of the chromosomes determines the sex of the individual. One of the 23 single chromosomes from the mother is an "X" chromosome. The corresponding chromosome from the father may either be an "X" or a "Y." If the sperm which fertilizes the egg carries an "X" chromosome, the pair of chromosomes is "XX" and the child will be female. But if the sperm carries a "Y" chromosome, the pair is an "XY" and the child will be male.

There is often a question about *sex-linked inheritance* such as color blindness and hemophilia (a bleeding disorder). These are conditions that women do not generally have themselves, but they inherit these condition from their father and pass them on to their sons. The explanation lies in the fact that the "Y" chromosome is not a full sized chromosome; it is short. Some of the genes on the upper end of a full sized "X" chromosome do not have a corresponding gene on the shorter "Y" chromosome. If a woman has a *recessive* gene for hemophilia on one "X" chromosome, it would normally be matched with a *DOMINANT* gene on the other "X" chromosome. She would not be hemophilic; however, she could carry the recessive gene and pass it on to her children. When a women has this condition, she has two recessive genes. When a male inherits a recessive gene for hemophilia, he will be hemophilic, because there is no gene on the missing part of the "Y" chromosome to dominate the recessive gene on his "X" chromosome.

THE BEGINNING OF LIFE

After conception, the fertilized egg divides many times so that when it reaches the uterus, approximately seven days later, there are over a hundred cells formed into a hollow ball that attaches to the nutritious endometrium lining of the uterus. There cell division continues, and cell specialization takes place. Some cells become part of the placenta attached to the wall of the uterus, and other cells become part of the embryo. Oxygen and nourishment from the mother's blood supply pass through the placenta along the umbilical cord to the developing infant. Further cell specialization takes place in the embryo as organs start to form. Harmful substances, such as drugs consumed by the mother, have a high potential for interfering with the embryological development and causing deformities in the developing infant. At five weeks, the embryo is about the size of a grain of rice.

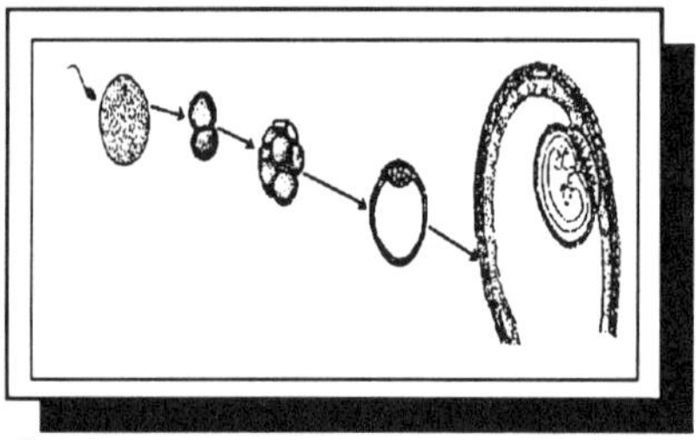

A

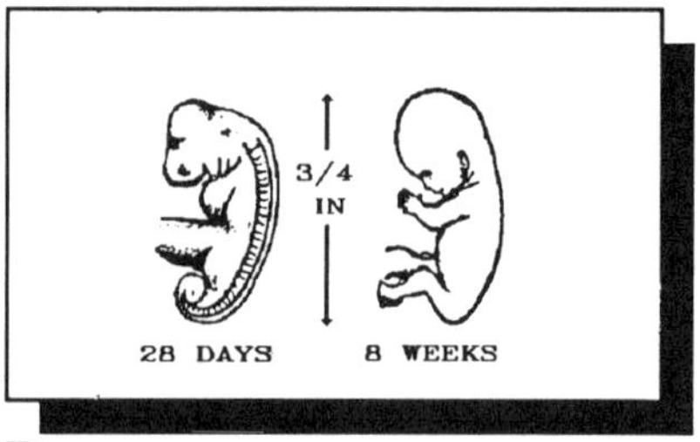

B

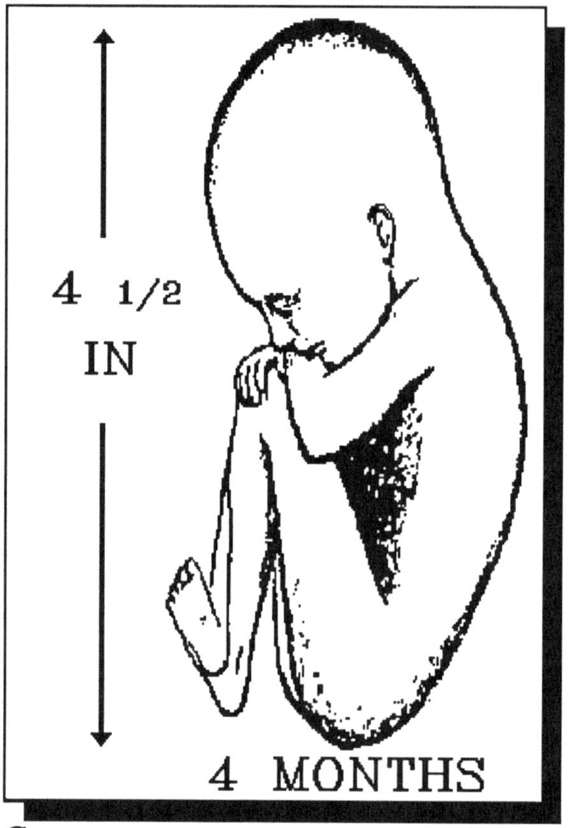

C

The question as to when life begins is controversial, and so is the question as to when life ends. If one of the traditional indications of death, cessation of heartbeat, is applied as an indication of life, it would be at approximately 28 days. A primitive heart starts to beat in the fourth week of pregnancy, blood cells form, and circulation begins. At eight weeks, the embryo becomes known as a fetus, and it has distinguishable human features though it is still only about an inch in length. At twelve weeks, its external genital organs could be recognized as either male or female. It is now about three inches in length and weighs about one ounce. At 20 weeks, it may be ten inches long and weigh about 11 ounces. The fetal heartbeat can be heard through the mother's abdomen. At 24 weeks, it may be a foot long and weigh one and one-half pounds. If born at this point with modern technology, it has a fair chance of survival. By 36 weeks, full term, it may be about twenty inches long and weigh about seven pounds.

When the child is born, it brings with it a variety of hereditary potentials good and bad. It also may bring some congenital abnormalities resulting from its life in the uterus. In spite of the risks, most infants are normal and have tremendous potential.

SEX DIFFERENCES

While it is important to recognize the similarities between males and females in regard to growth and development, there are some recognizable differences. At the time of conception, the ratio of female to male is significantly higher for males, but by the time of birth, the numbers are almost equal, 105 males per 100 females. By the time infants reach one year of age, the ratio has survived so that for every 100 surviving females there are 95 surviving males. For any given age group, there is a higher death rate for the males than the females.

There is a difference in developmental levels between boys and girls. At birth, girls on the average are considered to be about a month more mature in spite of the fact that boys on the average are larger in size. This difference in maturation level continues to expand. As students enter school, in kindergarten the girls are about a year more mature than boys. Most girls are toilet trained earlier, they learn to do physical skills earlier such as skipping, and they develop communication skills earlier. When there is competition for grades and teacher approval during the early years of school, girls may have an advantage and boys may develop an inferior self-concept.

Boys and girls differ greatly in the age at which they enter puberty, the period which marks the beginning of physical changes leading to manhood and womanhood. Girls enter puberty about two years earlier than boys and experience an earlier growth spurt. This is very noticeable in the seventh grade as girls on the average are about a half foot taller than the boys. Information reported in *Life and Growth* by Alice V. Keliher printed by Appleton Century Company in 1941 indicated the following:

About twenty percent of the eleven-year-old girls have entered puberty while all of the boys that age are still in childhood. By age thirteen, all but ten percent of the girls have entered puberty, and half of them have passed puberty and are physically capable of bearing a child. In comparison, sixty percent of the thirteen year old boys are still pre-pubescent, thirty percent are in puberty, and ten percent are physically capable of fathering a child. Two years later by age fifteen, only ten percent of the girls are in puberty and the rest are post-pubescent. At age fifteen, still ten percent of the boys are pre-pubescent, thirty percent are in puberty, and sixty percent are post pubescent. By age seventeen, only ten percent of the boys are still in puberty, and all of the rest are post-pubescent.

More recent statistics indicate that the beginning of pubescence may be moving slowly downward, and that there is an earlier onset of puberty in populations in the more tropical regions of the world.

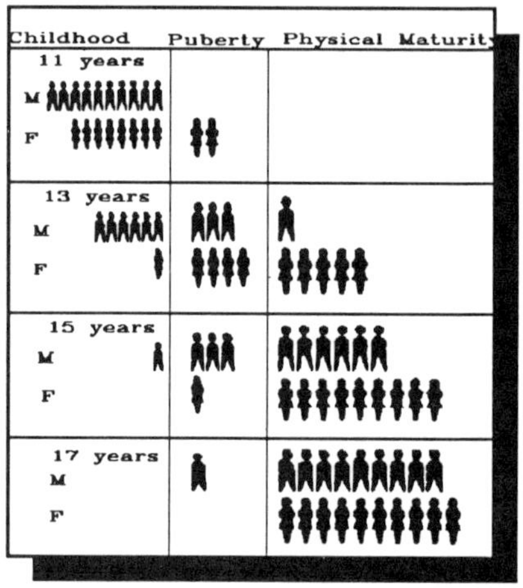

During the high school years, boys catch up and pass the girls in growth but remain behind the girls in development. Also during the high school years, boys tend to catch up intellectually. Women reach full physical maturity at about age 21, men at age 24. Women on an average die at a later age then men. Currently the average length of life for men in the U.S. is in the low seventies while the average length of life for women is in the high seventies, about a seven year difference.

People are well aware of differences in what is referred to as the secondary sex characteristics, but there are some other differences that might be of interest. Men usually have more red blood cells, women more white blood cells. The arm structure is noticeably different when they stand with their arms to the side with palms forward--men's arms tend to be straight from the shoulder to the writs while women's arms tend to bend outward. There is a difference in overweight patterns. In typical male type obesity, weight tends to accumulate around the waist, while in typical female type obesity, the weight tends to accumulate at the hips. Women generally have a higher percent body fat and a faster heart rate. Men have a higher basal metabolic rate. Muscular development is also different. Men are better prepared for large muscle activities such as lifting while women tend to be better prepared for small muscle activities referred to as manual dexterity such as is required for manipulating small objects.

Vital statistics are different for males and females of all ages. Life-expectancy, mortality, and morbidity rates are different for men and women. Some of the differences are based on biological factors, and others are based on cultural differences. There appear to be differences in behavioral patterns between boys and girls, men and women. For example, parents are all too aware of the difference in auto insurance premiums for their sons and daughters. Women are more to prone to certain medical problems, and men are more prone to other problems. People continue to speculate on what makes the difference. While it may be important to recognize that there are differences, it is more important to realize that there are many more similarities than differences. There are greater differences within one sex than there are between the averages of the two sexes. Every effort should be made to avoid sex role discrimination in the school setting.

The changing roles for men and women in this society seems to be diminishing some of the traditional differences.

CHARTING GROWTH PATTERNS

Growth patterns are difficult to predict. Growth does not take place evenly. There is not a steady pattern of growth, or a predictable unit of growth for a unit of time. There are spurts and plateaus. Nevertheless, height and weight measurements are important indicators of overall health. Schools should maintain such records. Growth

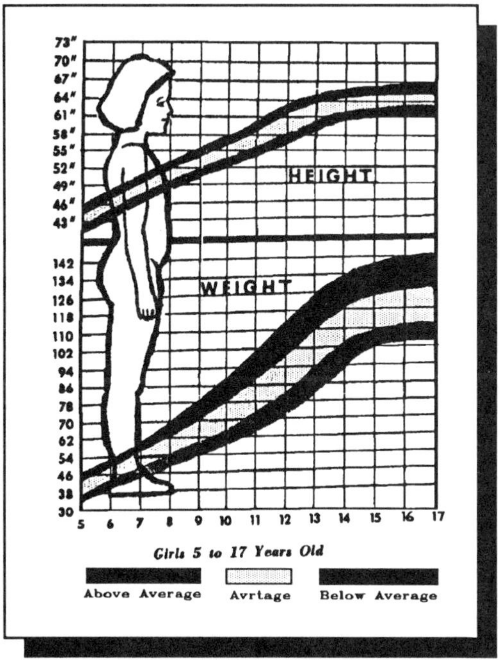

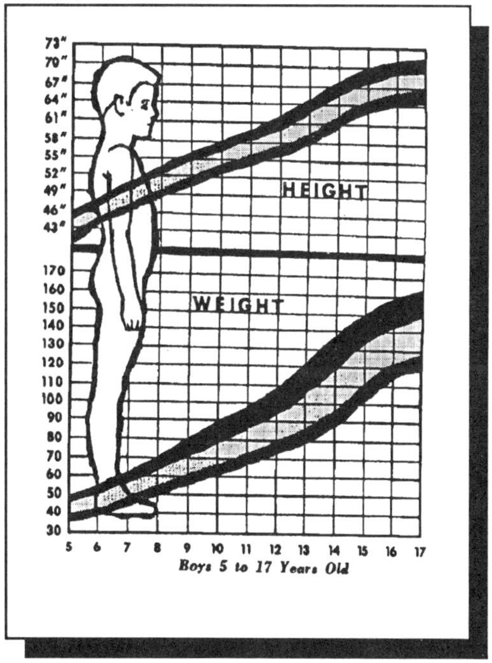

data to be meaningful, however, must be plotted on a grid along with other factors such as age and body type. Various grids have been devised scientifically to record that information. These grids, showing a channel of expected growth based on age, body type, and past performance, are useful as a basis of referral. A deviation from the channel may indicate malnutrition, an allergic reaction, an endocrine disturbance, or some type of disease. The Wetzel Grid is based on the following principles:

- Growth is a sensitive indication of the general state of health.

- Growth of healthy children of a given body type follows a predictable pattern.
- Once the pattern of growth has been established, a chart of the expected growth could be plotted.
- Departures from the expected may indicate a health problem.
- Nutritional needs can also be determined from some charts.

Many elementary schools use the Wetzel Grid or the Meredith Growth Record. If growth profile charts are transferred to the junior high school, teachers, particularly physical education and health teachers, counselors, and the school nurse, should know how to use them. Many parents with the help of their physician maintain growth records for their children.

THE BODY'S SYSTEMS

A school teacher should have a basic understanding of the normal structure and function, as well as abnormalities, of the various systems of the human body. The body is uniquely organized with a single cell being the basic unit. The function of the cell is determined by both internal and external factors. The genetic codes are the chief internal factors. The availability of oxygen and nutrients, the influence of the endocrine and nervous systems, and the presence or absence of harmful substances are a part of the external factors.

A group of similar cells working together to perform a function is called a *tissue*. A group of tissues working together to perform a function is called an *organ*. A group of organs working together to perform a variety of functions is called a *system*. In the human body, several systems work together to perform related functions. The skeleton, the skeletal muscles, and the skin work together to provide structure for the body. The digestive, circulatory, and respiratory systems provide for body maintenance, and the reproductive system provides for the continuation of new life. The endocrine system and the nervous system work together to regulate the body. The following will provide a basic summary of these systems.

BODY STRUCTURE

SKELETAL SYSTEM

The skeletal system provides a rigid framework to support soft structures of the body, and it furnishes a system of levers to provide body movement. The skeletal system is made up of 206 bones of varying sizes and shapes. Some bones, such as the skull and rib cage, are flat to provide protection for the brain and organs of the chest cavity. Some bones, such as the vertebrae, have irregular shapes for slight but specialized movements. Some bones, such as in the legs and arms, are long and are used for moving parts of the body. The marrow in the hollow core of the large bones serve as a site for the manufacture of blood cells: white cells, red blood cells, and platelets.

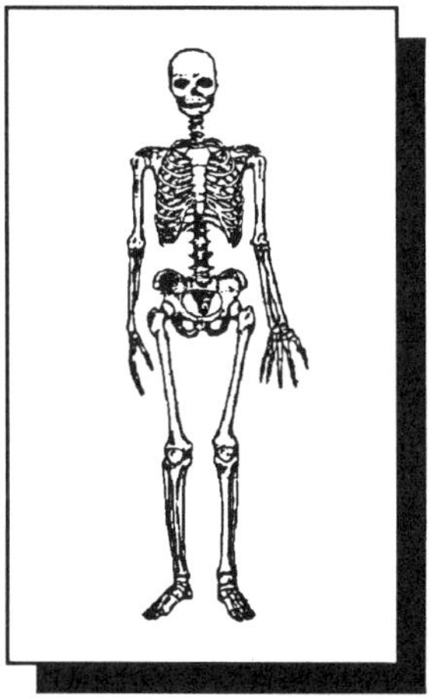

Besides bones, the skeletal system also includes joints, cartilage, ligaments, and tendons. Joints are the points where bone ends meet and articulate. Although some joints such as the skull are fixed, most joints are movable. Cartilage or soft bone covers the bone ends at joints and protects the bone ends during movement. Cartilage is also found in other places such as the nose. Ligaments are straps which connect one bone to another at the joints. They keep the bone ends together at the joints and restrict the direction of movement. Tendons connect the muscles to the bones to provide a system of levers so that bones are moved when muscles contracts.

Bone growth is divided into three periods. The formative period lasts from the fifth to twelfth week of life in the uterus. The growth period lasts to puberty. The consolidation period lasts from puberty to maturity, the attainment of full physical stature. An adolescent's maturation status is determined by a part of the long bones called the *epiphysis.* It is an area between the long shaft of a bone and the bone end at a joint. Bone growth takes place in this area. The epiphysis remains soft until maturity when it becomes ossified or hardened. If an x-ray of a teenager shows the bone end floating apart from the bone shaft, the youngster is still growing, but if the bone is solid, full growth has taken place.

Skeletal injuries include fractures when bones are broken, dislocations when bone ends are forced out of their sockets, sprains when ligaments are torn, strains when tendons or muscles are torn, and cramps when a spasm occurs in a muscle. Teachers should know how to provide first aid for these types of injuries. (This will be discussed in lesson 18.) There are also a number of medical problems that affect both the muscles and the bones. Posture problems are one thing that teachers should be aware of. Poor posture in the teenage years can cause much more serious problems years later. Other disorders of the bones, joints, and muscles include arthritis, osteoporosis, and cancer.

MUSCULAR SYSTEM

There are over 600 muscles in the body. The muscles are composed of muscle cells bound together to form muscle fibers, and a series of muscle fibers work together to form a muscle. The function of muscles is to move bones and other parts of the body. Muscles are either voluntary or involuntary. There are three different types of muscle: skeletal muscle, cardiac muscle, and smooth muscle. The skeletal muscles are controlled voluntarily by impulses along nerve pathways from the brain. Cardiac muscles are involuntary muscles of the heart that contract rhythmically without impulses from the brain. Smooth muscles are also involuntary and allow movement of the internal organs.

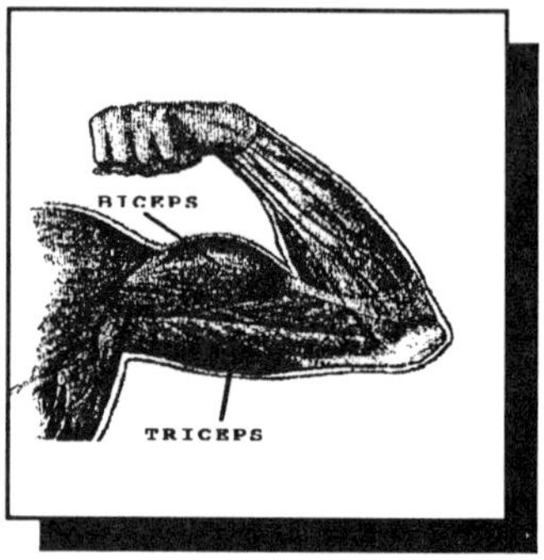

Skeletal muscles are anchored on one end by a tendon to a bone that cannot move. The other end is attached to a bone that is intended to move. The tendon extends across a joint which provides a point of leverage. Usually muscles work in pairs such as in the upper arm where the *biceps* muscle flexes the arm and the *triceps* muscle extends the arm. Physical fitness training and body building does not increase the number of muscle cells in a muscle, but it can increase the size and efficiency of the cells. A person's capacity for speed or endurance may be partially determined by the type of muscle cells he or she inherits.

THE SKIN

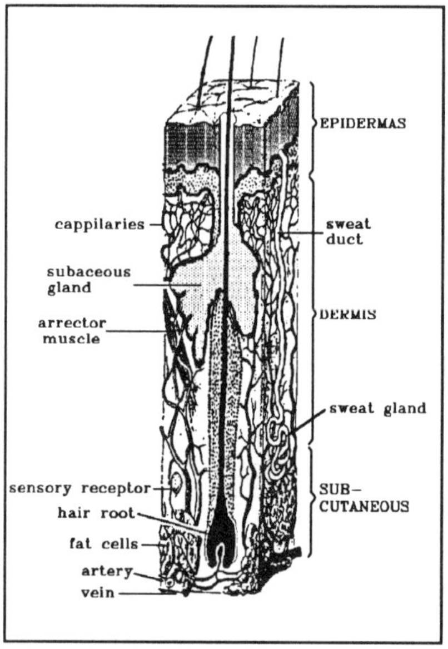

The outer covering of the body, the integument system, plays an important protective function for the body. The skin is the largest single organ of the body. It weighs about six pounds and if spread out flat may cover about 16 square feet. The structure of the skin is composed of three layers. The outer layer, called the *epidermis*, is made of dry, flattened, dead cells. The next layer is the *dermis* where the sebaceous glands, sweat glands, nerve endings, and hair follicles are located. The blood and lymph vessels, fat cells, and hair roots are located in the *subcutaneous tissue*. As cells in the epidermis continuously slough off, they are replaced by cells moving up from the dermis. *Melanin pigment* in the skin determines the color of the skin. Sunlight stimulates the production of melanin which causes tanning or freckles if the melanin is not distributed evenly. The hair, nails, and membranes at body openings are a part of this system.

In addition to providing protection, the skin also helps control body temperature. In hot weather, the small blood vessels in the skin dilate to radiate heat away from the body; in cold weather, they constrict to conserve heat. The sweat glands produce perspiration which cools the body as it evaporates. The sebaceous glands produce waxy oils which help keep the skin soft and keep it from drying out. Also imbedded in the skin are many nerve ending receptors which sense touch, pressure, heat, cold, and pain.

Acne is a skin disorder which frequently affects teenagers. Acne occurs when the sebaceous ducts become plugged. Sometimes a dark plug called a blackhead can be seen from the surface. When the sebaceous ducts are plugged, sebum accumulates within the gland, and this pressure leads to a localized inflammation called a pimple. If the pimple becomes infected, the glands may become filled with white pus and may be observed at the surface as whiteheads. Hormones secreted during puberty may cause the sebaceous glands to become more active. Most cases of acne are mild and can be taken care of with self-treatment. Usually, the best treatment is a medication which acts as an irritant to the skin and causes the outer layer of skin to slough off. This may help keep the sebaceous ducts open. Greasy creams and makeup should be avoided. The skin should be washed normally twice a day. Squeezing or picking at pimples should be avoided. Some cases of acne are severe and must be treated by a physician, perhaps a specialist in dermatology, to avoid permanent scarring. Other skin disorders teachers may observe among their students include: boils, warts, eczema, allergy type dermatitis, hives, and contagious skin infections such as athlete's foot, impetigo, and ringworm. Schools may have special policies for dealing with students with communicable skin disorders.

BODY MAINTENANCE

DIGESTIVE SYSTEM

The digestive system includes all of the organs that receive food and break it down into smaller and smaller molecules until the basic nutrients are small enough to be used by the body. People require about forty different chemicals for body growth and maintenance, and the nutrients are extracted from the food as it passes through the digestive system. These nutrients will be discussed in the next lesson, but the digestive process will be discussed briefly here.

There are two types of digestion, chemical and mechanical. The chewing action of the teeth in the mouth and the peristaltic or squeezing actions of the tubes through which the food passes provides mechanical digestion. Enzymes from the saliva glands in the mouth, gastric juices from the stomach, bile from the liver, and pancreatic juices from the pancreas are used in chemical digestion. Digestion starts in the mouth and continues in the esophagus, stomach, duodenum, and small intestine. Except for fats, the nutrients are absorbed through the walls of the small intestine into the blood vessels. Fats are

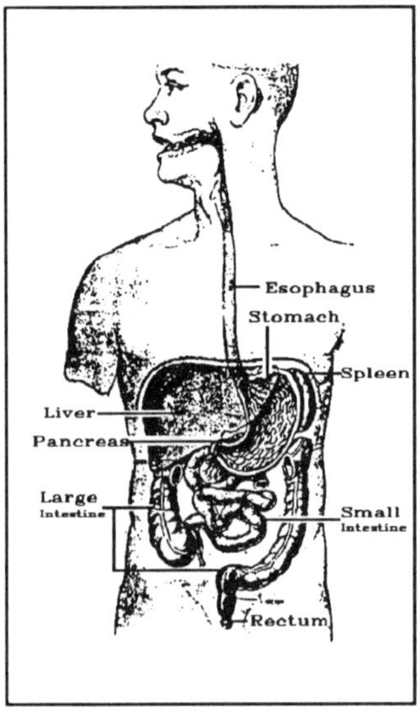

absorbed into the lymphatic vessels and are taken to the liver for further processing before entering the blood stream. Water is absorbed in the large intestines. The unusable waste products are eliminated through the rectum.

Once in the blood stream, the nutrients are transported to the cells. Proteins and minerals are used for cell structure and maintenance. Minerals and vitamins are used to help regulate other body processes. Sugars, fats, carbohydrates, starches, and proteins not used to build and repair the body are converted into simple sugar to be used by the body as fuel for heat and energy. But first the sugar must get into the cells. Insulin from the pancreas facilitates the transport of sugars through the cell membranes. Sugars in the cells are metabolized for fuel. Waste products from metabolism are transported by the blood from the cells to the kidneys and lungs where they are eliminated from the body.

Disorders of the digestive system include dental problems, indigestion, ulcers, gastritis, appendicitis, colitis, cancer, hemorrhoids, and many others. There is often a link between emotional problems and many disorders of the digestive system.

RESPIRATORY SYSTEM

The respiratory system consists of the air passages, the lungs, and the blood vessels of the lungs. The air passes through the nasal cavity, past the pharynx and larynx, past the epiglottis and vocal cords, through the trachea and bronchi, through the tiny bronchiole, and into the alveoli or air sacks. The air sacks are surrounded by blood vessel-filled membranes porus enough to allow the exchange of oxygen and carbon dioxide gases. Oxygen inhaled in the air is carried from the lungs by the blood to the various parts of the body. At the same time, carbon dioxide, a waste product of metabolism in the cells, is carried to the lungs and exhaled from the body. The diaphragm is the muscle that makes possible the breathing process.

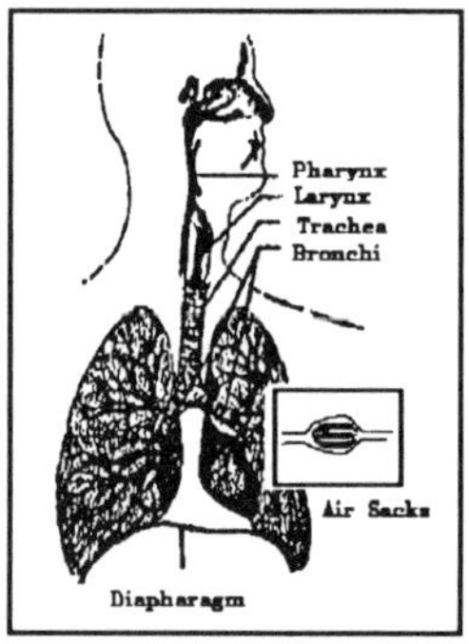

Asthma, bronchitis, emphysema, cancer, tuberculosis, and the various respiratory diseases such as whooping cough, hay fever, influenza, croup, and the common cold are diseases of the lungs and respiratory system.

CIRCULATORY SYSTEM

The purpose of the circulatory system is to transport substances from one part of the body to another. It transports nutrients, oxygen, hormones, white blood cells, antibodies, carbon dioxide, and other body wastes. The blood circulatory system consists of the heart, vessels, and blood. The blood is pumped from the heart to the lungs, from the lungs back to the heart, from the heart to the body, and from the body back to the heart. Arteries carry the blood away from the heart under pressure. Blood flows back to the heart through veins. Between the arteries and the veins the blood passes through tiny capillaries. This is where the substances transported by the blood are distributed to the cells.

The lymphatic circulatory system is also involved in transporting fluids and other substances from the extremities to the central areas of the body where they enter the bloodstream. The lymphatic system is an important part of the body's immune defense system. The lymphatic system consists of the lymphatic vessels, lymph glands, and the spleen. Lymphatic glands or nodes along the lymphatic vessels throughout the body trap and destroy infectious agents. Lymphatic glands often become swollen when there is an infection. The lymphatic glands produce lymphocytes, a type of white blood cell which recognizes foreign substances and reacts against them.

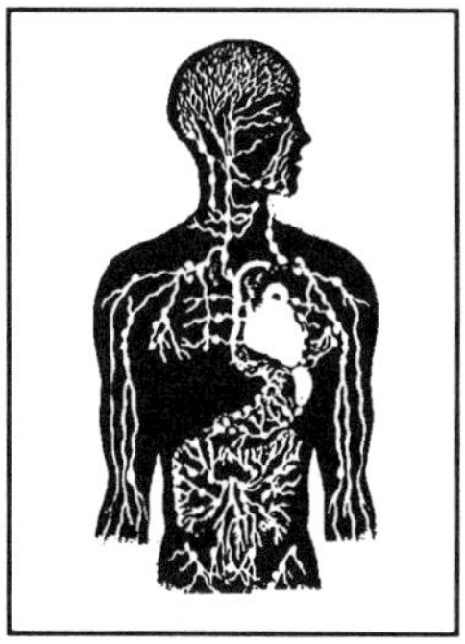

Diseases of the blood circulatory system that are most apt to affect students are congenital heart defects and rheumatic heart disease. Other diseases of the circulatory system are high blood pressure, atherosclerosis, arteriosclerosis, blood clots, varicose veins, gout, stroke, and uneven heart rhythms. Although these conditions may take place later in life, lifestyle patterns established by students may increase or decrease the risk. Various types of cancer such as leukemia and Hodgkin's disease are examples of disorders of the lymphatic system. Anemia and hemophilia are examples of blood disorders.

EXCRETORY SYSTEM

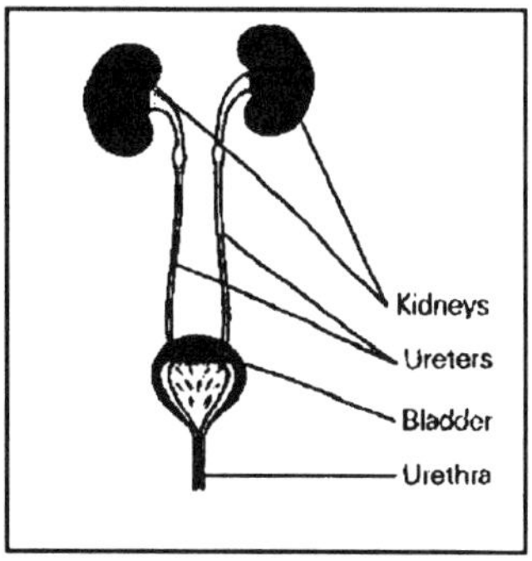

Some of the body's waste products pass through the pores of the skin. Fluid also passes through the skin as perspiration to help control the body's temperature. These fluids, oils, and wastes combine with surface dirt and bacteria to cause body odors and other unhealthy conditions that should be removed through regular bathing and washing of the skin and hair. Waste gases such as carbon dioxide are removed from the body by the circulatory and respiratory systems. Indigestible food that remains in the intestines is excreted as semi-solid waste, fecal matter, or stool through the rectum and anus. The kidneys remove a variety of waste products, along with fluids, from the blood. Much of the fluid is reabsorbed into the blood, leaving the concentrate urine which passes through the ureter tube to the bladder where it is stored until it is excreted through the urethra.

BODY REGULATION

NERVOUS SYSTEM

The nervous system is composed of the brain, the spinal cord, and the peripheral nerves throughout the body. It has two portions--the sensory portion and the motor portion. The sensory portion consists of sense receptors for sight, hearing, taste, smell, and feel. The motor portion consists of motor neurons that stimulate voluntary muscles and the autonomic nerves which control involuntary muscles. The brain consists of the cerebrum, cerebellum, and the medulla. The cerebrum is divided into two hemispheres and each has centers for thinking, memory, vision, hearing, sensory perception, and a voluntary motor center. The highly developed frontal lobe of the cerebrum is the center for making judgments, establishing values, and providing inhibitions. The cerebellum coordinates muscular activity. The medulla controls the automatic functions such as the beating of the heart.

Diseases such as polio, cerebral palsy, epilepsy, encephalitis, meningitis, multiple sclerosis, and injuries to the spinal cord affect the nervous system. There are also several congenital disorders of the nervous system.

ENDOCRINE SYSTEM

The endocrine system serves as the body's chemical factory. Hormones are secreted from the various endocrine glands through the blood to all tissues of the body, but only certain tissues of the body will respond to a particular hormone. The endocrine system works along with the nervous system to regulate body activities. But, while nervous impulses begin and end instantaneously, glandular action begins and ends more gradually and provides longer or sustained effect. Nerve impulses are directed to a few places at a time, but glandular secretions reach all parts of the body and tissues that are capable of responding, thus producing a whole system of responses. While nerve impulses either start or stop an action, hormones either speed up or slow down an action that is already in progress.

The endocrine system provides internal regulation for many of the body functions and has significant influence upon growth and development as well as personality and

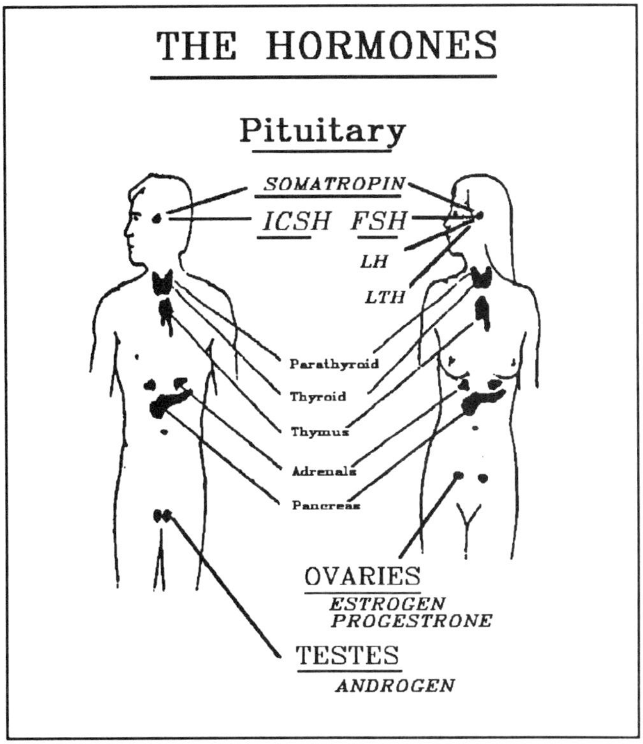

temperament. The endocrine system itself is influenced by factors such as heredity and environment. The endocrine system's function starts when the endocrine glands secrete hormones (chemical messengers) to the blood stream for transportation throughout the body. Each hormone controls one or more physiological functions of the body, including growth and development. Normal secretion of hormones results in normal growth and development, but occasional over or under secretion of the hormones may result in abnormalities in growth and development.

The pituitary, or master gland, is located at the base of the brain. Although it is very small, about the size of a garden pea, it secretes several hormones which in turn control the functions of other glands. It secretes somatropin, the growth hormone which regulates growth patterns prior to puberty. Under the influence of somatropin, the silhouettes of boys and girls are very similar. Too little results in dwarfs, and too much produces giants.

SEX HORMONES

At puberty, the pituitary gland secretes a hormone that, although chemically the same, has different names in males and females. In females it is called *follicle stimulating hormone* (FSH). It is a hormone that stimulates the follicle cells in the ovaries. In males it is called *interstitial cell stimulating hormone* (ICSH). It is a hormone that stimulates the interstitial cells in the testes. At puberty, FSH will cause the ovaries to secrete the hormone estrogen which causes the body to develop the secondary sex characteristics of the female. FSH also causes the ovaries to produce eggs. Similarly at puberty, ICSH causes the testes to secret the hormone androgen which causes the body to develop the secondary sex characteristics of the male. ICSH also causes the testes to produce sperm.

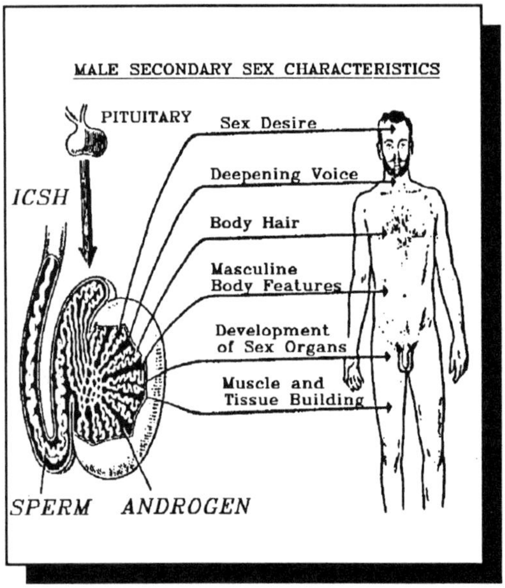

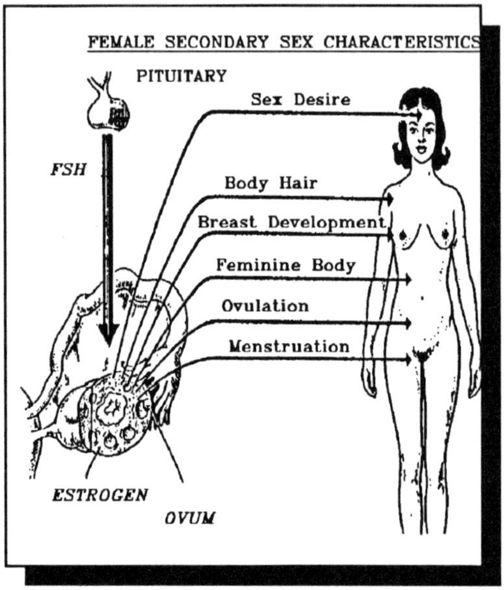

The secondary sex characteristics of the male are the development of body and facial hair, changes in the larynx (voice box), and the development of the male body shape. The secondary sex characteristics for the female are breast development, growth of pubic and axillary hair, and development of the female body contour. The female sex organs also mature, and the menstrual cycle begins.

Each month after puberty girls and women experience the menstrual cycle. The length of a cycle may range from 18 to 36 days, but are normally 28 days, a lunar month. The menstrual cycle is initiated by the secretion of FSH from the pituitary. FSH causes the eggs in the ovaries to mature and the endometrium lining in the uterus to start to develop. FSH also causes the ovaries to produce estrogen, but when the quantity of estrogen in the blood is high enough, the pituitary stops producing FSH. At about the fourteenth day of the cycle, less if the cycle is short or more if the cycle is long, ovulation occurs. A mature egg erupts from the follicle in the ovary and starts to descend through the fallopian tube. The cavity remaining in the ovary when the egg was discharged is called the corpus luteum. It is lined with some special cells which produce the hormone progesterone. The purpose of progesterone is to maintain the endometrium lining of the uterus. Under the influence of progesterone, the endometrium becomes thick with materials intended to provide nutrition for a developing zygote if the egg is fertilized. However, within a few days the corpus luteum dries up and no longer produces progesterone to maintain the endometrium. If the egg is not fertilized by about the twenty-eighth day of the cycle (14 days since ovulation), the blood-like endometrium sloughs off and is discharged through the vagina. This discharge signals the beginning of the next cycle.

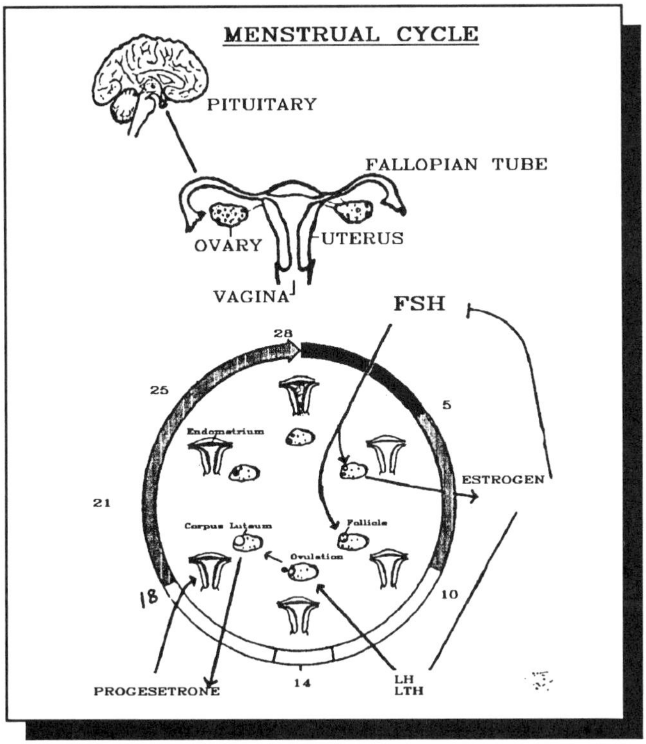

There are a number of menstrual cycle dysfunctions. There are painful periods, *dysmenorrhea*, heavy periods, and missed periods. While a missed period may be associated with pregnancy, it may also be due to other problems. Premenstrual tension is also associated with abnormal production of estrogen and progesterone.

OTHER ENDOCRINE GLANDS

Other glands produce hormones which affect the body's functioning, but are not so closely related to changes in body structure and function associated with puberty. Thyroxin from the thyroid gland regulates metabolism, the rate the body uses energy foods and oxygen. The parathyroid glands produce parahormone which helps control blood-calcium levels which influence bone strength and neuromuscular coordination. The adrenal glands produce hormones which are important to metabolism, healing, shock control, and providing extra energy in times of emergency. Insulin from the islet of Langerhans helps transport sugar into the cells. Undersecretion may result in sugar diabetes.

The endocrine system is concerned with regulating biological processes such as mustering body reserves for emergency defense, promoting the sexual stimulus to ensure the reproduction of the species, controlling the use of food by the body, and maintaining the balance of salts and water in the body. Since it helps regulate our comfort, our sense of security, and our various appetites, our endocrine system has an important influence on our emotional health.

The thyroid gland is located in the neck. An enlargement of this gland is goiter. Thyroxin is the hormone produced by the thyroid, and it helps regulate metabolism or the use of food by the body. Insufficient thyroxin or *hypothyroidism* before birth may result in mental retardation and a type of dwarf known as a *cretin*. Hypothyroidism later in life produces toxedema, a condition that gives a swollen appearance to the face, arms, and legs. Students with hypothyroidism may appear disinterested, chronically slow, and sleepy. The parathyroid glands are embedded in the thyroid glands in the neck. They produce *parahormone* which helps maintain the calcium and phosphorus balance in the blood and bones. Insulin is a hormone produced by many island glands located in the pancreas. Insulin is needed to transport sugar from the blood clots faster, and strength is increased.

REPRODUCTIVE SYSTEM

Some of the same body organs involved in excretion of wastes and the endocrine system are also used in the reproductive process. In the embryological stage, the tissues of the male and female reproductive systems started out the same but gradually specialized to become the male or female genital organs and primary sexual characteristics. In the female, these organs include the ovaries, fallopian tubes, uterus, cervix, vagina, hymen, and labia. In the male, these organs include the scrotum, testes, epididymis, vas deferens, prostrate gland, seminal vesicles, urethra, and penis. Note, in the male, the urethra serves a dual purpose in excretion and reproduction, but in the female the vagina and urethra are separate organs.

Diseases of the reproductive, urinary gastrointestinal systems include kidney and bladder infections, cystitis, diarrhea, constipation, cancer, hemorrhoids, dysmenorrhea, sterility, and sexually transmitted diseases (STDs).

CONCLUSION

This Chapteer has dealt in a general way with the growth and development patterns in children from conception through adolescence. Hopefully, this information will help teachers better understand their students and help the schools carry out their disease prevention and health promotion responsibilities.

STUDY HELPS

Distinguish between growth and development and between male and female growth patterns.

Match the body systems in the first column with the organs in column two and the diseases in column three.

1. CIRCULATORY
2. DIGESTIVE
3. ENDOCRINE
4. EXCRETORY
5. MUSCULAR
6. NERVOUS
7. REPRODUCTIVE
8. RESPIRATORY
9. SKELETAL
10. SKIN

Terms related to conception, sex determination, growth and development, heredity, secondary sex characteristics, and sex-linked inheritance.

prenatal
puberty
precocious
latent
conception
recessive
dominant
X and Y chromosomes
genes
growth channels

1. alveoli
2. autonomic
3. bronchi
4. capillaries
5. cardiac
6. corpus luteum
7. duodenum
8. endometrium
9. epididymis
10. epiglottis
11. epiphysis
12. esophagus
13. fallopian tube
14. FSH
15. hormones
16. ICSH
17. insulin
18. lymphatic system
19. ovaries
20. pituitary
21. progesterone
22. prostrate
23. scrotum
24. sebaceous
25. semen
26. skeletal
27. smooth
28. sperm
29. stomach
30. testes
31. thyroxin
32. urethra
33. uterus
34. vagina
35. vas deferens
36. voluntary

1. acne
2. anemia
3. appendicitis
4. arthritis
5. asthma
6. bronchitis
7. cerebral palsy
8. colitis
9. congenital heart defects
10. cystitis
11. dislocations
12. dysmenorrhea
13. emphysema
14. encephalitis
15. hemophilia
16. Hodgkin's disease
17. hypothyroidism
18. influenza
19. leukemia
20. meningitis
21. osteoporosis
22. polio
23. premenstrual tension
24. rheumatic heart disease
25. sterility
26. tuberculosis
27. ulcers
28. whooping cough

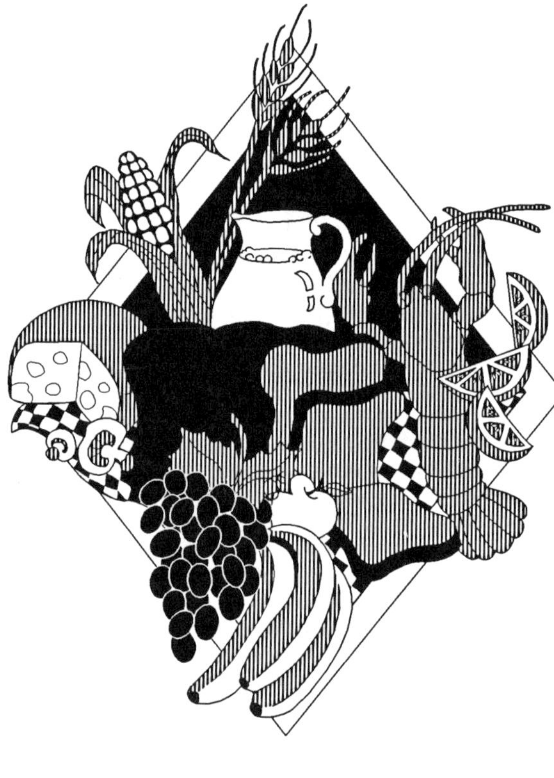

Chapter 11

MAINTAINING HEALTH AND FITNESS

You may be able to cite examples of students who have performed well academically in spite of apparent physical handicaps. However, such instances are probably exceptions, since poor physical health usually has a negative effect on learning. Good health is essential to the maximum utilization of educational opportunities. While student health is a major concern, the health of teachers is also important.

MAINTAINING PHYSICAL HEALTH AND FITNESS

The physical health of students is also a teacher's concern. What students know and do about their health will not only relate to their learning effectiveness today, it may also relate to the quality of their future life. This lesson deals with the basic requirements for maintaining physical health. This is an area in which many fads and fallacies continue to prevail, and teachers should do their part to try to combat them, particularly in the areas of nutrition, weight control, and fitness. Teachers teach more about health by what they do than by what they say.

A number of procedures have been employed to indicate the general level of a person's health. An example reported in the text *School Health Principles and Practices* by C.L. Anderson compares levels of health to school grades.

LEVELS OF HEALTH

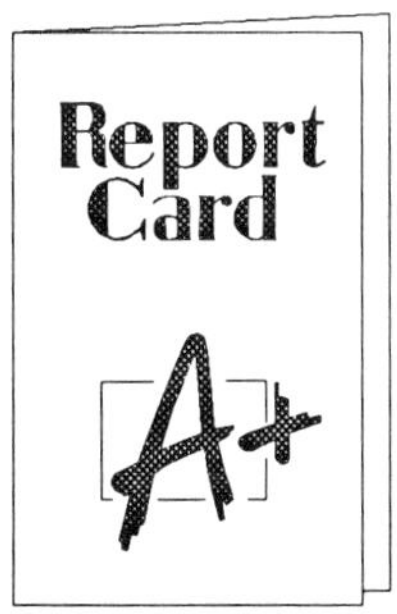

A A high level of health, but not perfect health, is indicated by this classification. A person with this quality of health may have an occasional cold, minor infection, headache, or other mild disturbance. Freedom from disabling remediable defects is an obvious requirement. Youngsters in this category display pronounced vigor and buoyancy and sufficient vitality to carry on the demands of life. This does not connote great muscular power and endurance, but more than enough strength and endurance for any likely venture. It does not include physical size. A child in this health category enjoys life, participates wholly in normal activities, and adjusts well to social situations.

B Freedom from disabling defects is a primary requirement in this category. Persons in this group do not have quite the vigor and buoyancy of level A. Many in this classification can attain the higher level of health by conscientious application of health principles.

C Persons in this classification pass as well, but lack the vitality for a dynamic mode of living. They go through life functioning at a minimum--not sick, but dragging rather than buoyant like people with good health. Many can attain an A level of health, and most can attain at least a B level of health. There should be no school child with a C level of health.

D Children in this classification attend school regularly, but are not well. A chronic infection or some other apparent or concealed factor is the basic cause of the low level of health. Until the cause is discovered and remedied, these children are not likely to improve their level of health. The teacher or other school personnel should be aware of the state of health of these children and take the proper steps to safeguard their welfare. School obviously is not the place for them. Even children with a low level of vitality, but without specific defects or diseases, should be under the care of a physician.

E Children in this classification are obviously ill and should not be in school. Usually they are not.

GENERAL INDICATORS

The following are indicators of general physical health. Their absence may be observed and considered by a watchful teacher.

- Buoyancy. Body movement conveys the im-pression that it carries no weight.
- Unawareness of body. A healthy body does not call attention to itself. The person does not concentrate on a physical problem.
- Pleasure in activity. Pleasure is gained through physical action.

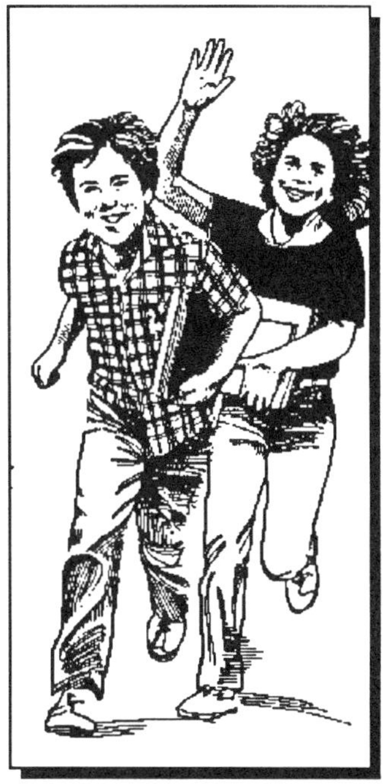

- **Vigor**. Sufficient energy is possessed to do the things one wants and can be expected to do in a normal day.
- **Zest**. A desire to continue working on a project even after much time has already been spent.
- **Recovery**. Ability to recover from fatigue. Adequate rest is important.
- **Relaxation**. Occasional tension is fine, but constant tension indicates a departure from normal health.
- **Appetite**. Steady but not suddenly changing. The teacher should be concerned about the student who always has a poor appetite.
- **Steady weight**. No appreciable variation in weight. A small degree of fluctuation is normal.
- **No remediable defect**. Absence of disabling remediable defects. Any remedial defect such as loss of hearing or poor eyesight has been remedied by hearing aids or glasses.

GOOD HEALTH HABITS

Listed below are ten health habits that can help people enjoy good health. This list comes from *The Homemaker's Guide to Home Nursing* by Alice M. Schmidt, R.N., and it applies to students and teachers as well as all family members.

1. **Good posture**. This health habit allows body organs to function properly and eliminates many minor aches and pains. It also leads to a better self-image and allows for higher self-esteem.

2. **Adequate rest**. Adequate amounts of rest vary from individual to individual; each must determine for himself the right amount. Illness, pregnancy, and other factors may increase the need for rest temporarily.

3. **Adequate exercise and relaxation**. Relaxation helps to restore mental equilibrium and provides social interaction. We also need sufficient exercise to allow our bodies to function optimally. How this exercise is obtained may vary considerably. This program should include some aerobic exercises, which improve cardiovascular-pulmonary functioning by forcing the heart and lungs to become

more efficient. If you are interested in developing a personal aerobic exercise program, remember the following rules:

a. Have a complete physical examination before embarking on a strenuous physical exercise program.

b. Wear good shoes if your program involves running or jumping.

c. Increase the amount of exercise gradually each week.

d. Be consistent. The most effective exercise program includes exercising four or five times a week.

e. Make it a lifetime effort.

4. Regular medical and dental checkups. Every family should have a physician. All family members should be encouraged to maintain adequate immunizations against communicable diseases in their area. Regular yearly physicals can do much to prevent or detect such problems as cancer, heart and lung disease, diabetes, and other chronic conditions. Dental checkups should be part of the family routine. Many communities now have dentists who are specifically interested in preventive dentistry and are anxious to help families prevent dental problems as well as remedy them.

5. Awareness of safety hazards. There is no way to make a home completely safe, since many complex factors enter in. Although some accidents are due to lack of knowledge, especially among children, the majority occur to individuals who knew the safety hazards and ignored them. Psychological factors such as fear, anger, nervousness, or anxiety often have a strong influence on our behavior. During such periods, we tend to be less attentive to what we are doing.

6. Avoid pollutants. Environmental pollutants such as excessive noise, improper waste disposal, and contaminants in the air are all around us. We all cannot manage to move from the cities to the mountain tops, but we all can become conscious of the need to support government measures intended to give us cleaner air, less noise, and adequate water supplies and waste disposal.

7. Avoid harmful substances. Avoidance of smoking can help to lessen the danger of cancer and emphysema. Other harmful substances containing drugs of various kinds should also be avoided. Tea, coffee, and colas contain harmful stimulants. Alcohol can cause severe problems in many areas of the body. Laxatives, some pain relievers, tranquilizers, or sedatives can cause the user to develop a

dependence on them. It is best to use medicines only when they are necessary or when they are recommended by a doctor.

8. <u>**Personal hygiene**</u>. Cleanliness among family members can do much to help prevent the spread of infection. Clean hands, individual drinking cups and silverware, daily bathing, clean clothing and hair--these are some of the things members of a family can do to help themselves remain healthy.

9. <u>**Good mental health**</u>. All of us need to be useful and independent, to love and be loved, to accept what we cannot change. When one has good mental health, he can face the world and work out solutions to his problems. Family members should be encouraged to develop a good self-image, to feel good about themselves and their relationships with other people. Good mental health includes the ability to cope with the recurrent stresses of life and to live comfortably with oneself and others in all types of situations.

10. <u>**Good nutrition**</u>. We are what we eat, and adequate diet is extremely important if we are to remain healthy. By making the appropriate selections from the basic four food groups, one can plan adequate daily menus that will supply the necessary daily nutrients.

NUTRITION

Although nutrition is an important part of health maintenance for people of all ages, it should be particularly important for teenagers. Good nutrition is important during the time of rapid growth, yet teenagers frequently have poor eating habits. Sometimes school policies and practices tend to contribute to these problems. This section should help you as a teacher to be aware of the nutritional needs of adolescents and some of the special nutritional problems they experience. It will help you distinguish between nutritional facts and fallacies so that you will be able to give your students sound nutritional advice.

The American people as a whole are better off nutritionally than most people throughout the world, yet many young Americans could improve their nutritional status significantly. Nutritional science has discovered that in order to be healthy, the body requires specific amounts of certain chemicals which are referred to as nutrients. A number of factors determine our eating habits. Food availability, group customs, individual preferences, and the hope for some magical or special power in foods may be the basis of food selection. Prior to the advent of nutritional science, one person's opinion was as good as the next person's about food selection. But today the difference between fact and fallacy has been established by science. Yet among the nutritionally ignorant, the wishful thinkers, and the gullible, the food fads and fallacies persist.

Certainly teachers in the public schools should not be among those who promote nutritional nonsense.

WHY STUDY NUTRITION?

More than 40 chemical elements, nutrients found in food, are needed by the body. Some nutrients are needed to build parts of the body, some are used to supply energy, and others become part of chemical processes that regulate the body's functions. The amount of nutrients required by the body varies with age, sex, and other conditions. With some nutrients, the difficulty may be avoiding excessive consumption. Other nutrients (trace elements) are required in such small quantities it is impossible to measure the amount needed each day. The following are seven good reasons why we should study nutrition.

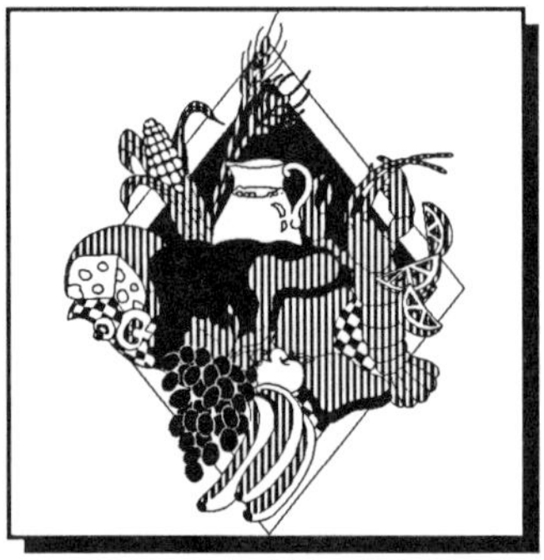

To Know What Is an Adequate Diet

The lack of knowledge is one reason why many college students don't eat properly. People need to study about nutrition in order to have an adequate diet. We require over 30 separate chemicals in their right amounts and at the right times for proper growth and body maintenance. The knowledge about how to provide those nutrients does not come automatically, people must learn it. A nutrition unit in a college health course is a good place to study nutrition.

To Develop Proper Attitudes About Nutrition

Poor attitudes and the lack of self-respect is another reason why some college student don't have an adequate diet. Knowledge of nutrition does not guarantee that people will eat properly. Poor attitudes are frequently the problem. This nutrition lesson may not provide any new information, but it might prompt an attitude adjustment. College is often a time when nutrition becomes more relevant.

To Be Able To Eat Well and Still Save Money

To save money is an often mentioned reason why college students do not eat properly. Students operating on minimal financial resources frequently skip meals and eat just a few inexpensive and nutritionally limited foods. A good reason for studying nutrition is to learn how to select foods that are less expensive, but nutritionally adequate.

To Be Able To Eat Well and Still Save Time

To save time is another frequently mentioned reason college students give for not eating properly. The "quicky" meal, eating on the go, skipping meals, or eating the same thing day after day is all too frequent on a college campus. An increased awareness of the importance of nutrition might help students plan their eating patterns better.

To Be Able To Properly Control Weight

Some students say they skip meals, because they are already overweight. Many people modify their food consumption because they are conscious of weight problems. Frequently, their concern is not justified and their approach is irrational. Knowledge of nutrition is essential to an effective weight modification program.

To Be Able To Avoid Food Fads and Fallacies

Sometimes students' eating habits are based on fads and fallacies. A lot of information about foods and nutrition is printed, but unfortunately about half of it is false. It is not unusual for a class on nutrition to have to spend as much time overcoming misinformation as it does in teaching new information. Not only should misinformation be avoided because of its association with fraud and quackery, but it is also dangerous in some instances. People should study nutrition to be able to distinguish between nutritional facts and fallacies.

To Understand the Social and Emotional Roles of Food

Some students say depression is the reason they either eat too much or too little. Food consumption is not only associated with physical needs, but it is also tied to social and emotional expressions. Often people turn to food as a substitute for social and emotional gratification and this may be good, but it frequently is bad. The potential for this becoming a problem is particularly high on a college campus, and students should learn how to avoid it.

THE SEVEN BASIC NUTRIENT GROUPS

The nutrients required for good health are found in seven basic nutrient groups. Some of these nutrients are used to build body structure such as muscles, bones, connective tissues, and body organs; some provide fuel for body heat and energy; and some are used to help regulate body processes.

PROTEINS

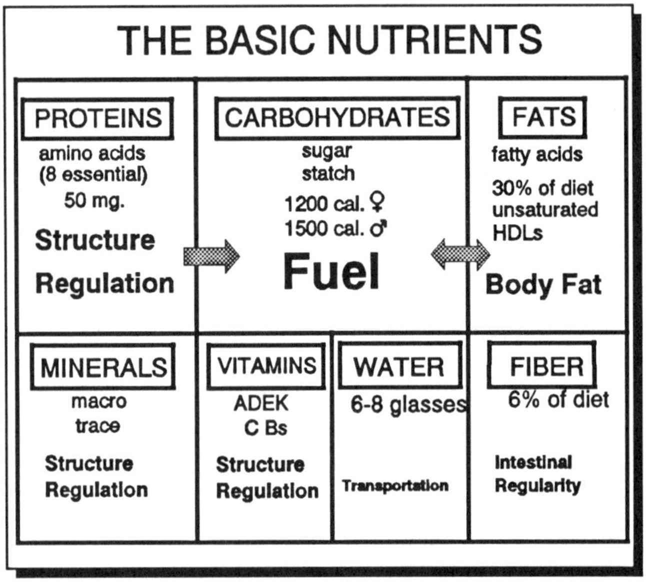

Proteins are important parts of the cells of all living tissues. They are needed for cell growth and repair and to form enzymes to regulate body processes. Proteins are made up of amino acids. The human body requires 22 different amino acids. Some of the amino acids can be synthesized in the body; that is, some amino acids can be broken down and rearranged to form other amino acids. However, there are eight amino acids, referred to as *essential* amino acids, which cannot be synthesized. Foods that contain all eight essential amino acids are called complete proteins; those foods that supply only some of the essential amino acids are called incomplete proteins. People have no problem in getting sufficient quantities of most amino acids, but getting the eight essential amino acids can require some special attention in meal planning. Most proteins of animal origin such as meat, milk, and eggs are complete proteins. As little as two ounces of meat (45-65 grams) when combined with milk, fruits, grains, and vegetables will supply the protein needed each day.

Vegetables are generally incomplete proteins; however, a combination of certain grains, red beans, and corn, for example, can supply the essential amino acids. Soybeans are complete proteins by themselves. All of the essential amino acids can be obtained from plant sources by combining two incomplete proteins such as nuts, grains, or legumes. With careful selection, all protein needs can be satisfied from plant sources. It does not take a lot of food to supply the body's protein needs. Athletes need no more protein than less active people. Excessive amounts of protein each day are converted by the body to blood sugar to be used as fuel or stored as fat. Excess proteins become an expensive source of fuel. Only about fifteen percent of our diet should be protein.

CARBOHYDRATES

The food we eat contains calories or fuel for the body. A calorie is a unit for measuring the amount of fuel that is in food. All food contains calories, but some contains much more than others. The body requires calories for heat and energy. The daily caloric requirement varies from person to person based on age, sex, activity level, and metabolic rate. For example, a teenage boy may require 2800 calories per day and a girl may require 2400. If they are very active, they will require more.

The main source of body fuel for heat and energy should be carbohydrates. Carbohydrates should supply about 55 percent of our calories, proteins 15 percent, and fats 30 percent. Most carbohydrates come from vegetable starches and sugars; the only animal source of starch is sugar from milk. The starches and sugars are converted to glucose or blood sugar. The glucose is taken from the blood into the cells to be used as fuel. Starches or complex carbohydrates are preferred for health reasons to sugars or simple carbohydrates because the sugars contain only calories while starches contain other nutrients as well.

It is easy to consume more calories than the body requires for fuel, and the excess is stored as body fat. The normal range for daily calorie consumption for males is 1500 - 3000. Because females have a lower metabolic rate, they only require 1200 - 2100. If the daily calorie consumption drops below 1500 for males and 1200 for females, the person will probably not get the other needed nutrients. A 900 calorie-per-day diet would probably be dangerous. On the other hand, increased physical activity may require more calories than the ranges listed above indicate.

FATS

Fats and oils are the most concentrated source of calories. When a molecule of dietary fat is digested, it forms one molecule of glycerol and three molecules of fatty acids (triglycerides). The glycerol is used by the body as fuel or stored as body fat. There are several kinds of fatty acids. Some fatty acids are essential to life, but there are problems associated with an excessive intake of certain fats such as cholesterol, which is linked to coronary artery disease. Thus, fat in our diet is sometimes a controversial issue.

To avoid confusion, we should distinguish between dietary fat that we eat and body fat that is the storage place for extra calories. Body fat is the accumulation of extra calories whether consumed in the form of proteins, carbohydrates, or fats. Extra fuel is stored as body fat. A small amount of body fat, 15 percent for men and 20 percent for women, is needed to provide protective padding and insulation.

The fatty acids are essential to life. They become an essential part of various body cells and are an essential ingredient in various body processes. Fatty acids are either *saturated* or *unsaturated.* A saturated fat is a chain of carbon atoms all linked to a hydrogen atom. A monosaturated fat has one pair of carbon atoms that are free or not linked to a hydrogen atom. A polyunsaturated fat has many free carbon atoms.

Animal fats are usually saturated fats, and most vegetable oils are unsaturated fats. Polyunsaturated fats are usually liquid at room temperature; however, there are some exceptions. Poultry and fish are high in unsaturated fats, and coconut and palm oil are saturated. Hydrogenation is the process of adding hydrogen atoms to polyunsaturated fats to make them solid and more stable at room temperature--margarine and peanut butter for example. Nutrition experts recommend a reduction in the consumption of saturated fats and an increase in polyunsaturated fats in the diet.

Cholesterol is a saturated fatty acid. If the amount of cholesterol in the blood exceeds 200 milligrams per 100 milliliters of blood, a person should consider limiting their cholesterol consumption. There are two types of cholesterol. Cholesterol combined with certain types of protein form High Density Lipoprotein (HDLs) and cholesterol combined with other proteins form Low Density Lipoprotein (LDLs). LDLs tend to promote heart disease by keeping large quantities of cholesterol in the blood. Cholesterol in the blood combines with calcium and other substances to form atherosclerotic plaques which block the coronary arteries of the heart. HDL's seem to protect the heart against heart disease by transporting excess cholesterol to the liver where it is metabolized and eliminated from the body. Some studies suggest that the proportion of HDLs to total cholesterol can be increased by eating certain foods such as fish and maintaining an exercise program.

MINERALS

The required minerals are used for building and repairing body tissues and regulating certain body activities. The body requires a few minerals in fairly large quantities (100 to 6,000 mg per day) and a few other in much smaller or trace amounts (1.5 to 20 mg). Although only trace amounts may be needed, serious health problems will result if they are deficient in the diet. Health problems will also result if excesses occur. Calcium, phosphorus, iodine, and iron are needed in identifiable amounts. Smaller amounts of copper, sodium, potassium, chlorine, magnesium, sulfur, zinc, manganese, chromium, molybdenum, cobalt, and selenium are needed in the body and are available in ample supplies when a person eats a variety of foods. Most people who eat a balanced diet will not require mineral supplements. Any mineral supplementation should come through the advice of a physician. People who take mineral supplements on their own may be inviting health problems. There may be a question about the availability of iodine, fluorine, and iron in the diet. Foods grown in certain areas of the world may lack sufficient iodine, but a good supplemental source of iodine is iodized salt. Iron comes from a variety of meats, grains, fruits, and vegetables. In some areas of the country, fluorine supplementation may be advisable in the drinking water (one part per million). Fairly frequently, women are advised by their physician to obtain a supplemental source of iron. Calcium is another mineral that may require dietary supplementation for some people, if advised by a physician. Calcium may also be needed in some areas to help form strong teeth.

VITAMINS

Vitamins are not structural components of the body. They are substances which work with various enzymes to help the body utilize other nutrients. Vitamins help regulate certain body functions, and although the quantity that is needed is very small, they are essential. Fat soluble vitamins (A, D, E, and K) are absorbed through the intestines with the help of fats, and excessive amounts are stored in the fat cells. An excessive buildup of fat soluble vitamins in the cells may become toxic. Water soluble vitamins (B-complex vitamins and Vitamin C) are easily dissolved in water, and excessive amounts are excreted. Excessive consumption of water soluble vitamins is a problem. The Recommended Dietary Allowance (RDA) indicates approximately how much of each vitamin is needed each day, and that amount varies for each vitamin. The fat soluble vitamins are measured in International Units (IU), and the water soluble vitamins are measured in milligrams (mg). Vitamins in the RDA quantities are obtained from a variety of plant and animal sources, the same sources that supply proteins, carbohydrates, and fats. Rarely do people need additional vitamins unless they have a health problem that requires medical supervision. The practice of taking large doses of supplemental vitamins without medical supervision is not only a waste of money, but it may also be harmful.

Vitamin D is produced by action of sunlight on the skin or is provided from fortified milk. Vitamin B_{12} is primarily available in meat and may be difficult to obtain from other sources. The daily need for Vitamin C can be satisfied by a small orange or other citrus fruit, cantaloupe, tomato, or potatoes. The rest of the vitamins are available through a variety of fruits, vegetables, and grain products as well as meats and milk products.

WATER

Water is probably the most essential nutrient. People can survive for weeks without other nutrients, but dehydration can become a critical problem in a few hours. Water accounts for over 50 percent of body weight, and it plays an important role in keeping the body's chemistry in delicate balance. It is the major component of the blood which transports oxygen, nutrients, and hormones to the cells. Although the amount of water needed each day varies with a number of factors, for optimal body functioning, a person should consume at least eight glasses of fluid per day. Part of that amount may come in food. Probably more Americans' diets are short of water than any other nutrient. Much of the time we cannot rely on thirst to prompt us to drink enough fluids.

FIBER

Fiber is a nondigestible carbohydrate that is important for intestinal regularity, sometimes called cellulose, roughage, or bulk. It is the part of whole grains, fruits, vegetables, and nuts that cannot be digested in the human gastrointestinal tract. Type I fiber absorbs much water, swells in the intestinal tract, and produces a soft stool that passes easily and quickly. This reduces the transit time for waste products through the intestines and shortens the exposure of the bowel to possible irritants. People who consume foods high in fiber have fewer incidents of intestinal cancer, constipation, and other intestinal problems. Type II fiber acts to prevent the absorption of certain chemicals into the bloodstream. The fibers found in oats, fruits, and vegetables seem to reduce blood lipids and cholesterol. People on high fiber diets seem to have fewer incidents of heart disease, and high fiber diets may help in weight control. High fiber foods are low in fat content. They absorb large amounts of water (causing a sense of fullness), and they are chewed more slowly, remain in the stomach longer, and thus provide a sense of satisfaction. Since the recognition of the health benefits of fiber, a number of fiber supplements have come into the health food market. Generally, these fiber supplements are not necessary and can be dangerous. Eating whole raw foods that contain the other nutrients is much safer than consuming fiber concentrates.

THE BASIC FOUR FOOD GROUPS

The essential nutrients have been distributed among the four food groups, so that if a person eats a variety of foods from each group, he will receive a proper balance of all the needed nutrients. The balance of nutrients for energy, body structure, and regulatory processes can be obtained from the basic four food groups whether a person is attempting to gain, lose, or maintain weight. A regular food diet is best for most circumstances. The size of the servings may vary with age, sex, and level of activity, but the ratio among the servings should remain the same. It is important to maintain the balance among the groups and variety within the groups.

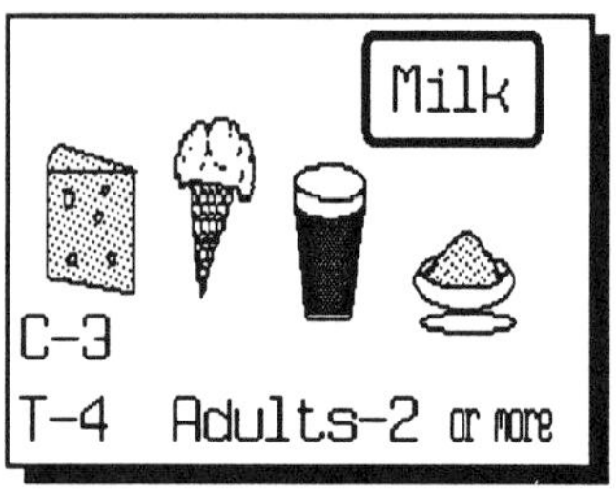

- <u>Milk group</u>. Adults should have two servings each day from milk and milk products. For people who are concerned about calories or dietary fat, skim or 2% milk is best. Children and teenagers should have three or four servings per day. A cup of milk, eight ounces of yogurt, or two ounces of cheese is a serving.

- **Meat group**. People should have two servings from the meat group each day. Two ounces of cooked lean meat, fish, poultry, or cheddar cheese is one serving. Two eggs, one-half cup cottage cheese, one cup dried beans or peas, or four tablespoons peanut butter is a serving.

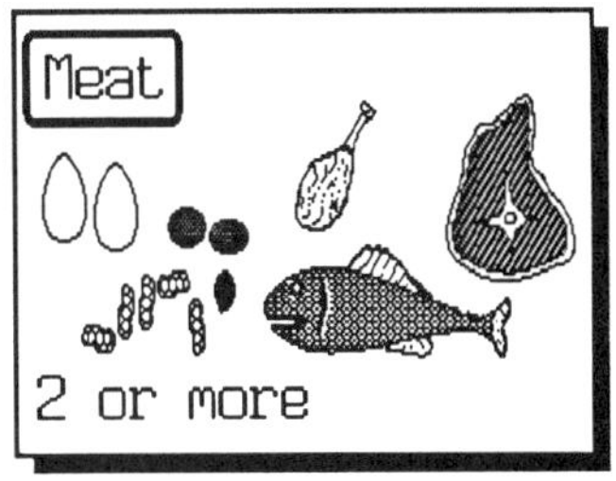

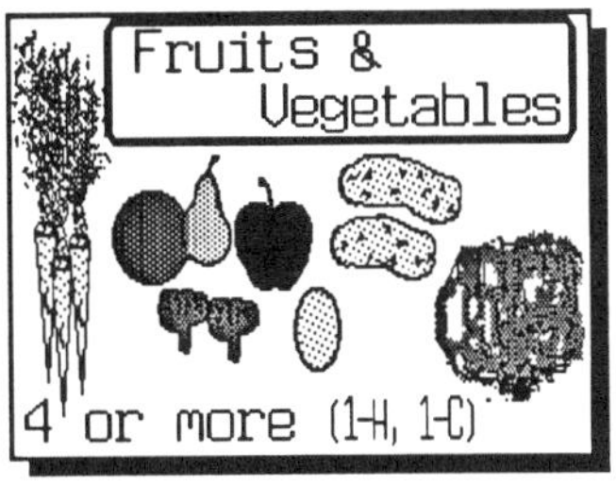

- **Fruit and vegetable group**. Adults should have four servings each day from the fruit and vegetable group. One of those servings should be a source of Vitamin C, and another should be a source of Vitamin A. One-half cup of cooked or chopped vegetables or fruit equals a serving; if raw, one serving would be one cup. A whole apple, orange or banana, a half grapefruit, a melon wedge, or one-half cup berries is one serving.

- **Grain and cereal group**. People should have four servings from the grain and cereal group. A slice of bread, a roll, a muffin, or a biscuit, one-half cup of cooked cereal, rice, or pasta, or one ounce of dry cereal is one serving. It is best if one or more servings come from a whole or enriched grain product.

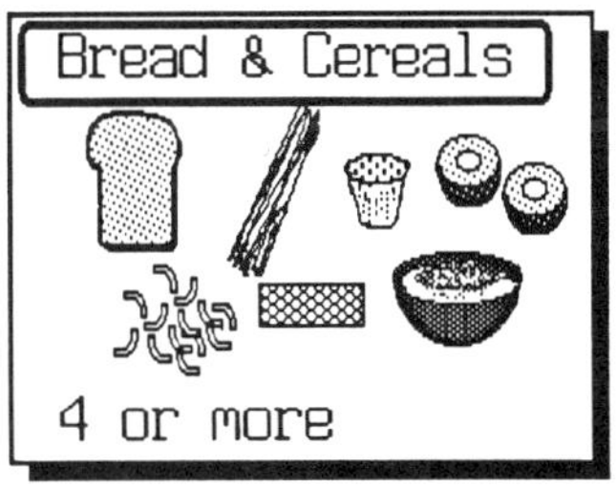

DIETARY GUIDELINES

These guidelines were published jointly by the U.S. Department of Agriculture and the U.S. Department of Health and Human Services and are based on the most frequent dietary problems in the United States. These guidelines are intended to provide healthy Americans with sensible, uncomplicated guidance on the kinds of foods they should be eating. These guidelines are based on current scientific information and this evidence does not support more specific advice for the general public. These guidelines are suggested for most Americans and do not apply to people who need special diets because of disease or conditions that interfere with normal nutrition.

> **DIETARY GUIDELINES**
> For Americans
>
> 1. Eat A Variety of Foods
> 2. Maintain Ideal Weight
> 3. Avoid Too Much Fat, Saturated Fat, & Cholesterol
> 4. Eat Foods With Adequate Starch and Fiber
> 5. Avoid Too Much Sugar
> 6. Avoid Too Much Salt
> 7. Don't Drink Alcohol
>   If You Drink, Do So In Moderation

1. Eat a variety of foods. You need about 40 different nutrients to stay healthy. These nutrients are in the foods you normally eat. Most foods contain more than one nutrient. No single food supplies all the nutrients you need; therefore, you should eat a variety of foods. There are no advantages in consuming excess amounts of any nutrient. You will not need to take a vitamin or mineral supplement if you eat a variety of foods. Important exceptions are infants, the elderly, pregnant women, those who are breast-feeding, or those who have an iron deficiency.

2. Maintain ideal weight. If you are overweight, your chances of developing some chronic disease are increased. To lose weight, you must take in fewer calories than you burn. This means eating less or increasing activity, or both. Increase activity gradually. Do not try to lose weight too rapidly--no more than 1 to 2 pounds per week. Avoid crash diets; eat smaller portions of normal food. A pound of fat contains 3500 calories. If you burn 500 calories a day more than you consume, you will lose a pound a week. To improve eating habits, eat slowly, eat smaller portions, and avoid seconds. To lose weight, increase activity and eat less fats and sweets.

3. Avoid too much fat, saturated fat, and cholesterol. A person who has a high blood cholesterol level has a greater chance of having a heart attack. Reducing the intake of total fat, saturated fat, and cholesterol tends to lower the blood cholesterol level. This is especially appropriate for people who have high blood pressure or who smoke. This does not prohibit any specific food items as long as they are eaten in moderation and as long as the overall cholesterol intake is not excessive. Choose lean meat, poultry, fish, and dried peas and beans. Moderate your use of eggs. Limit cream, butter, coconut oil, shortenings, and hydrogenated margarine. Broil, bake, or boil; don't fry. Trim excess fats off meat. Read labels to determine the type and amount of fat.

4. **Eat foods with adequate starch and fiber.** Carbohydrates have less than half as many calories per ounce as do fats. Complex carbohydrates are better than simple carbohydrates. Simple sugars have many calories, but few other nutrients. Complex starches have additional nutrients besides calories. Complex carbohydrates also contain dietary fiber. The average American diet is low in fiber. Substitute starches for fats and sugars. Select foods which are good sources of fiber and starch such as whole grains and cereals, fruits and vegetables, and beans, peas, and nuts.

5. **Avoid too much sugar.** The major health hazard from eating too much sugar is tooth decay. Although there is no strong evidence that sugar causes diabetes, heart attacks, or blood vessel disease, there is no conclusive evidence that it does not. Therefore, since sugar serves no real need (except as a source of calories), and since it may cause some harm, it is foolish to use much of it. To avoid too much sugar use less of all sugars--white, brown, raw, honey, and syrups. Use less food containing sugar--candy, soft drinks, ice cream, cake, and cookies. Read food labels for sugar--sucrose, glucose, maltose, dextrose, lactose and fructose. Select fresh fruits or fruits canned in light syrup.

6. **Avoid too much sodium.** Table salt contains both sodium and chloride--both are essential elements. Although a small amount of sodium is needed, too much is bad. The major hazard of excessive sodium is for people with high blood pressure, and in the U. S. high blood pressure is common (17%). Since there is no good way to predict who will develop high blood pressure, and since a low sodium diet might be a way to help prevent it and an important way to treat it, it may be wise to learn how to avoid too much sodium. Learn how to enjoy the unsalted flavor of food. Cook with small amounts of salt and add no or little salt at the table. Read the labels and limit the intake of salty foods such as potato chips, pretzels, salted nuts, popcorn, cheese, pickled foods, cured meats, and soy or steak sauce.

7. **If you drink alcohol, do so in moderation.** Alcoholic beverages are high in calories and low in other nutrients. Drinkers may need to drink less if they wish to lose weight. Heavy drinkers may lose their appetite for food. They get too many calories from the alcohol, but not enough of the essential nutrients. Heavy drinking may cause a variety of serious conditions such as cirrhosis of the liver and neurological disorders. Excessive alcohol consumption by pregnant women has caused birth defects. Therefore, it is better not to drink alcoholic beverages, or if you do drink alcohol, do so in moderation.

NUTRITIONAL QUACKERY

People who are overweight have a higher rate of illness and death. Weight should be fairly stable after age 25. For optimum health, it is important to maintain approximately one's ideal weight. However, fad or crash diets where weight is lost and rapidly gained back again may be worse than remaining overweight.

When one's weight begins to increase above the ideal, it is time to taper off in how much is eaten. But whether controlling or reducing weight, it is wise to follow a sensible plan. One should continue to eat a variety of foods from the four food groups, the same foods he will want to eat throughout life, but modify the amounts. The calories should be low enough to cause a weight loss. A person should find out how many calories he is eating normally, and then cut it back 500 to 1000 calories per day, making sure to eat at least 1200 calories daily. Foods which are high in calories but provide few other nutrients should be eliminated.

Characteristics of

Nutritional Quackery

1. Distrusts the "Establishment"
2. Promotes a "Special" food product.
3. Says "Disease is due to Faulty Diet."
4. Speaks of "Subclinical Deficiencies."
5. Speaks of "Soil Depletion."
6. Says "Processing removes most nutrients."
7. Promotes Vitamin and Mineral "Supplements."
8. Claims "Natural or Organic" foods are Better.
9. Promotes Products with "Testimonials."
10. Claims Persecution by "Orthodox Medicine."

People who have or suspect an accompanying illness and people who need to lose a great deal of weight should consult a physician before starting a weight reduction plan. Two pounds per week of actual fat weight loss, not water or lean muscle, is considered maximum without a physician's supervision. Likewise, a diet of less than 1200 calories per day for women or 1500 calories per day for men should not be attempted unless one is under the careful care of a physician. An exercise program is also an important part of a weight loss program. It burns a few calories, adds tone to the muscles, and provides an emotional stimulus to the program.

It is generally not necessary to take special nutritional supplements. It is better to get the nutrients from the foods than from a pill or other form. So-called health foods are not only more expensive but may provide a false sense of security that may actually lead one to poorer nutrition. If one has a special health problem, he should be under the care of a physician and not left to the follies of self-medication or improvised nutrition. Claims for health foods, natural foods, or organic foods are difficult to substantiate. It is estimated that only about half of the information printed about nutrition is accurate, the rest ranges from fallacy to quackery. Food choices should be based on scientific information, not fads and fallacies. Vitamin pills, herbs, and other food supplements are legally marketed as foods not medications, but people usually take them for medical benefits. Such medical claims cannot be advertised or placed on the label. Teachers have the right to personal food choices that may not be based on scientific evidence, but the promotion of such choices among their students would verge on quackery.

EATING DISORDERS

There is an apparent link between self-concept in relationship to sexuality and eating disorders. Eating disorders may be considered as a type of psychosomatic disorder. There is an emotional problem that is often well hidden as well as the physical complications. The eating disorders that will be dealt with here are anorexia nervosa, bulimia, and obesity.

ANOREXIA NERVOSA

Anorexia is not a new phenomenon, though most people had not heard of it ten years ago. It was described in the 1600s and again in the late 1800s, but in the last decade it has come on like an epidemic. Anorexia is a disease of the affluent; few cases have been reported among the poor. Most of the cases are among young women of high school and college age. A 1985 report said there were at least 300,000 and perhaps twice that number of anorexics in the United States. One out of every 250 adolescents are anorexics, and as many as 15 percent of victims die from it. At least 85 percent of the anorexics are girls and women. The few male victims get involved through such pursuits as trying to meet weight for wrestling competition or to maintain an appropriate figure for a college dance team. Drill teams and pep squads have also triggered their share of anorexia.

Some experts say there are no typical cases of anorexia; each case is unique. But if there were a typical case, it would be a middle-class or well-to-do female, a second or third child in the family, and a quiet, cooperative, high achiever. What begins with a desire to lose weight turns into an obsession with food. She develops a fascination with food, reading recipes, and counting calories, but a revulsion toward eating. She may also exercise fanatically. No matter how thin she becomes, she sees a distorted image of herself and believes she is still too fat. For this, she feels guilty, so she exercises even more and accepts less food. Her condition is marked by a terror of getting fat or a desire to achieve extraordinary thinness.

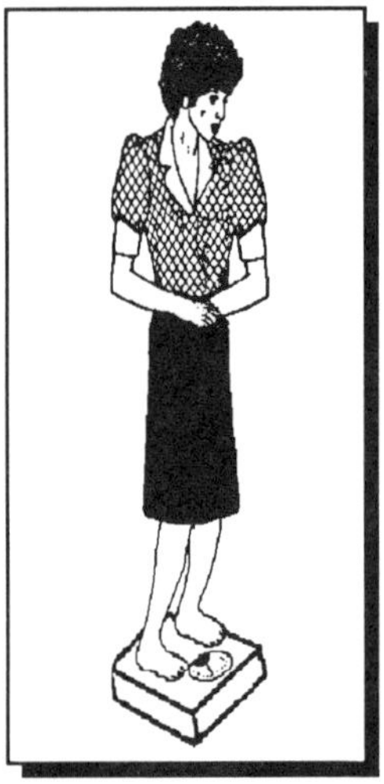

The anorexic often was a child who desired very much to please others, was highly motivated to achieve, was obedient, well liked, accomplished academically, and one with special talents. Still, the anorexics felt some difficulty in reaching a vague level of expectation. No matter how hard they tried or how successful they became, they felt their performance remained a few steps below the accomplishments of a sibling or other rival. Yet they show no signs of rebellion against siblings, peers, parents, or other people in authority. They remain overly compliant and anxious to please.

Most cases of anorexia are associated with an identity problem. The anorexic is trying desperately to create a new image. She may be striving for achievement. She may be in silent competition with a sibling whose achievements, she feels, are more recognized than her own. Or she may be in competition with an image she feels her parents are trying to make her into. Perhaps the mother is trying to live out her own dreams through her daughter. While on one hand she tries valiantly to achieve, on the other hand she feels like her life is out of her control. She tries desperately to retain one area of control, what food enters her body. She would rather give up her life than surrender that area of control. Anorexia becomes a deep-seated emotional problem that requires expert help and much family cooperation. Even with expert help this condition is difficult to treat.

The acute stages of anorexia are painful even to imagine. It is very much like starvation. There is a loss of at least 25 percent of body weight and an electrolyte imbalance occurs. Her body becomes emaciated, and her hair becomes thin. Her skin becomes dry, flaky, and covered with a downy hair called lanugo. Menstruation stops (amenorrhea), and she may become permanently sterile. Constipation occurs, and she is unable to move her bowels. Her pulse, temperature, and blood pressure become abnormal. She loses so much weight and padding that it becomes painful to walk or sit. Kidney disease sets in and this may be the cause of death.

Some of the physical problems begin once the amount of fat in the body gets approximately 20 percent below normal. An electrolyte imbalance results in the following physical conditions:

- Constipation --loss of ability to move the bowels.
- Amenorrhea --the cessation of menstruation.
- Change in hair, skin, and nails.

- Change in heart rhythm and metabolic rate.

- Kidney disease (often the cause of death).

The anorexic needs expert medical and psychological help, the sooner the better. She needs help for the medical complications and help in resolving the underlying psychological problems. Because of the psychological complications and the newness of the disorder, anorexia is difficult to treat. Few psychologists have real expertise in dealing with this disease. Often the whole family needs to be involved in the treatment, not that the family is at fault for the problem, but their help is needed to deal with it. It often requires a long term follow-up, but approximately half of all diagnosed and treated anorexics recover fully within two to five years.

No doubt society's infatuation with thinness today contributes to the problem. So much has been said about the problems of obesity that there is a strong tendency for some people to go overboard in the other direction. Again the problem deals with a distorted image, this time somewhat imposed by society. Schools must do what they can to remedy society's misconception about thinness and help prevent the problem. School activities, such as drill teams, should not contribute to the problem. Schools also need to be alert to recognizing potential victims so that intervention may take place.

BULIMIA

It is estimated that 1 million Americans suffer from bulimia. About 95 percent of these are women, and most of them are between age 13 and 40. However, instances of bulimia and anorexia among men is on the increase. Some anorexics use bulimic methods to achieve their anorexic state. Bulimia is characterized by episodes of voracious eating or binging followed by purges to get rid of the food and avoid weight gain. They may get rid of the food by inducing vomiting or by using laxatives, or both. There is a distinction between bulimia and bulimic behavior. For example, wrestlers sometimes engage in bulimic behavior to try to meet weight requirements without having the psychological characteristics of a true bulimic.

Bulimics often have the same motivation and background as anorexics, an overwhelming desire for thinness. They both share a desire for perfection, and both are found primarily among young women, although there are a few male bulimics and fewer anorexics.

While anorexics consume incredibly small amounts of food, the bulimic consumes incredibly large masses of food. Some bulimics mimic anorexics between episodes of binging. Anorexics have tremendous control over their eating, but bulimics are noted for their overwhelming loss of control. They gorge to the point of pain, purge, and start over. Another important difference is their perception of their eating habits. The anorexics do not regard their eating habits as abnormal. The bulimic recognizes his abnormal eating patterns and carries a great burden of guilt. Deception and dishonesty to keep others from finding out becomes a part of their life.

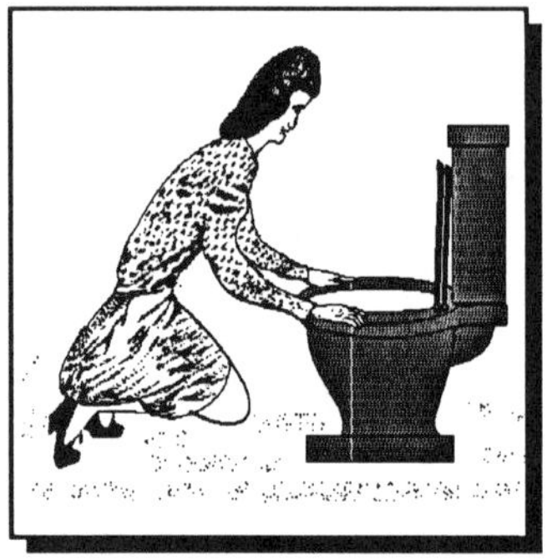

The bulimic is usually at normal weight or slightly above; therefore, they do not have the physical problems associated with starvation. But they do have many other physical problems associated the fluid loss due to either method of purging. There are also problems associated with frequent vomiting.

- Rapid tooth decay and ulcers in the gums and mouth due to the acid in the vomit.

- Puffiness in the face and ruptured blood vessels around the eyes as a result of forceful vomiting.

- Constipation due to the loss of mobility in the bowels because of the extensive use of laxatives.

- Dilation and stretching of the stomach due to the severe gorging and purging.

- Dehydration or fluid loss from the frequent purging causes an electrolyte imbalance in the body.

Bulimics frequently suffer severe depression, anxiety, stress, guilt, and low self-esteem. Treatment must be multifaceted to help the victim learn how to deal with these feelings. The family may also need to be involved. Hospitalization may be needed to stabilize the physical problems. If this is followed by competent psychological counseling, most bulimics can be helped to overcome their problems.

OBESITY

Overweight and obesity conditions are also associated with emotional problems and a negative self-concept; not that they are motivated to become overweight, but because eating becomes an emotional outlet. Then they become depressed because they are overweight, but the outlet for this depression is still eating. The problem is cyclic--

the poor self-concept contributes to obesity and obesity contributes to the poor self-concept.

On the average, obesity causes three times the normal risk of death. Obesity may be associated with the following physical health problems:

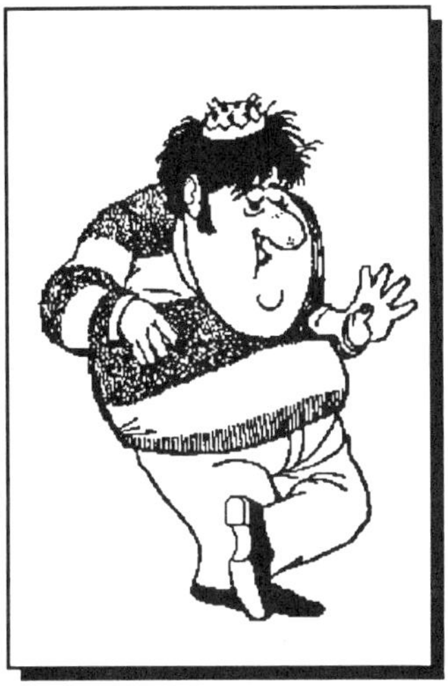

- High blood pressure. If a person is under the age of 45 and is obese, he stands a 5.6 times greater risk of developing high blood pressure.
- Heart disease. Overweight conditions, even a few extra pounds, increases the risk of heart disease.
- Cancer. People who are 60 percent above ideal weight have twice the cancer rate.
- Diabetes. Obesity increases the risk of adult onset type diabetes.
- Other. Obesity is associated with an increased risk of developing orthopedic and other health problems.

Most people sooner or later in life will have some concerns about weight control. It is important for them to avoid the unrealistic expectations that are often promoted by magazine articles and advertisements about ideal weight and about diets and weight control. One should develop a realistic expectation of what your body build ought to be. Realize that most models are not as thin as they appear to be; they rely on trick photography and photographic touch up work. Many of the height/weight charts may be unrealistic for your body build. The current emphasis on thinness is dangerous. Accept the body build nature and genetics has blessed you with.

One should also set a long term main goal for next year, not next week. The goal should be, "take it off and keep it off." Then set intermediate goals so you can monitor your progress, but have the goals far enough apart so you can see some progress. It is realistic to expect an average one and a half to two (1-1/2 - 2) pounds loss per week on a long term weight modification program. It is unrealistic to expect much more. One should keep the total body composition in mind. Some programs may produce water loss, but that is negligible at best and very dangerous if dehydration occurs. Some programs may result in the loss of proteins found in the lean body mass, and that is not only undesirable, but also dangerous. An effective body weight management program will involve both diet and activity. Why are most overweight children overweight? Not because they eat too much, but because they do not exercise enough. They do not eat any more than their healthier classmates, but they do not exercise as much. Exercise has many benefits, but perhaps the most important is the improvement in emotional health. Exercise can do wonders for the self-concept.

WHAT CAN THE SCHOOLS DO?

The role of the school in dealing with eating disorders includes all three phases of the school health program.

- Providing a healthy school climate which promotes the development of a healthy self-concept and thus helps prevent these problems.
- Providing health and nutrition education gives the students specific information about proper nutrition, the existence of eating disorders, how to prevent and recognize them, and how to get help.
- Provide health services that will--through teacher observation, screening procedures, and medical examinations--be able to recognize possible eating disorders and provide proper counseling and referral.

PHYSICAL FITNESS

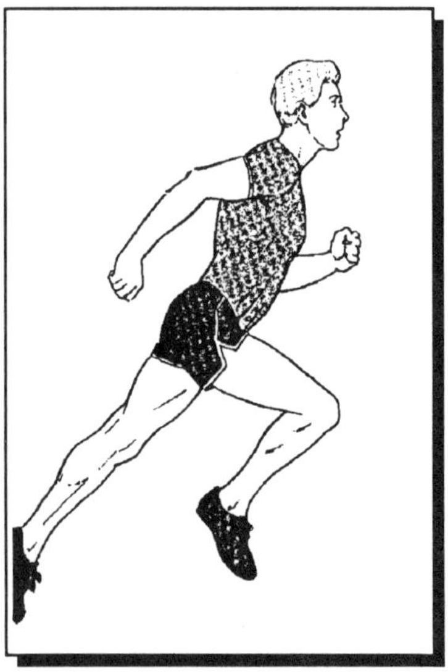

Physically active people of all ages tend to be healthier than their sedentary counterparts. Physical fitness is an important component of total health. Although a person can be physically fit and still have a serious physical or physiological disorder, a person cannot have optimal health without being physically fit. Health is more than the absence of a negative, it is the presence of the positive. Physical fitness is a positive. It is achieved not by passive avoidance of problems, but by actively pursuing life at its fullest.

A person who is physically fit has sufficient energy to perform life's normal tasks with vigor left to meet emergencies and enjoy leisure. A physically fit person not only stands straight and moves with power, but also thinks alertly, has a bright outlook on life, and relates well with other people. Physically active people have fewer incidents of disease and disability. Inactivity, on the other hand, seems to increase the eventual risk of the following diseases: hypertension, heart disease, osteopetrosis, adult onset diabetes, muscular atrophy, being overweight, depression, and other emotional problems.

USE IT OR LOSE IT

The statement "Use it or lose it" refers to a principle of nature sometimes called *The Law of Use or Non-Use.* It means that the body tends to maintain those parts that are being used and get rid of those that are not used. This principle of use or non-use applies more to some parts of the body than to others. A sad but dramatic example would be an athlete with well-developed leg muscles who suffers an accident and becomes paralyzed. Soon the unused leg muscles atrophy and become smaller. Although a person does not lose muscle cells, the size of each cell diminishes and the muscle becomes weak. But this affects more than the leg muscles. When the legs are not used, the heart is not exercised and cardiovascular fitness will also be diminished. Other examples of how the level of use may affect body parts and processes include the following:

- The number of red blood cells decreases with inactivity.
- The metabolic rate increases with activity.
- Bone thickness and density increases with exercise.
- Activity increases the ratio of High Density Lipoprotein.
- Fitness training tends to increase artery size and profusion.

TYPES OF FITNESS

Of the four major types of fitness, cardiovascular fitness is most important to total health.

Cardiovascular Endurance

Cardiovascular endurance is the ability of the heart, lungs, and circulatory system to provide the cells of the body with the substances necessary to perform work for an extended period of time. The term *aerobic*, meaning with the use of oxygen, has to do with the capacity to utilize oxygen. Aerobic fitness occurs as a person engages in exercises requiring hard breathing for an extended period of time. Some of the benefits of fitness training are the following:

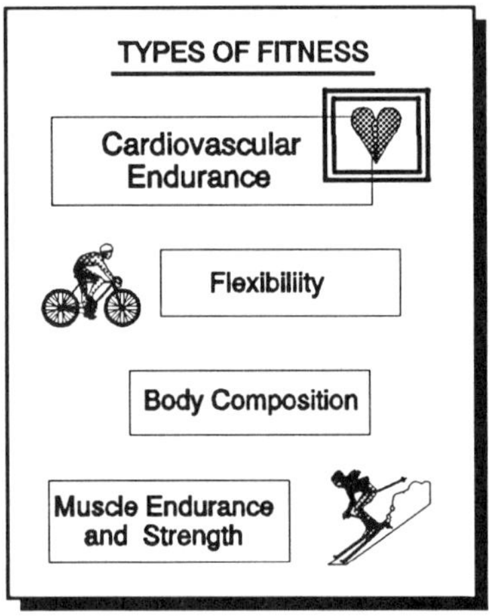

- The resting heart rate is decreased.
- The heart can rest longer between beats.
- The respiratory rate decreases.
- The breathing recovery rate following exercise is decreased.
- The number of capillaries in the body is increased.
- The size of the coronary arteries increases.
- The red blood cell count increases.
- The length of the exercise period can be extended.
- The heart stroke volume increases as the heart becomes stronger.

Muscular Endurance and Strength

Strength is the ability of a group of muscles to exert a force against resistance. Endurance is the ability of a group of muscles to repeat performances over a period of time. Sufficient muscular strength and endurance should be maintained to perform everyday tasks efficiently. An increase in muscle cell size, called *hypertrophy*, occurs with exercise which increases resistance. Without maintenance exercise, *atrophy*, or the decrease in size of muscle cells, occurs.

Flexibility and Agility

Flexibility is the range of movement of a joint or joints. Inflexible people are accident prone. Agility is the ability to move quickly and gracefully. Stretching exercises and activities using all muscle groups and a full range of movement at all joints is important.

Body Composition

Body composition is the ratio of fat to lean muscle and bone. It deals with shape and proportion of the body. Achieving proper body composition requires a combined diet and exercise program.

PRINCIPLES OF CARDIOVASCULAR FITNESS

A person will benefit to some extent from even a small amount of exercise. Inactive older people can benefit a great deal if they start to do just a small amount of exercise. In spite of its benefits, exercise is not without its risks. Each person should try to find a level of exercise where the benefits are greater, and the risks are lower. This level varies from person to person and from time to time. Experts agree that exercise is beneficial, but they do not agree as to precisely how much exercise is needed to protect the heart from coronary disease. The majority agree on the following principles of cardiovascular exercise:

START — Start out slowly and work up gradually. Warm-ups and cool-downs are important. Inactive people beyond age thirty-five should have a medical evaluation including an electrocardiogram before starting an exercise program.

EXERCISE — Mode: -- large muscle groups, legs.
Frequency: -- 3 to 5 times a week.
Duration: -- 15 to 60 minutes.
Intensity: -- heart rate at 60-80% of maximum.
(maximum = 220 minus age)

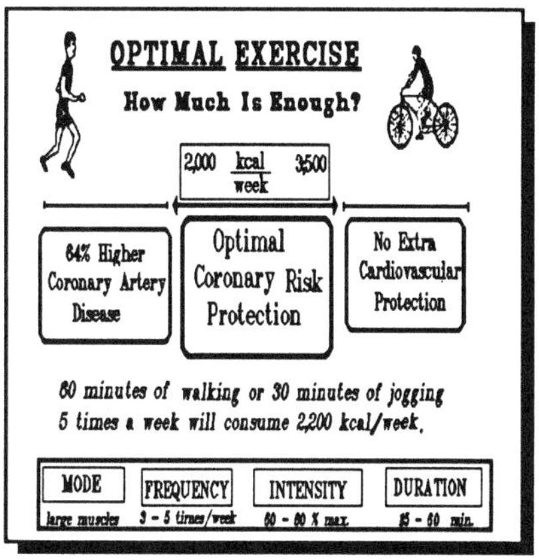

There seems to be an *optimal* level or *window* of exercise with maximum benefits and minimum risk. Exercise below that level will not produce significant improvements in cardiovascular fitness. Consistent moderate exercise will reduce the risk of coronary artery disease; but more than moderate exercise confers no additional benefits and may engender greater risks.

A Harvard study correlating levels of activity and coronary artery disease found that a 2,000 kcal/week was optimal. Men who exercised at that level had fewer incidents of coronary artery disease, but no further significant reduction occurred with exercise above that level. The threshold for lowering risk starts at 150 kcal per day and continues to 400 kcal per day. Sixty minutes of brisk walking or thirty minutes of mild jogging five times a week will consume approximately 2,200 kcal per week. Optimal exercise benefits can be obtained by walking or jogging 10 to 15 miles per week.

There are also a number of fallacies associated with exercise. The following list may expose some of them:

- Newspapers tell of people who die while exercising, but this can be misleading because usually the death is not due to exercising. There may have been a pre-existing condition, and exercising may have prolonged their life.

- Muscle development will impair flexibility--you will be muscle bound (not if you do stretches as well as lift weights).

- Exercising causes unwanted muscle definition in women (not unless they take male hormones).

- Muscles will turn to fat when you stop exercising. (Muscle cells do not turn to fat cells, but muscles will get smaller and fat deposits larger if a person stops exercising and continues to eat the same.)

- No pain, no gain. (There is a distinction between pain and discomfort. Pain is a warning sign of an injury that needs possible medical care.)

- Joggers are always getting hit by cars. (Perhaps the euphoria experienced by exercisers distracts them from following safety precautions.)

- Some people become addicted to exercise. (There are compulsive exercisers. They lose perspective and exercising becomes an end in itself, rather than a means. Instead of exercise being a balancing factor in their lives, it becomes a way of escaping. But this may be better than some other forms of social and emotional maladjustment.)

- Fitness centers are a big rip-off. (Many people spend a great deal of money for little benefit at fitness centers, but that may be more their fault than a problem with the fitness center. They may be motivated by social status, or succumb to a fancy but unrealistic sales pitch. We must be wise consumers. Often people get caught up in fancy apparel. Good shoes are a justifiable expense. Physical fitness need not be expensive. It is exercise--not money spent--that brings fitness.)

- People who exercise are always getting hurt. (Sometimes the excitement of the competition gets in the way of common sense. Often it is the weekend athlete--not the regular exerciser who works into condition gradually--who gets injured. Common sense, good equipment, and proper rest are important. Wisdom and moderation are the keys.)

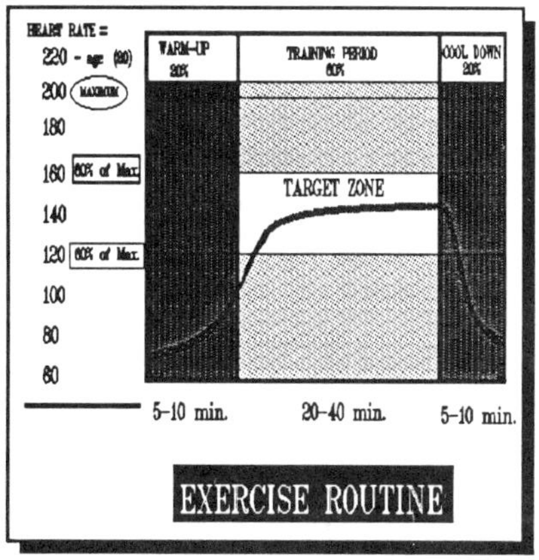

EXERCISE ROUTINE

While all of these types of fitness are important, for most people cardiopulmonary endurance is most important. It is the ability of the body to provide adequate nutrition and oxygen to the cells and to carry the waste products away from the cells over a sustained period of time. This results from being aerobically fit. To achieve this, a person needs exercise that will make him breathe hard. Swimming, jogging, rope jumping, running in place, and bicycling are good examples of aerobic exercises. A person needs at least 15 minutes of vigorous exercise of this type at least four times a week. Vigorous exercise is when the heart rate exceeds 150 beats per minute. The pulse is taken in the groove at the side of the neck. Take the pulse for 10 seconds and multiply by six to get the beats per minute.

A person who is not in shape needs to start out gradually. If he has been out of shape for long, he should have a physical examination and get a doctor's advice for an exercise program, particularly if he is over age 35. If he is going to jog, for example, he should start out walking a half hour a day to get his leg muscles in shape. After a month, he will be ready to jog and walk alternately. A formula for determining the exercise level he should follow is:

> Subtract your age from 220 and then multiply that figure by .60 and by .80 (percent). The numbers you get are the minimum and maximum rates for the exercising heart.

Soon he will be able to keep right on jogging and be able to complete a mile and a half in 15 minutes. The 15 minutes of vigorous activity should be preceded by a warm-up activity until the person begins to sweat and followed by a cooling-down period of activity until his breathing is at a normal rate.

TEACHERS' HEALTH

Teachers should not only encourage their students to maintain a physical fitness program, but they should also maintain good physical health themselves. The best teaching is by example. Any teacher, no matter what the subject, can find opportunities to give students instruction on the "whys" and "hows" of maintaining physical fitness. Physical fitness is also important for teachers. Teachers with a high level of health will usually do a more effective job than those who have a low level of health. Poor physical fitness is a chronic problem of teachers. A physical fitness program for teachers is important therapy for emotional stress. It is a means of getting their otherwise sedentary bodies going. A teacher may feel at the end of a hard day that he or she is too tired to exercise; however, exercise will usually make him or her feel less tired. Waste products that have accumulated in the body through a day of inactivity make a person feel tired. The increased heart rate of exercising will get the waste products into circulation and out of the body. It will also get the oxygen and blood sugar into the cells and make the person feel less tired.

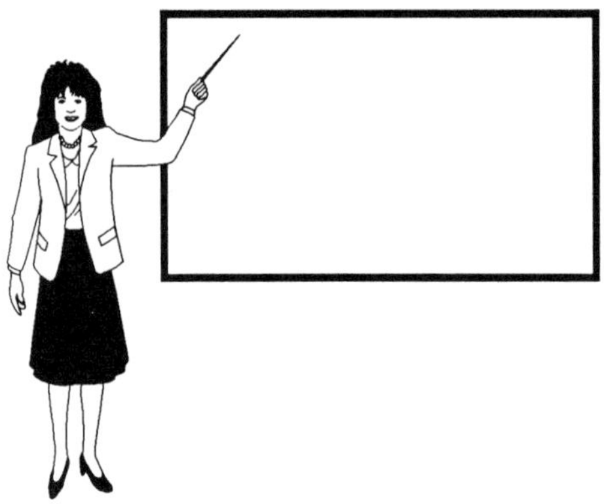

Statistical evidence suggests that the health of teachers as a group compares very favorably with that of other groups of workers and of the general population. The death rate of teachers is consistently among the very lowest recorded for any occupation. The disorders which rank highest in causing illness among teachers are respiratory infections (particularly colds), digestive disorders, and nervousness.

It has been estimated that colds are responsible for more than half of all absences from work due to sickness and injuries. Colds spread rapidly because most people are susceptible and few people isolate themselves. Parents are urged to keep their children home from school at the first signs of respiratory illness, both for the sake of the child and for suppression of the spread of airborne infection in the school. Unfortunately, most people, including teachers, are prone to ignore a cold as a legitimate cause of absence from work. It may be difficult for young people to reconcile what they learn from teachers and health textbooks about colds with what they see many teachers doing--or not doing--about their colds.

An article in the *Instructor*, September, 1976, asks the question in its title "Is Teaching Hazardous to Your Health?" The following quote was taken from that article. It illustrates the teacher's daily routine.

If you're the average teacher, you get up at 6 a.m., grab coffee (possibly toast and juice), tend to home tasks, and then with books in hand rush out the door. While battling traffic, you review lesson plans, remind yourself of details that must be attended to once you arrive, and make notes to yourself at stoplights.

Once at school you shove desks and chairs into place, haul 20 kilos of books off the shelves, rearrange learning centers, cart science equipment to your room, balance yourself on a chair to put finishing touches on a bulletin board--all before the kids arrive.

Your morning is productive but hectic. At lunch you eat with 25 kids and worry about your weight as you bolt down your food. No time to slip off to the teachers' lounge to relax--you have playground (or hall) duty in five minutes. The afternoon rushes by in spite of your headache. The kids leave--all except Stuart, who has lost his lunch pail (or book). You find it, send him off, and hope to have five tranquil minutes before Mrs. Webster arrives for a parent conference. But Mrs. Webster, anxious to discuss . . . this or that, is always early.

After she finally leaves, you stay another hour preparing for tomorrow. Preparations can't be made in an hour, so you drag the work home. You'll finish after dinner.

By the end of your day, you've made as many decisions as a Fortune 500 executive. You've directed as many comings and goings as an air traffic controller at O'Hare. You've walked X miles around the school treating your feet like those of an umpire who calls a 27 inning game. Your vocal cords have been worked out not unlike those of Beverly Sills (an opera star) in a rehearsal. Your eyes have performed like those of a Tiffany gem cutter. The physical energy you have expended would wear out a construction worker, and the mental stress and strain matches that of a family doctor except that he sees one person at a time and by appointment only. Do you still wonder about your headache? Is teaching hazardous to your health?

The term "nervousness" covers a multitude of unpleasant symptoms, such as indigestion, headache, and serious personality disorders of various kinds. Some of them are caused by conditions that teachers themselves can remedy by improved personal health practices. The continual adjustment of a mature mind to what is going on in each of many immature minds is bound to consume nervous energy. But the healthy, well-adjusted teacher seems to have a little spring of fresh water which continuously replenishes his reserve of physical energy and intellectual enthusiasm. Healthy minds and bodies possess reserves of strength and recuperative powers. These reserves are needed to compensate for the normal wear and tear of mind and body. These reserves can be conserved by sensible regard for health practices that permit the body and mind to replenish depleted stores of energy.

Mental health problems are one of the most common reasons for teachers missing work. A teacher's emotional problems can also have the most negative effect on students. *Emotional problems* can be manifest in a variety of conditions including feeling tired and blue, moodiness, headaches, depression, and anxiety. Too much pressure, or an inability to cope with problems, may bring tension-related aches and pains.

According to some observers, the problem of *alcoholism* appears to be on the increase among teachers. Co-workers are sometimes guilty of overlooking and covering up the signs of a drinking problem. Alcoholism is also on the increase in other professions. Programs to help the alcoholic employee have been developed in many businesses but not so in schools.

The *common cold and respiratory problems* are a frequent cause of teacher absence, particularly among first-year teachers who have not been around children enough to be exposed and build up an immunity. A cold may be the body's subconscious way of demanding rest and relief. It is also more acceptable for the teacher to say "I have a cold" than to say "I can't cope, and I need rest."

Another frequent complaint of teachers is *stomach problems*. Many teachers start to develop ulcers and colitis after a few years of teaching. They start to rely on antacids to keep down the stomach pain. The more hectic the day, the more antacids are needed. At the same time, they become more impatient with students and less able to work cooperatively with fellow teachers.

Foot problems and orthopedic conditions are also a frequent complaint of teachers. In this category are problems ranging from corns, bunions, bursitis and arthritis, and protruding intervertebral discs. Being overweight, having poor muscle tone, poor posture, and ill-fitting shoes can contribute to this problem. These pains can also make a teacher tired and short-tempered.

Many teachers have *vision and hearing problems* without realizing it. Hearing loss particularly can go unnoticed because it occurs so gradually. Stressful efforts to see may cause tension. Classroom activities may be hampered if the teacher has difficulty hearing his students.

Many teachers are *overweight*, and this can put a greater burden on the heart, blood vessels, and lungs. Overweight teachers are frequently tired in class. The daily hot lunch in the school cafeteria is often overlaid with calories, and the friendly lunchroom manager often invites the teachers to have extra dessert.

Even things as wonderful as *pregnancy* can cause its problems. School policies cannot discriminate against women because they are pregnant. Absence because of pregnancy, childbearing, and child care requires a well-planned substitute placement program to minimize the disruption caused by teacher absence.

The school administration can do much to help teachers stay healthy. The American School Health Association says that each district should have:

1. Explicit personnel policies with regard to health as it affects employee hiring, continuing contracts, and termination.

2. Pre-employment evaluations of employees by questionnaire and physical examination.

3. A school district physician or medical consultant to deal with employee health problems and medical reports.

4. A preventive health program including screening and referral programs, health counseling and workshops on specific health problems, and fitness and exercise programs.

The school principal can be the best ally or worst enemy to a teacher's health. If a teacher has a principal who criticizes, never compliments, and creeps around corners rather than being open, then morale will drop and absenteeism will increase. If a teacher works with a principal who cares, who cooperates with the faculty, and who creates a supportive environment, then the teacher will feel positively reinforced and emotionally rewarded. Administrators should encourage a number of activities and conditions which will promote teacher health.

Teaching loads should not be excessive and teachers should have mid-morning and mid-afternoon breaks. Teachers should also have a lunch hour with minimum responsibilities. Teachers should have access to a teachers' lounge and restrooms for relaxation. Good breaks yield better quality of work. The schools should have a required periodic health examination for all employees. Teachers should have adequate sick leave with pay and health insurance. Teachers should be able to earn tenure and have good retirement provisions. The schools should make gymnasium facilities available to teachers, and there should be opportunities for sports activities between teachers and teachers and between teachers and students.

A teacher can help keep himself physically and mentally fit by following these suggestions:

- Have regular medical and dental examinations.
- Eat nutritious and well-balanced meals and maintain the recommended weight.
- Exercise daily.
- Get sufficient rest.
- Maintain good posture.
- Maintain a positive attitude. Don't let personal problems carry over to the classroom, and don't let school preoccupy your life.
- Be good to yourself. Make time for hobbies and friends.
- Analyze your feelings about your job. If you are not happy, do something positive and within channels to make it better.

Teachers should seek opportunities to renew their vitality. Some teachers are inclined to neglect recreation that takes their minds off their work and helps to fulfill the need of all individuals to have a corner of life where they can be themselves and do what they as individuals enjoy doing. One of the obstacles standing in the way of free choice of recreation has been the goldfish-like existence which teachers in many communities have to lead, especially in small towns and rural areas. The recent emphasis on the individual rights and needs in a democratic society has made it easier for teachers to break out of the goldfish bowls and to swim more freely in community life. A teacher who can express himself in other interests besides his school work can return to his professional activities renewed and invigorated. A person should not build his life on only one interest. Nor should he or she have to select a form of exercise or recreation or hobbies because it is good for him or her; to do so turns leisure into work. Those things may be needed, but the recreation should be in addition.

Medical determination of the teacher's health status after certification and employment varies throughout the United States. Depending upon where the teacher is employed, an annual medical examination may be required, urged, mildly recommended, or not even mentioned by the school authorities. Left to their own devices, most teachers--like most other people--admit the importance of the periodic health examination but do not always appreciate its value fully enough to have one.

The social importance of teaching, no less than a proper regard for the protection of their own health, calls for the taking of a health inventory of teachers at regular intervals. The fact that they are in constant close contact with the students imposes, at the very least, the obligation to make sure they are not sources of infection. Authorities in tuberculosis insist, for example, "that all school personnel should be unequivocally certified as being free from communicable pulmonary tuberculosis before embarking upon the profession which brings them into close contact with numbers of children." They consider it equally important for teachers in service to be re-examined periodically to rule out the development of this infection.

Health in all its aspects is now considered to be fundamental to success in teaching. Health standards have been set up for admission to most professional schools for teachers, and good health is one of the requirements for teacher certification in a number of states. Many local school systems have established even higher health standards for employment than states require for certification. Although these standards deal with physical fitness and mental stability for the most part, there are numerous other virtues which are considered essential by almost everyone for sound ethical character--intelligence, honesty, emotional stability, and the ability to work well with others. These come under the heading of health in its broadest interpretation.

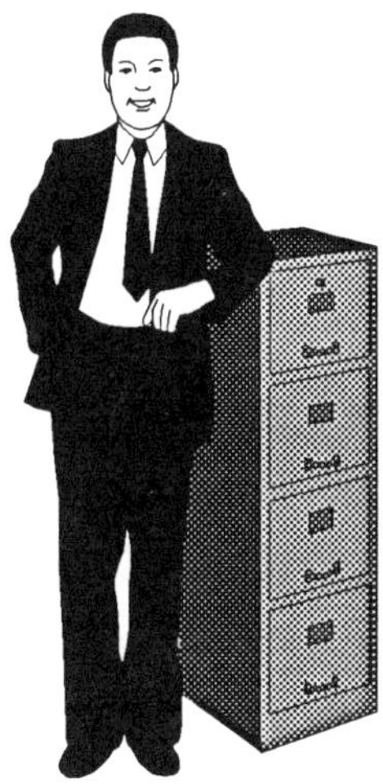

STUDY HELPS

1. What are the indicators of general physical health?
2. What are the ten habits that can help people enjoy good health?
3. What are some good reasons why we should study nutrition?
4. What are the seven nutrient groups and why are they required for good health?
5. What are the basic four food groups and what nutrients do they contain?
6. What are the seven points in the dietary guidelines?
7. What is wrong with most fad or crash diets?
8. Why is it best to get nutrients from food rather than from pills and supplements?
9. What is the problem associated with so-called natural, organic, or health foods?
10. How reliable are the printed sources on health information? What is quackery?
11. What is anorexia and what are the harmful physical consequences of anorexia?
12. What is bulimia and what are the harmful physical consequences of bulimia?
13. What problems might occur when a person becomes noticeably overweight?
14. What are some realistic expectations in respect to planned weight loss?
15. What is meant by the statement "Use it or lose it"?
16. What are the four major types of fitness, and which is most important to health?
17. What are the benefits associated with physical fitness?
18. What principles should be considered in planning a physical fitness program?
19. How does the health statistics for teachers compare with other professions?
20. What are the health problems experienced most frequently by teachers, and what can teachers do to avoid or minimize these problems?

Chapter 12

MATURATION AND ADOLESCENT SEXUALITY

The question of sex education has been one of the most controversial questions in the school curriculum. This chapter may help the prospective teacher deal with this question in his or her own mind; but more than that, it should help the teacher gain a perspective of the problems experienced by youth related to sexual development. The material which follows deals with the questions: "What is meant by sex?" and "What is the basis of sexual morality?"

UNDERSTANDING SEXUAL DEVELOPMENT

Learning about sexuality is a constant process. Beginning at birth, as the infant interacts with humans, he or she develops a sexual self-concept. A person's biological structure is inherited, but attitudes are learned. It is generally believed that children begin to develop their sexual attitudes early in life. Even before infants understand spoken language, perhaps they are able to register subtle feelings or attitudes. Perhaps their sexual self-concept starts to be influenced by the attitude displayed by their parents as they change a soiled diaper. Is this a messy, disgusting event, or is it a dispassionate hygienic routine? Throughout life, much of a person's sense of worth as an individual is tied to his or her sexual self-concept. Early in life, that concept is gleaned as they identify with the adults who serve as models. The amount of love, warmth, and affection displayed is reflected in the child's ability to become an affectionate, uninhibited adult.

When a child enters puberty, he or she experiences rapid growth, the appearance of the secondary sex characteristics, and new strong emotions. This may shatter the relatively stable self-image and breed insecurity. It is like sitting on a volcano full of needs, impulses, and drives without a means of understanding, preventing, or controlling the eruption. This highly volatile state of conflicts and confusion is expected during the teenage years. Adolescence is a time to resolve those feelings and questions. That is a part of maturation, but many teenagers grow into adulthood without resolving these issues, and their attitudes about sex remain out of balance throughout life.

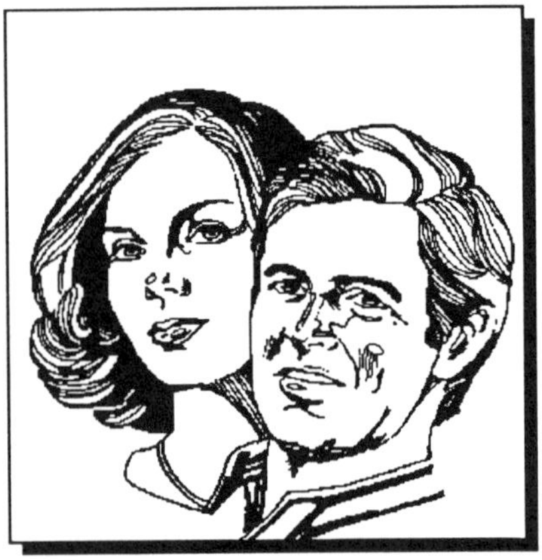

During the years of childhood and adolescence, there is a conflict between the hunger for adult guidance and the pressures to be independent and grown up. Despite this longing for parents' help, the child often breaks ties with them. He may turn to another adult, perhaps a teacher, for help; he may try to work it out by himself; or he may follow the path of his peers. This apparent rebellion is more correctly a searching for self.

If parents or other responsible adults are able to be of help, the best help might be to broaden rather than limit the young person's perspective of what sex is. It might be helpful to look at the various meanings and dimensions of sex. The word sex or sexuality means different things to different people at different times. Some people are preoccupied with sex; it is the biggest thing in their life, but it gets in the road of other important things. Other people attempt to ignore the fact that sex in its many facets is an essential part of each stage of life. The better adjusted individuals understand their sexual nature and impulses and have found a harmonious way of living with them.

Sexuality might be viewed as having four dimensions, and each dimension influences and is influenced by the other three. The *biological* dimension involves such topics as human growth and development, puberty, the sexual response, and pregnancy and reproduction. The *psychological* dimension reflects attitudes and feelings towards self and others. The *social* dimension involves the cultural influences on sex role relationships while dating, in the work-place, and in other social environments. The *moral* dimension deals with the basic questions of what is right and wrong, what is fair, and what should I do. For some people the moral dimension is derived from a particular religious philosophy, for others it is derived individually based on what seems to be most humanistic or pragmatic.

WHAT IS SEX?

The fact that the word sex means different things to different people at different times can be illustrated by the following answers to the question, "What is sex?"

1. **Sex is a designation of gender.** Sex is the most readily observable characteristic about a person. You don't meet a person one day and forget what sex she or he is the next day. The whole area of physiology and anatomy relating to maturation may be included under this heading.

2. **Sex is a designation of role.** Many roles in life are based on gender. Because of biological and cultural differences, various roles are based on sex; some roles are performed generally by males, some by females, some by either, and some roles require both. The roles change as the culture changes.

3. **Sex is a feeling of arousal.** Certain feelings within the body are defined as sexual responses. These feelings are based on a combination of both physical and psychological stimulation. The stimulation of certain parts of the body give rise to erotic activity, and in this sense, sex is defined as using those parts of the body for purposes of pleasure. Psychological stimuli that produce sexual feelings are described as "sexy." But there is a big difference between sex and sexy.

4. **Sex is a physical language.** Some forms of communication are based on physical relationships. Erotic activity is a means of expressing the degree of personal involvement. Sometimes this physical language can be more meaningful and more eloquent than verbal language. In this language, the degree of physical involvement should correspond to the degree of total involvement. However, irresponsible use of this language can result in failure to communicate accurately.

5. **Sex is a means of reproduction.** To reproduce his own kind has been described as man's greatest power. Biologically, the process of sexual reproduction provides for an exchange of chromosomes so that there is a variety in the species, and we all do not look alike.

The communications media and talk among peers have presented a limited and distorted answer to the question, "What is sex?" The media provides a constant exposure, in many cases overexposure, to sexual material. Current emphasis on sexual experimentation makes many young people feel very unsure of themselves. They may think they have to prove themselves by engaging in early sexual relations. Vulnerable as young people always are to pressures from peers, they may have friends who claim that anyone who espouses traditional morality is a "square" or anyone who finds any subject more engrossing than sex is probably not developing properly in sexual and/or personality areas. These pressures can become very strong and very frightening, particularly if the young person does not have good support from his family in dealing with them.

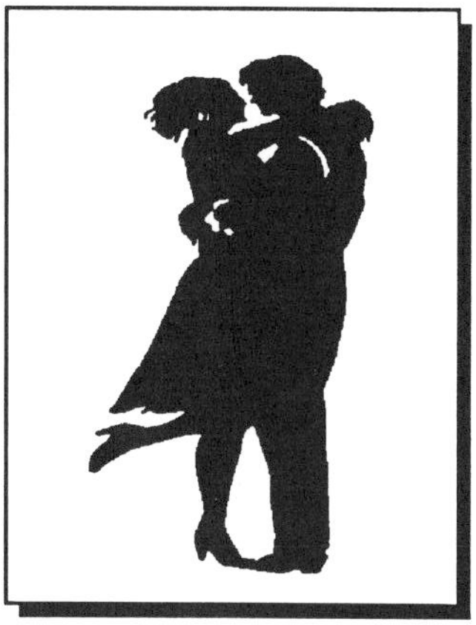

Some young people have rejected the whole concept of sexual morality in favor of free and uninhibited behavior, with much encouragement from those who are in a position to exploit or influence them. But many youth have discovered that relationships with no standards have been equally, if not more, unsatisfying than relationships conducted according to the older standards. The majority of young people remain idealistic, hopeful for their future, and concerned with developing sensible and nonhypocritical standards of sexual behavior. Their question is: What kinds of relationships between the sexes are most conducive to true satisfaction?

Today's statistics make it obvious that many young people have not fully considered the legal, political, or moral consequences of apparent sexual freedom. They have seen sex exploited, sold as a commodity, and portrayed as fulfillment. At the same time, it is banished from the topics of appropriate discussion in a responsible setting. Young people are intrigued by it, yet fearful of discussing questions about sex with those whom they should trust the most.

SEXUAL ROLE IDENTITY

No aspect of life is more rewarding and important to the quality of life than our interpersonal relationships, and no interpersonal relationships are more significant than those involving one's family and one's own sexuality. The development of human potential is dependent upon the acquisition of the feminine or masculine behavior patterns which society considers appropriate for each sex. It seems strange that a society that can make such tremendous scientific achievements as putting man on the moon can be so inept when it comes to family and man/woman relationships. Difficulties in learning and accepting one's sexual roles are fundamental to this problem.

The sex of the child is one of the first factors determining the child's acceptance or rejection within the family. Of course the sex of a child has been determined at the time of birth depending on whether the mother's egg was fertilized by an X or Y sperm cell from the father. If the sperm contained an X chromosome, the child became a female. If the sperm contained a Y chromosome, the child became a male. Whether the baby is a girl or boy is the first question at birth. The external genital organs, of course, indicate the difference at first, but the differences become most apparent with the development of the secondary sex characteristics at puberty.

Emotional and social factors are important in role identity. Some sectors of society still expects little boys not to cry and to develop the "John Wayne Syndrome," and little girls to assume the "Little Miss Muffet Syndrome." A common emotional response to a little girl is "I love you," but to a boy it is "I'm proud of you." The question is: would the double standard continue to exist if little boys and little girls received similar moral training? Inappropriate sex-role behavior is more acceptable for a girl than a boy--sissies are more frowned upon than tomboys. It becomes apparent that each area of the child's development is influenced by his sex.

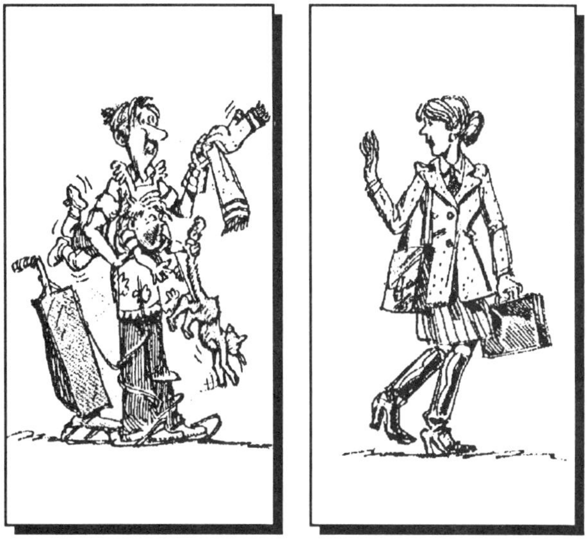

In adolescence and adulthood, sexuality may be the most vulnerable part of the self-concept. Tell a man that he is not a real man or a woman that she is not feminine or that either will not be attractive to the opposite sex, and you are threatening their role identity. Confusion often exists over the apparent conflict between proving one's femininity or masculinity and maintaining one's standard of morality. Both are important parts of one's identity, but fewer traditionally, mutually acceptable methods remain in our society to do so. Even the role models found in the work market have been integrated. Young people feel that they are left only with intimate sexual behavior to prove their identity, and if they can't prove it through heterosexual behavior, they may try to prove it through homosexual behavior. In some segments of today's society, it appears that even homosexual identity is preferable to no sexual identity. In any illicit or promiscuous behavior, any sense of achievement may be overshadowed by the associated feelings of guilt.

Even on the conceptual level where there is no overt behavior, the acceptance of ideas, attitudes, and feelings may carry the same consequence as threats to the identity. Each person must shift through a variety of proposed identities and come up with a sexual identity that is compatible and integrated with his central value system and general identity. To be able to successfully do so is a sign of maturity. To take it one step further, convergence or divergence between the expected identity and actual behavior is a basis of good or poor mental health.

The following are false concepts that sometimes cause conflicts:

- One is a "square" if one embraces traditional morals.
- Necking, petting, and intercourse are the key to popularity.
- Sex is the only way to hold a girl's or boy's interest.
- Sex is the only way to prove one's love.
- Sex is the only way to prove one's manhood or womanhood.

Obviously, acceptance of one's sex is a prerequisite to a healthy sexual identity. Parents and teachers can help by sharing with the young child their feelings that it is good to be a boy or a girl, and that there are unlimited opportunities for either. We should not confuse them by putting on them our concepts of masculinity or femininity. We should help them discover that it is first and most important to accept their identity as a person. As is true in other areas of development, children and youth learn most of their concepts of masculinity or femininity through identification with significant adults in their environment. Educators and other adults should learn to avoid subtle, unconscious influences which may limit young people in terms of future self-concepts and interpersonal relationships. Individuals, families, and society can ill afford to limit the development of human potential.

WHAT PROBLEMS DO ADOLESCENTS FACE?

While it is true that a rapidly changing society brings with it different kinds of problems, it is interesting that the basic problems are still just the same for the teenager of today as they were for the teenager of past decades. An analysis of student opinions in one study revealed that the big problems, the things that really bothered children, were not related to sexual intercourse, conception, contraception, homosexuality, or any of these things that adults often view as problems.

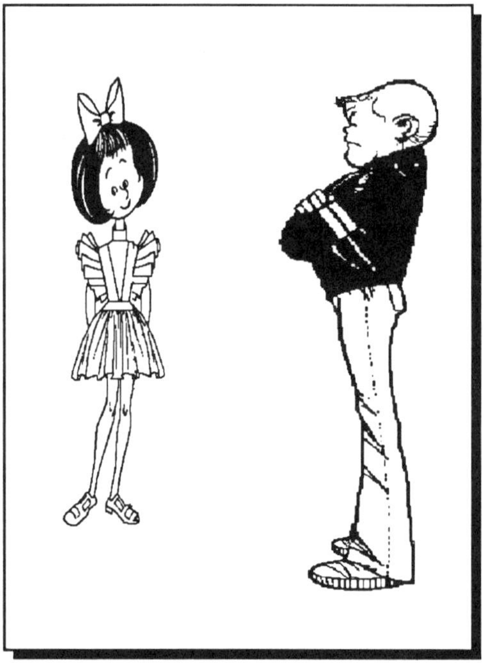

1. **The most common problems were related to self-understanding**, including the physical and emotional changes and reactions which are often unexpected, frightening, and difficult to deal with.

2. **Next in importance were problems of interpersonal relationships**; learning how to understand and get along with peer group members of the same and of the opposite sex. Also, within the home, relationships with parents, siblings, and other family members and with authority figures posed problems. For example, "How can I get my mother to see I can be trusted and stop her nagging?"

3. **The third problem area dealt with establishing a value system and a code of ethics by which to live.** They did like class sessions which dealt with morality; however, they did not want to be preached at. They did want to have some guidelines but preferred open discussion and the opportunity to look objectively at the many different ways that other people behave. They then wanted to have the freedom to evaluate and choose for themselves.

Adolescents have asked about problems or anxieties which have to do with normalcy of their sexual organs and their ability to perform sexually. Many of the anxieties of adolescents are the result of either lack of information or misinformation, but they may lead to sexual behavior that society considers abnormal and that may increase the anxieties.

DEVIATIONS IN SEXUAL EXPRESSION

Sexuality is an important component of identity, but for some people sexuality seems to take on undue significance. If some basic needs are not met in the normal ways, they may try to compensate by exaggerating some type of sexual behavior. If their needs to love and be loved and their need to feel a sense of worth are not met through normal interpersonal relationships, they may turn to some abnormal sexual relationships to try to meet those needs. A teenage girl who may feel starved for affection may become involved in promiscuous relationships to try to satisfy her needs. A teenage boy who feels a need to prove his manhood may engage in sex as a mark of conquest with associated bragging rights. For many young people, sexual behavior becomes the arena for proving their worth, but later they find it did not prove anything. In fact, it frequently makes the situation much worse.

No wonder young people searching for identity are having difficulties. American teenagers today seem to have inherited the worst possible worlds regarding their exposure to messages about sex. The media (movies, music, television, and radio) tell them that sex is romantic and exciting. Premarital sex, extramarital sex, cohabitation, and homosexuality are viable ways of life and viable choices. At the same time, their exposure to traditional sources of morality and values is being reduced. Religious views on morality, even prayer, cannot be expressed in the public schools. Educational sources have given up on teaching abstinence. The fear of a "shotgun wedding" is no longer a deterrant or a solution to the problem.

PORNOGRAPHY

Pornography implies literature or art designed to invoke sexual arousal, often a neurotic arousal. Current legal attempts to define what is pornographic stress that a pornographic work is one that has no redeeming social worth and is designed to arouse

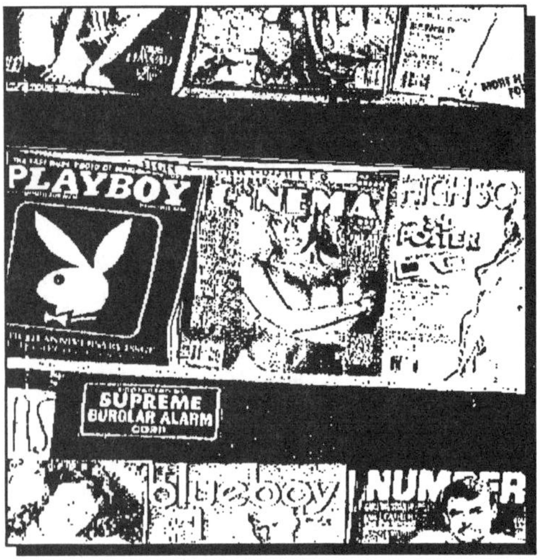

prurient feelings in the average person. Prurient refers to a negative or immoral way to incite or arouse sexual desire. Society's concern is that once sexual feelings have been aroused, the individual is inclined to act in a lewd or licentious manner. Lewd implies coarseness of sexual appetite without affection or tenderness. Licentious emphasizes the active satisfaction of desire in a manner that goes past legal or moral bounds or violates customary standards of behavior.

Pornography includes writings, photographs, drawings, videos, and films designed to produce sexual arousal. The distinction between "soft-core" and "hard-core" is not clear, but respective examples might be photographs featuring nudity and erotic poses in contrast to photographs featuring sexual abuse or exploitation of children. Both are under attack. Feminists are fighting pornography, because it exploits and degrades the role of women. Church and civic organizations accuse pornography of contributing to the growing rate of sexual violence.

Although questioned by some researchers, the 1986 report of the Attorney General's Commission on Pornography linked hard-core pornography to sex crimes. Statements in 1989 by serial killer Ted Bundy supported the case against pornography. Bundy admitted before his execution in Florida that he had killed dozens of girls and women (perhaps over a hundred) in several states from Washington to Florida. He said that his passion started with soft-core pornography.

Pornography is big business. Based on the most reasonable definitions, it runs into the hundreds of million dollars. The U.S. Postal Service estimated as early as 1960 that over one million school children (1 in 35) received unsolicited pornographic materials by mail, and the problem has increased since then. Some psychologists and police workers believe there is a link between exposure to pornography and sex crimes. We have no way of knowing how many youth who are habitually exposed to pornography do not commit sex crimes, but police investigation find that many adolescents arrested for rape and child sex abuse were collectors of pornography. J. Edgar Hoover said, "The destruction of moral character caused by pornography cannot be overestimated." Psychologists, educators, and welfare workers point out that a majority of youthful criminals have had a background impacted by more than a casual exposure to pornography.

Much of society is becoming less critical of pornography. For example, movies contain scenes that a few years ago would have been called pornographic and rated "X" are now rated "R" or "PG-13." Photographs that may be considered borderline pornography are found in abundance in commercial advertisements. This use of sex to sell merchandise may also be selling a dubious standard of morality and contributing to an amoral society.

Whether young people having difficulty with their self-concept are prone to became infatuated by pornography, or whether pornography leads to identity problems, or both; there seems to be a relationship. In either case, efforts that may have a positive influence on the self-concept may help.

TEEN PREGNANCY

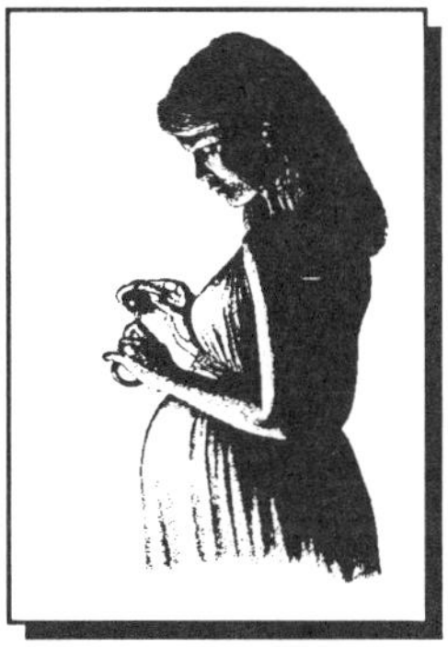

The Spring 1987 issue of *Educational Horizons,* indicated that annually in this country nearly 350,000 girls under age 18 become pregnant. Of these pregnancies, over 85 percent were unintended. About half become mothers, and half choose abortion. Only 30 percent of the these young mothers were married. Double the number to account for the fathers, and there are three quarters of a million kids who should be in high school who are going through the complex processes surrounding pregnancy and childbirth. The majority of these pregnancies were not wanted.

These are kids who are too young to vote, and many are too young to drive a car and get a job. Besides the disruption in their personal lives, government welfare costs for families started by adolescents is estimated to be 16 billion dollars per year. Teenage pregnancies are costly to society. Babies born to teenagers tend to be smaller and are more likely to die within the first year of life. The negative implications of pregnancy among adolescents are immeasurable. Adolescents who become pregnant forfeit a critical portion of their own childhood. The November/December 1988 issue of *Update*, published by the American Association for Health Education indicated that 50 percent of teenage mothers and 30 percent of teenage fathers quit school early. That article also indicated that 82 percent of teens who become pregnant are also daughters of adolescent mothers.

Teenage pregnancy stems from and contributes to a complex set of social problems: poverty, racial discrimination, lack of education, drug and alcohol use, and the commercialization of sex by the media. Political leaders are reluctant to take on these social problems. Teenage sexual activity is on the increase. A multitude of socioeconomic, cultural, and educational factors influence sexual activity and the use of contraceptives. It seems that today this country needs to discover an effective means of reducing teenage sexual activity, unwanted pregnancies, venereal disease, and deviant sexual behaviors.

Because the family has been the basic unit for preserving society throughout history, society has condoned behavior that strengthens the family and condemned behavior that weakens the family, particularly in regards to sexual behavior. Society accepts sexual behavior that by tradition is considered normal, but censors by law and taboos those behaviors considered to be abnormal. Deviant sexual behavior is not only a social problem, but also a psychological problem.

The sexual norms in society today are changing. The apparent freedom in sexual expression is accompanied by serious social and psychological problems. The integrity of the family and the self-esteem of its members are threatened by various forms of sexual abuse and infidelity. Psychologists, psychiatrists, and social workers have to deal with the damaging effect of deviant sexual behavior on their client's personality.

Sex is a very important aspect of everyone's personal well-being. Sex is much more than physical gratification. It is much more than a shared emotional experience. Sexuality is a significant component of a person's self-concept, and it is not without conflicts. What one may do to be socially acceptable may run counter to what one should do to be morally acceptable. Sometimes people who are thought of as being physically attractive, having all of the right curves in all of the right places, are not recognized for their intellectual capabilities. For many young people, sexual behavior becomes the arena for proving their worth. They get caught up in the challenge and lose sight of the proper role of sex for the well-balanced individual. A particular sex act must be evaluated as either right or wrong depending on how it contributes to the harmony of the total individual. Sexual maladjustments do not seem to exist by themselves; they affect the total personality.

Who knows which experiences may tend to color a child's sexual self-concept. A child may become confused if its parents think it is cute for it to play with its toes, but show their displeasure when it plays with its genitals. If such interest is harshly condemned, the child may associate sex with evil and wrong doing. If such associations are reinforced, a person's sexual self-concept may be crowded by feelings of guilt, fear, disgust, and avoidance. Then a natural and healthy interest in sex may be side-tracked into some deviant sexual preoccupation that would be detrimental to the person's social and emotional well-being. Unless these misconceptions are corrected, they may give vent to misdirected sexual expression that may prove detrimental not only to the individual but also to others. A person may not be able to express love in an intimate sexual manner. Preoccupation with pornography, voyeurism, exhibitionism, sexual abuse of children, rape, incest, homosexuality, and other forms of deviant sexual behavior that are harmful not only to individuals, but also to society, may result.

HOMOSEXUALITY

Homosexuality is an example of an extreme identity problem. Until recently, homosexuality was considered an embarrassing topic. It was not discussed in high school health courses, and it was rarely mentioned in college health or psychology courses. But the AIDS epidemic has brought the topic and participants "out of the closet." Today, proponents of AIDS education insist that AIDS education start with young children. Although the need for all people to know how to prevent AIDS is real, it appears that some groups promote AIDS education in order to publicize and thus seemingly legitimatize homosexual preference.

Many psychiatrists, psychologists, and social workers have seriously disturbed homosexuals as clients. These therapists may characterize their clients as anxiety-ridden and often tormented persons who have difficullty achieving self-fulfillment. Critics ask if the efforts of homosexuals to organize and campaigning for civil rights are not a manifestation of a groups refusal to confront a serious personality distortion. Homosexuals have been accused of attempting to spread the propaganda that they are healthy members of a "third sex." Rather than to try to change, they try to relieve their own burden by convincing themselves that heredity or glandular factors have made their condition unalterable.

One investigator reported in 1970 that 54 percent of his married men respondents admitted to some homosexual practices during adolescence. Kinsey reported that 37 percent of the men and 13 percent of the women he studied reported at least some homosexual experience. Some of these are people isolated from contact with people of the opposite sex. Most of these would be heterosexual by choice. Some of these are bisexual by choice. About 4 percent of males and 2 percent of females remain exclusively homosexual after adolescence.

The AIDS crisis has challenged society's ability to deal with complex social, emotional, moral, and biological issues. The schools have become involved in this controversy on a number of levels. Old issues have been renewed and new issues have emerged.

SEX EDUCATION

Public officials frequently try to deal with social problems by making the schools responsible for preparing the next generation to solve its problems. There are two weaknesses with this approach. First, once society shifts the buck to the schools, other methods of solving the problem are ignored. Second, all problems cannot and should not be prevented. The child or the adolescent who has not been allowed to work his way through problems of interpersonal relation-ships will be poorly equipped to face the continuing problems which the young, middle-aged, and older adults face until the day they die.

Nevertheless, although the role of the schools is limited, they can make some important contributions. The schools cannot do everything, but the things they can do, they should do well. The contributions of schools and individual teachers in two major areas are really the keys to learning and growth of any type. The first is accurate information and wide knowledge of all aspects of human sexual behavior. The second is skill in problem solving, in collecting all the facts, evaluating objectively, and reaching a decision on the basis of rational discussion and thought.

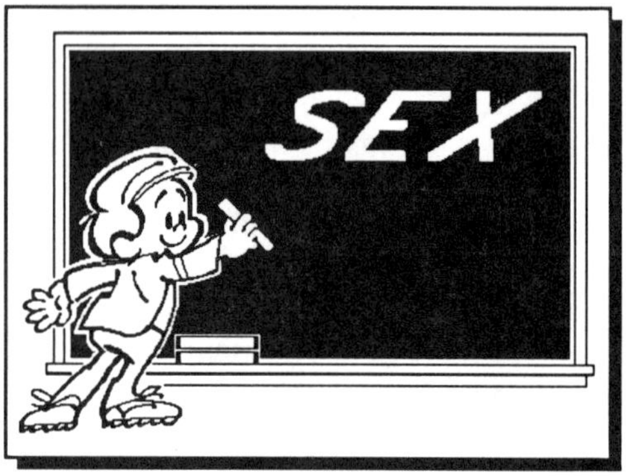

One of the first things to do is to arrive at a consensus regarding what the schools should do. This is the biggest problem because of the different opinions of various segments of the community. Some community groups are opposed to sex education in the public schools for opposing reasons. Some are afraid the schools will go to far. Others are afraid the schools won't go far enough, and once the "buck" is passed to the schools, no one else will do anything.

Some groups feel that sex education should emphasize abstinence, and other groups feel the use of contraceptives should be emphasized. Some feel that effective education must deal with attitudes and values, but others feel that the schools have no business in teaching sexual values. It is a controversial topic, and every teacher should be familiar with their state laws and regulations and local policies regarding sex education.

The assumption that sex education will solve the problem may be erroneous. The *Journal of School Health* in its December 1985 issue published an article by Douglas Kirby called "Sexuality Education: A More Realistic View of its Effects." Several well-designed studies to measure the impact of sex education were reviewed in the article. In summary, the findings answered the following questions:

- **Did the course in sex education increase knowledge?** The findings were nearly unanimous that instruction in sex education increases knowledge.

- **Did the course in sex education change attitudes?** The analysis showed that sex education had little impact on the students values regarding their own sexual behavior. The programs did not have a measurable effect on self-esteem. However, several studies suggest that a course in sexuality increases tolerance in the students' attitudes toward the sexual practices of other people.

- **<u>Did the course in sex education change behavior?</u>** Although the sex education courses selected for the studies were exemplary and represented a variety of approaches, the findings indicated that sex education did not affect whether or not participants engaged in sexual intercourse. One study found that sex education programs may increase the use of birth control among some groups, but not among others. Another study found no measurable impact on the use of birth control. There was no indication that the sex education programs had any measurable effect on the number of pregnancies.

The sex education programs did not appear to have the effect on behavior that educators hoped. Students who were knowledgeable about the probability of becoming pregnant were neither less nor more likely to engage in sexual intercourse than students with less knowledge. Similarly, students who were more knowledgeable about birth control were neither more or less likely to use birth control. Evidently factors other than knowledge affect teenage sexual behavior.

Does this mean that sex education should be abolished? Those who say no give two reasons. First, even when information does not change behavior, people should still have access to information. The principle of informed consent applies. Some educational theorists raise the question as to whether changing behavior should even be the goal of any program in the public schools. Instead they believe the goals should be to: 1) provide accurate information, 2) provide opportunities for value clarification, 3) improve decision-making skills, and 4) allow the students to make their own decisions. Second, if the programs do not change behavior, they should be modified and improved until they do.

Some suggest that the programs should be more comprehensive. One way to make sex education more comprehensive is to make it a part of a coordinated health education program that includes appropriate material on all grade levels from kindergarten through the twelfth grade. In such a program, sex education would not be an isolated single course approach, but an integrated approach that treats sexuality as merely one component of total well-being. Another way to make sex education more comprehensive is to organize it on a community-wide basis involving all interested parties such as the public health department, state welfare agencies, and family planning services.

In some ways, the regular classroom teacher, not the sex education specialist or health educator, might have more opportunities to deal effectively with certain sex-related topics. In some states, teachers cannot include such topics as contraception in the planned curriculum, but these same topics can be dealt with in response to questions asked by students. A literature teacher may be in the best position to teach moral values. Class discussions about reading assignments may be an ideal time to examine the various sides of moral issues. The task of education is not to make judgments about specific acts of commission or omission, but to help students find a value framework which will enable them to interpret all behavior in context. A major concern should be to develop effective interpersonal relationships. Lester A. Kirkendall wrote:

> Whenever a decision or choice is to be made concerning behavior, the moral decision will be one which works toward the creation of trust, confidence, and integrity in relationships. It should increase the capacity of individuals to cooperate and enhance the sense of self-respect in the individual. Acts which create distrust, suspicion, and misunderstanding, which build barriers and destroy integrity, are immoral. They decrease the individual's sense of self-respect and rather than producing a capacity to work together, they separate people and break down the capacity for communication.

If students could absorb and use this principle in distinguishing between what is right or moral and what is wrong or immoral, it might do more for reducing the number of unwanted teenage pregnancies than instruction about birth control. Every teacher can help promote such principles. Every teacher should be an exemplary role model for their students in matters of morality. Every teacher should find opportunities to help students improve their self-concept. But going beyond that in teaching or counseling students about sexual matters, teachers must be extremely careful. They must be careful in discussing sensitive issues and realize that what is sensitive may vary from community to community. Sometimes a referral to the school nurse may be appropriate.

National leaders in the field of sex education for adolescents have emphasized the following points. If the goal of sex education is to help young people learn how to make responsible health decisions, it will be based on building self-esteem. Effective sex education will find ways to optimize contributions from parents and enlist community support. The educational experience will help students explore expectations about dating, going together, and love. It will help teenagers develop positive relationships and mutual respect. It will help teenagers clarify their values. It will deal with strategies for putting teenagers in control of their own feelings and dealing with peer pressure and other social pressures.

The adult best equipped to help the adolescent will be one who: (1) is aware of the stages of heterosexual development through which the normal child passes from infancy to adolescence, (2) is cognizant of the pressures placed upon individuals in a changing society, (3) recognizes the influence of the family and of adults upon the child, (4) is himself secure about his own sexuality, and (5) is burdened with a minimum of problems related to his own interpersonal relationships.

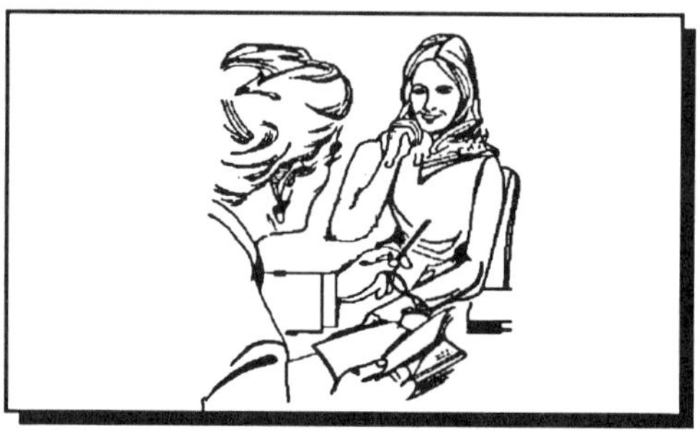

The controversy over whether there should be sex education is pointless. An informal course in sex education already goes on in the schools--and always has--taught by children to each other. The main difficulty with it is that so much of what children learn in their unsupervised experience is not true or reliable. Anyone who has taught a course in human physiology knows how much time has to be spent untangling the misinformation about sexual functions that young people have acquired.

The question schools must ask is not, "Should we have sex education?" Sex education will take place. The questions are: "When are we going to have it, who is going to teach it, and what will they teach?" The increased support for sex education in the schools is reflected in the fact that more than 40 states require or encourage sex education of some kind. Most teachers of sex education are specialists in health education, home economics, biology, or physical education. A majority of the sex education teachers are married women over age forty and have been teaching sex education for over eight years. Almost all sex education teachers have had coursework which has specifically prepared them for teaching the subject, although only three states (Michigan, Ohio, and Utah) require teachers to have completed a course in human sexuality before teaching sex education. There seems to be two basic approaches to sex education. One focuses on helping young people avoid unintended pregnancy and sexually- transmitted diseases (STDs). Others focus on the full range of family life and sex education topics.

When it comes to specific topics in sex education, some are more controversial than others. For example, some schools by law cannot teach about birth control, and other schools think that birth control is the most important topic. In some states, teachers can discuss birth control only in response to students questions. Most sex education teachers prefer to stress abstinence as the best method of preventing pregnancy and STDs. To do this, they emphasize the importance of taking personal responsibility for sexual behavior, and they discuss ways of resisting pressure from peers and boyfriends or girlfriends. Many teachers go on from there. Recognizing that many students are already sexually active, they teach their students to use contraceptives if they engage in sex. Because condoms have application for preventing both pregnancy and STDs, instruction in the use of condoms is fully detailed. Some parents, educators, church representatives, and community leaders are opposed to such frank discussions in the public schools. Some health authorities believe that topics such as STDs should be taught in the "Communicable Disease Prevention" unit rather than in a unit on "Maturation and Family Life".

Sex education programs, if they are to be accepted and successful, must be responsive to the individual families in a community as well as to the values of the community as a whole. Teaching about the anatomy and physiology of the reproductive system is less controversial than teaching about sexual values, attitudes, and morals. Within a community, one would probably find a variety of attitudes about sexual behavior including the following:

- **<u>Sex is a sin</u>.** (traditional) Sex is bad and shameful, but necessary. It is best to avoid it altogether; celibacy is preferred. If you can't avoid it, then confine it to marriage.

- **<u>Sex is free</u>.** (anarchy) There should be no restrictions whatsoever on sex. Anyone, any time, any place, anything goes. Sex is amoral.

- **<u>Sex is situational</u>.** (new morality) Let the relationship determine the standard. There is no predetermined right or wrong; it depends on the situation. A moral decision is one that enhances the relationship between people.

- **<u>Sex is sacred</u>.** (safeguarded) Sex is sacred because it enables a couple to join with God in the creation of life. Within the holy union of marriage, sex is good, beautiful, and pure because it brings couples together in greater oneness. Eternal, divine laws pertaining to sex exist to safeguard its sacredness.

If sex education is to be effective in the area of interpersonal relationships, it must deal with values and attitudes. The question is, whose values? If a parent had a strong feeling about any one of the four philosophies just discussed, and a teacher presented one of the other philosophies, the parent could become very unhappy. Can a teacher teach about sex without teaching values? It is questionable. Unless the teacher is very skilled at teaching about values, he or she will impose his own values. Although there have been some sex educational programs in the schools that have been widely accepted as good because they dealt delicately with non-controversial topics, others have dealt with sensational topics that are extremely controversial. That is why some people believe that sex education should not be in the schools and is a topic that should be left to the home.

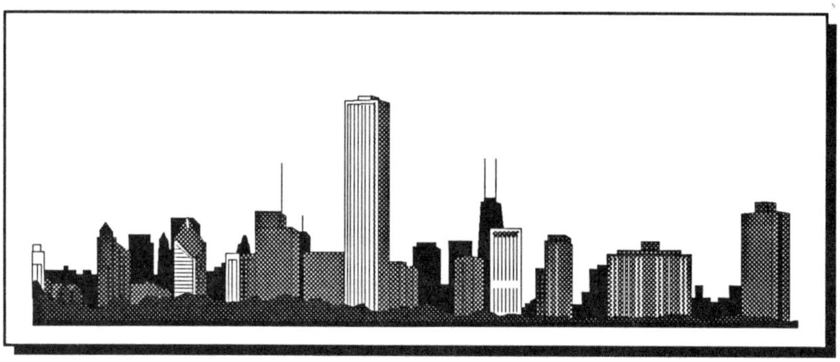

A sex education program should reflect the values of the community, but it may be hard to make everyone happy or to even come to some unanimity of opinion about what values are to be taught, particularly in the abstract. What some effective teachers do is to announce any controversial topics ahead of time and invite the principal, the superintendent, members of the school board, and members of the PTA to come to class that day. Usually, when they attend and see how the topic is handled, they become very supportive of the program.

The following is a list of topics selected at random that are taught in some parts of the country in courses related to family life and sex education. Based on values of each community, some of them can be taught and others can not.

- The Nature of Intimacy
- Marriage and Other Types of Commitments
- Reproductive Anatomy and Physiology
- The Human Sexual Response
- Sexual Preferences
- Masturbation
- Quality Sexual Relationships
- Sexual Dysfunction: Impotency, Infertility
- Sexual Abuse and Assault
- Prostitution and Pornography
- Variations In Sexual Behaviors
- Parenting Education
- Pregnancy and Childbirth
- Abortion, Birth Control, and Family Planning
- Dating and Marriage
- Family Living
- Diseases of the Reproductive System
- Sexually Transmitted Diseases
- Teaching Your Children About Sex
- Sex and the Aging Process

A person informed about the pros and cons of sex education would be familiar with the subtopics and concepts related to each item on this list and be prepared to defend, reject, modify, or restrict the content of each item.

The answers to the question," What is sex?" discussed earlier can be a basis of curriculum planning. The fact that sex is a designation of gender, a designation of role, a physical response, a means of communicating, and a means of reproduction can suggest a wide variety of concepts that might be taught at different school levels. Some are non-controversial, and others might be highly controversial. Deciding what is and is not appropriate is a difficult task. Some would take the irresponsible route and say "teach everything;" others would avoid the problem by saying "teach nothing."

The question is, "Who will teach it, and where and when and what will they teach?" Of more importance than "What facts should the young people learn?" is the question, "What attitudes will they develop while they are learning?" Attitudes are extremely important. It has been said that the quality of our existence is dependent on the quality of our interpersonal relationships. That is because it is through our interpersonal relationships that we fulfill our basic needs--the need to love and be loved, and the need to feel that we are worthwhile to ourselves and to others. Our most important personal relationships are those involving our families and our sexuality.

To feel worthwhile, we must have a standard by which we can measure that worth. But setting standards is difficult in a state of revolution. Society is experiencing a rapid sexual revolution, not necessarily a revolution of behavior, but a revolution of attitudes. The door to study and discussion in the area of sex has been thrown wide open. The freedom to talk about sex has in some ways created chaos. A teacher is in a position to help settle the confusion.

A TEACHER'S INFLUENCE

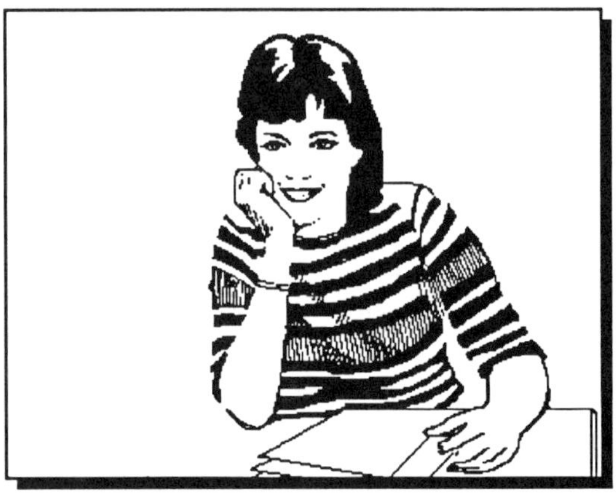

There are specific moments in everyday life which may be termed "teaching moments." This is a moment when a student is open and prepared to be taught. These moments must be recognized and utilized. If a teacher wishes to have a positive influence on the values his or her students select, he or she must first internalize these qualities. The teacher must also win the trust and respect of the student. The student will then feel free to confide in the teacher. Through these student-teacher interactions, the teacher has more opportunities for teaching moments.

The sense of right and wrong in a student is directly related to how the student perceives the world and himself. By treating the student with respect, the student can learn to respect himself and learn how to treat others with respect. Sex education should be taught as something uplifting as well as satisfying--an element that gives meaning and purpose to other things in life when participated in under wholesome conditions. It is not sex, but the use of sex for exploitation that is damaging. If it is the medium for the expression of the deepest affection, sex can be an aesthetic, emotional, spiritual, as well as physical experience. Some general principles that will guide the teacher as he attempts to have a positive influence upon the sexual moral values of his students are the following:

- Be a good example.
- Be sensitive to students' desires and problems.
- Inspire a classroom where morality is a legitimate discussion topic.
- Be aware of teaching moments.
- Do not reinforce negative behavior.
- As sex is an adult function, communicate as an adult to an adult.
- Know of what you speak! Make sure your own sexual conflicts are resolved before you try to help anyone else.

Teachers need to be prepared to deal appropriately with questions and situations that may come up regarding sex. If a teacher shows embarrassment when a question is asked, it might impair communication with a student who needs to have the help that can come from a confidential relationship with a trusted adult. The giveaway signs of embarrassment that may quickly appear on the face of a teacher may leave the teacher open to further attempts at embarrassment by mischievous students, and if this continues, it can seriously interfere with the teacher's effectiveness generally. While teachers should not become calloused to vulgar language nor allow offensive language to take place in the classroom environment, he should not become overly sensitized either.

Schools should have standards about language, conduct, and forms of pornography. Care should be exercised in the selection of literature and other teaching materials, and all school activities should be conducted so that they reflect the highest moral standards of the community.

A teacher should know the basic information about sex and interpersonal relations related to sex, as well as the misinformation frequently held and the problems often confronted by students so that he can provide effective help when students need it. There is a difference between knowing the information and knowing how best to share that information with young people. Advanced preparation may help.

The following are samples of questions that students have asked:

- What is the difference between masturbation and "wet dreams"?
- How can a girl tell if a boy wants to have intercourse with her?
- Can disease be spread during intercourse if rubbers are used?
- How come only one sperm enters the ovaries?
- Is it good for a girl to use a tampon?
- What should you do if you start to menstruate in class?

- How do you find out if you are going to have a baby?
- How much does a baby grow before birth?
- Can two eggs be fertilized in the same month?
- How old should you be before you start kissing?
- What should a girl do if a boy she likes very much tries to rape her?
- Everybody talks about making out. What does it mean?
- How do you get a date? How do you break up?
- What do you think of a girl who flirts when she is going steady?
- Should kids get married without their parents' permission?
- Should you let a date know you like her or keep her guessing?
- Is there a way to tell your mother to shut up without saying it?
- What can a person do when he hardly has a friend at all?
- Why does everybody think you are cheap just by the way you dress?
- What if a boy sees a tampon in your purse and asks what it is?
- What is intercourse and how do you go about doing it?
- How can you prevent having a baby if you are already exposed?
- How come mostly men are color blind?

A QUESTION OF MORALITY

Students may occasionally approach the teacher with moraly sensative questions regarding sexuality. They may be aware of the teacher's personal convictions and sincerely seek help with a moral dilemma. At such times a teacher must be very discreet in order to help the student, and at the same time, not go beyond propriety. It may be wiser to communicate to the student the need to talk to parents and other resources in the community inluding ecclesiastical leaders. A teacher should not presume to speak authoritatively on religious issues or family matters, yet should not bypass the opportunity to help young people clarify their values on matters of sexual morality.

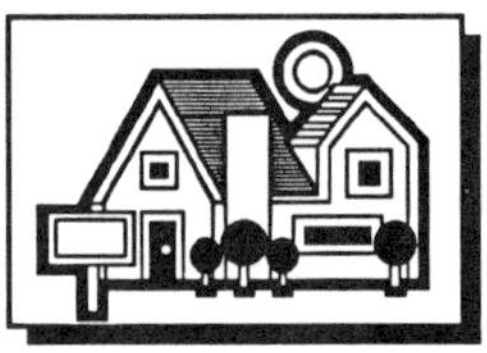

STUDY HELPS

Support or refute the following statements based on your personal opinion, information in the text, or other sources of information.

1. Much of a person's worth as an individual is tied to his or her sexual self-concept.

2. When a child enters puberty, he or she experiences changes that may fragment their self-image and generate insecurity.

3. Sexuality is much more than physical gratification; it is more than a shared emotional union; it is a significant component of a person's self-concept.

4. Sexuality might viewed as having four interrelated dimensions: biological, psychological, social, and moral.

5. There are five answers to the question, "What is sex?" What are they?

6. Sex is not without conflicts. What one may do to be socially accepted may run counter to what one should do to be morally acceptable.

7. The communications media and peer propaganda have presented an image of sex that is restricted, distorted, and overexposed.

8. Pressures regarding sex can become very strong and very frightening, particularly for young people who do not have good family support in dealing with them.

9. The majority of young people remain idealistic, hopeful, and desirous of developing sensible and nonhypocritical standards of sexual behavior. Their question is: What kinds of relationships between the sexes are most conducive to true satisfaction?

10. Today's statistics make it obvious that many young people have not fully considered the legal, political, or moral consequences of apparent sexual freedom.

11. It seems strange that a society that can make such tremendous scientific achievements as putting man on the moon can be so inept when it comes to family and man/woman relationships.

12. The sex of the child is one of the first factors determining the child's acceptance or rejection within the family. Whether the baby is a girl or boy is the first question at birth.

13. Sexuality may be the most vulnerable part of the self-concept. Tell a man that he is not a real man or a woman that she is not feminine and that they are not sexually attractive and you threaten their role identity.

14. Sometimes young people feel that they are left only with intimate sexual behavior to prove their identity.

15. American teenagers today seem to have inherited the worst possible worlds regarding their exposure to information about sex. The media tell them that sex is romantic and exciting, and that premarital and extramarital sex, cohabitation, and homosexuality are viable ways of life. At the same time, their exposure to traditional sources of morality and values is being reduced.

16. The apparent freedom in sexual expression is accompanied by serious social and psychological problems. The integrity of the family and the self-esteem of its members are threatened.

17. If negative sexual associations are reinforced, a person's sexual self-concept may be inflicted with feelings of guilt, fear, and disgust. Then the natural and healthy interest in sex may be sidetracked into either avoidance or some deviant sexual preoccupation.

18. Unless sexual misconceptions are corrected, they are not only detrimental to the person's social and emotional well-being, but they may also give vent to misdirected sexual expression that may also prove harmful to others.

19. No aspect of life is more rewarding and important to the quality of life than our interpersonal relationships, and no interpersonal relationships are more significant than those involving one's family and one's own sexuality.

Chapter 13

SCHOOL HEALTH APPRAISAL

School health appraisal is a process of determining the health status of students for the purpose of detecting remedial health problems, particularly those that may interfere with effective learning. Student health may be assessed in a variety of settings. Physical examinations can be performed by physicians. Screening tests can be performed by teachers, the school nurse, or trained volunteers. Dentists and dental hygienists can perform dental exams and screening procedures. Physical fitness may be appraised by specialists in physical education. But of all the appraisal techniques, the daily observation by the classroom teacher is probably the most important. An alert teacher will pick up possible health problems that other professionals may not be in a position to detect until much later.

SCHOOL HEALTH APPRAISAL

Most students are in the healthiest time of their lives. School health appraisal is a part of the school health program designed to help keep students healthy by detecting any problems early so they can be treated. All teachers should be aware of the various school health appraisal options, particularly those implemented in the districts in which they teach. Each teacher should be able to answer the following questions pertaining to school health appraisal in their district.

- Are student medical and dental examinations required?
- What screening tests are routinely given, by whom, when?
- What are the teachers' responsibilities for health observation?
- Are there policies to insure adequate referral and confidentiality?

HEALTH EXAMINATIONS

A health examination is conducted by a physician. In some districts, it may be referred to as a medical or physical examination, but the more modern and positive term is a health examination. In some states, the frequency of the exam is set by law; in other states, the frequency is determined by consultation between school and medical officials. The following options are typical:

- Students starting school for the first time.
- Students new to the school district.
- Students participating in vigorous athletic programs.
- Students entering middle school or junior high school.

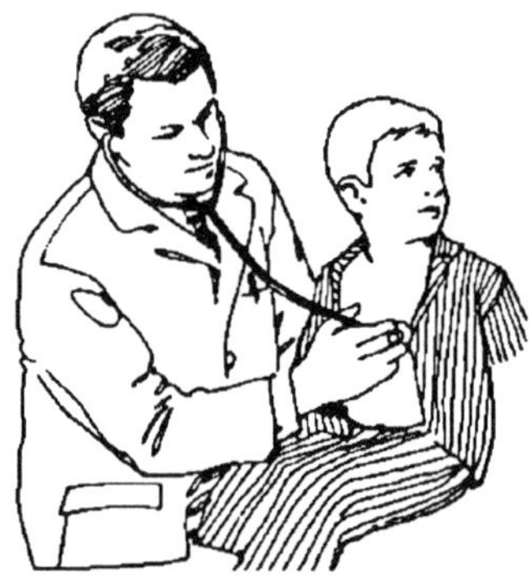

Some schools districts also require a medical examination in the senior year before graduation. Such examinations and any medical follow-up may give the student a better start on life and may be an important part of the student's health education as a reminder of the importance of routine health examinations. Others, including the American Academy of Pediatrics, suggest that a health examination should be considered when a student is identified as having special problems (academic, social, or emotional). A health examination may discover the basis for the problem.

Dental Examinations

Schools should require dental examinations at the same time they require medical examinations. Schools should also encourage students to follow good dental hygiene including brushing and flossing, a source of dental fluoride, and regular periodic dental check-ups.

HEALTH SCREENING

Screening is a test or procedure to identify unrecognized indications of possible illness or departure from normal. They can be administered rapidly and inexpensively to large numbers of people. They are used in schools to try to identify students who deviate from the average in a certain category of health. Screening tests are not diagnostic tests, they merely identify students who need more thorough examinations. Screening tests can be administered to a group or to an individual. That is, all members of a particular class may be given a screening test on a routine basis, or an individual student may be given a test because a teacher or nurse has noticed something that suggests the possibility of a problem. A number of screening tests can be given at the same time (multiphasic screening) or a single test can be given. Sometimes screening tests are conducted only for a portion of the population that is at high risk for certain problems. The amount of skill necessary to conduct a screening test varies from test to test, but nurses, teachers, and volunteers can be trained to administer most tests. The value of screening tests depends on the quality of the testing device, the care taken by those conducting the test, and the use made of the findings. Examples of screening tests include:

- Vision
- Hearing
- Dental
- Height and Weight
- Posture
- Tuberculosis
- Head Lice

TEACHER OBSERVATION

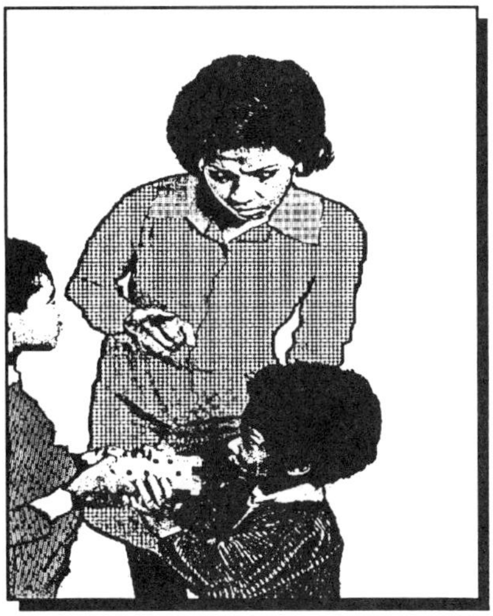

The daily observation by alert teachers is the most important part of school health appraisal. Some states have made health observations a legal responsibilities of the classroom teacher. Teachers should make an effort to be informed of and exercise such responsibilities according to the state in which they teach.

Teachers are even more likely than parents to notice indications of a possible health problem. This is because of their educational background, their more objective point of view, and their basis of comparison with other students. Prospective teachers have a responsibility both legally and professionally to develop the skills of observing students' health. The indications are not that hard to detect if teachers will only take the time and effort to notice them. Some teachers conduct health observations almost automatically without consciously thinking about it, but if a potential problem is observed, it is drawn to their attention. It is like a computer program that runs unnoticed in the background until a clue triggers a reaction to pop up on the computer screen. Other teachers have to regularly set aside a time to consciously make student health observations. It takes practice at first, but with enough practice health observation will become more automatic. The assignment for this lesson requires one practice session, but a prospective teacher should seek other opportunities in a variety of situations to improve their health observation skills. Although the list of health indicators for this assignment is not complete, it is a good sample. A teacher can start to develop the skills of health observation by trying to become alert to these conditions.

Some indications of a possible health problem require immediate response, and others provide time for extended observations. One of the important purposes of teacher observations is to detect the possibility of communicable disease. A student who shows the signs and symptoms of a communicable disease should be excluded from the classroom as soon as possible to reduce the risk of spreading the disease, if it exists, to other students. Another situation that may require relatively quick response is sudden illness. More specific information about communicable disease and sudden illness will be discussed later.

Usually a single observation is not as important as several observations. Any student can exhibit some questionable conditions on a one-time basis. But if a condition continues or changes for the worse, it may be appropriate to make a referral. A referral is usually made to the school nurse, but sometimes to a parent, or a school counselor depending on school policies. Some districts encourage a teacher to go directly to a parent, and other districts want the referral processed through the school personnel.

Sometimes school administrators get caught in a bind between what seems best for the students and what legal considerations dictate. A few years ago federal legislation regarding rights to privacy and confidentiality altered the way some schools handled student health records. Standardized procedures and forms encourage the inclusion of only the information pertinent to the student's educational development. All written records conveyed by physicians to schools receiving federal funds are open to inspection by parents. Also, because of the potential for students to be "harmfully labeled" by health information, it is important that schools develop clear policies on the procedures for handling health information.

The process of teacher observation will not catch all student health problems. And fortunately, not all potential problems a teacher observes and refers turn out to be problems, but teacher observation will catch some problems. Conscientious teachers, through health observations, have made a big difference in the lives of many students. Most college classes can think of several examples where, thanks to a teacher, a vision or hearing problem was discovered and dealt with before a student got too far behind, developed a poor self-concept, and stopped trying to learn. Teachers in the elementary level obviously have a much greater potential for impacting the lives of their students through health observations.

Most of the remedial problems have been spotted and corrected before the students get into secondary school. Also, as students get older, they take a greater responsibility for their own health. Nevertheless, secondary teachers still have an important responsibility for student health observation.

Effective Teacher Observation

Health observation. The teacher should evaluate each child's health at the beginning of the school year, and any health problems not previously observed or corrected should be resolved. Then after establishing each child's oral health pattern, day-to-day observations should be made so as to note any new deviations from this normal health.

Maintaining health records. Normal health should be recorded by the teacher on the student's health record as a means of comparison, and upon the discovery of an old or new abnormality, appropriate information concerning it should always be noted on this record. If there is no formal record available, the teacher should devise a process of keeping personal notes to serve this purpose.

Making student referrals. When a problem is observed, the teacher should definitely refer the problem to someone who is in the position to correct it. Depending upon school procedure and the seriousness of the problem, referrals should either be made directly to the parents or to a school authority such as a nurse or physician who can make further observations and evaluations and then refer it to the parents if needed. No matter who the referral is made to, the teacher should follow up on it by making sure action is taken and the problem solved.

Giving health counsel. When a teacher, particularly on the secondary level, gives students health counsel, he or she should try to help them develop a sense of responsibility in meeting personal and family health problems. The teacher should also try to help the students gain a clearer understanding of their health problems. When communicating with parents, the teacher should try to indicate the significance of health appraisal findings and to assist them in obtaining appropriate health care for their children. The teacher can also assist students in taking advantage of community resources which may provide help. When working with students with nonremediable defects, the teacher should try to help them adapt their programs, needs, and interests with due consideration for their disabilities. The teacher should try to impress the students with the value of a healthy lifestyle in helping them deal with their problem.

The teacher occupies a unique position in relation to the child's physical and emotional health as well as his academic accomplishments. It is with the teacher that the child spends his good days and his poor days, where he meets his successes and failures, where he reveals his reactions to other children, and where changes in his appearance and behavior may first be observed. Because of his familiarity with the usual appearance and conduct of each pupil and of members of the group, the teacher is in a strategic position to detect variations that may indicate deviations from health.

Problems Teachers Might Observe

As teachers observe students' appearance and behavior, they may note variations from normal, but do not make a medical diagnosis. A teacher is limited to what he or she can see objectively (*signs*) and how students may describe their feelings (*symptoms*). Based on these signs and symptoms, a teacher may suspect a particular health problem but may not draw conclusions. Nevertheless, these observations assist in health appraisal and may lead to the identification of a student in the early stages of a communicable disease or a student who is suffering from a physical defect or emotional disturbance.

It would be well for you to occasionally review the table listing the "Conditions Which Should Be Noted in Teacher Observations" found in this lesson. A more detailed discussion on some of these conditions will be found later in this lesson. If you still do not understand what is meant by some of these conditions, you might check with a health teacher or a school nurse. Conditions specifically related to communicable diseases will be discussed in that lesson, but a teacher should also observe for emotional problems, a topic covered in a previous lesson.

SCREENING TESTS

Like other appraisal techniques, screening tests are a means to an end. Not only should they help detect possible health problems, but they should also be a positive experience for the students and provide valuable health education. Teachers may be involved in administering screening tests, or at least they should be able to understand the value and meaning of the results. Therefore, information about the commonly used screening tests in the schools is given. Screening tests are administered to discover health deficiencies in students. Upon the discovery of such, general procedure is for the students to be referred to a competent source of correction and for follow-up visits to be made by a school nurse or teacher to be sure the correction is complete and accurate.

The discussion which follows deals with a number of common health problems. Some are discussed because you are likely to encounter them among your students; others are mentioned to provide a general health education background. The discussion will include the nature of the problem, some signs or symptoms that might be observed, and the procedures for conducting a screening test.

CONDITIONS WHICH SHOULD BE NOTED IN TEACHER OBSERVATIONS

EYES
1. watery, red, or inflamed eyes . ☐
2. styes or crusted eyelids ...... ☐
3. large or protruding eyes ..... ☐
4. crossed eyes or wall-eyes ..... ☐
5. squinting, frowning, scowling . ☐
6. rubbing or brushing of eyes .. ☐
7. twitching of the lids .... ☐
8. excessive blinking .... ☐
9. tilting head to one side ...... ☐
10. shutting one eye .... ☐
11. holds book too close .... ☐
12. repeated headaches .... ☐

EARS
1. discharge from ears .... ☐
2. failure to hear questions ..... ☐
3. picking at the ears .... ☐
4. turning the head to hear .... ☐
5. talking in a monotone .... ☐
6. inattention .... ☐
7. anxious expression .... ☐
8. creates excessive noise ...... ☐
9. earache .... ☐

NOSE, MOUTH, AND THROAT
1. persistent mouth breathing ... ☐
2. frequent sore throat .... ☐
3. recurrent colds .... ☐
4. chronic nasal discharge ...... ☐
5. frequent nose bleeding ...... ☐
6. nasal speech .... ☐
7. frequent tonsillitis .... ☐
8. enlarged glands on neck ..... ☐
9. cavities in teeth .... ☐
10. uneven bite .... ☐
11. irregular teeth .... ☐
12. inflamed gums or gum boils .. ☐
13. sores in mouth or on lips .... ☐
14. stained teeth .... ☐
15. offensive breath .... ☐

SKIN AND SCALP
1. unusual pallor of face .... ☐
2. excessive redness of skin ..... ☐
3. eruptions or rashes .... ☐
4. scales or crusts .... ☐
5. habitual scratching .... ☐
6. stringy, lusterless hair .... ☐
7. nits on the hair .... ☐
8. bald spots .... ☐
9. state of cleanliness .... ☐
10. cuts, scratches, bruises, burns . ☐

GENERAL APPEARANCE
1. underweight--very thin ...... ☐
2. overweight--obese .... ☐
3. tires easily .... ☐
4. chronic fatigue .... ☐
5. nausea or vomiting .... ☐
6. faintness or dizziness .... ☐
7. short of breath .... ☐
8. bluish lips .... ☐
9. excessive pallor, pale .... ☐

GROWTH AND POSTURE
1. undersized, failure to gain ... ☐
2. unexplained weight loss or gain ☐
3. a history of "growing pains" .. ☐
4. head tilted to side or forward . ☐
5. shoulders not square or level . ☐
6. hips not straight or level ..... ☐
7. knees pointed inward or outward ☐
8. feet pointed inward or outward ☐
9. peculiarity of gait .... ☐
10. obvious deformities of any type ☐

VISION

A student should be screened for vision problems each year they are in elementary and secondary school. Teachers should also observe students for vision problems on a continuing basis. Students with glasses should also be checked annually by the doctor who serves as their vision care specialist. The characteristics of the eyes change rapidly during childhood and adolescence. A problem that is not caught soon may seriously interfere with learning and emotional adjustments. There are a variety of vision problems, and some are more easily detected than others. Most schools screen for myopia, but neglect other problems.

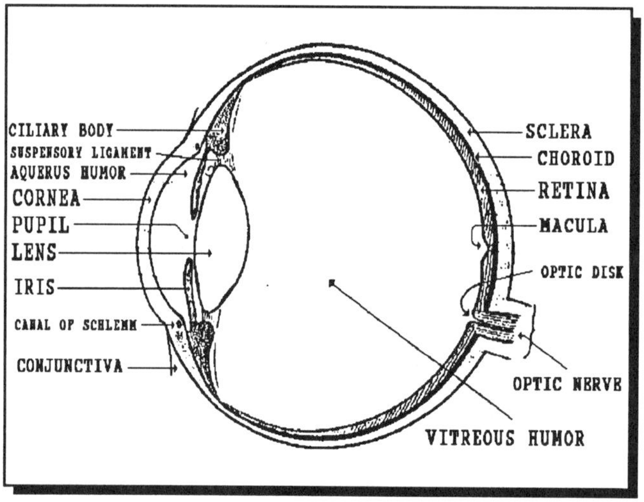

Structure and mechanism

The eye and the parts of the brain that work with the eyes are very interesting and adaptable organs. The skin type tissue around the eye is the conjunctiva. Most of the outside of the eyeball is the white membrum called sclera. The clear transparent front part of the eye through which light rays pass is the cornea. Behind the cornea is the iris which gives the eye its color. The iris contracts or expands according to the amount of light that passes through the pupil. Behind the pupil is the lens which bends the light to focus it on the retina. The lens is attached to the eye by tiny muscles (ciliary body) and suspensory ligaments. The retina is the part of the nervous system which receives the light images and transmits them to the brain through the optical nerve. For images to be seen clearly, they must be focused in the center part of the retina called the macula. The rods and cones are the nerve receptors in the retina which distinguish between light and dark and among colors.

The space in the eyeball cavity is filled with a thick jelly-like fluid or humor--aqueous humor in front of the lens and vitreous humor in back of the lens. Excess fluid flows out of the eyeball through the canal of schlemm. Muscles attached to the outside of the eyeball turn it in various directions.

Visual acuity problems

Visual acuity problems occur when the eye does not have a sharp, well-focused image projected on the retina. The three basic refractive errors (bending of light) are myopia, hyperopia, and astigmatism.

Normal

In normal vision, the light from the object is focused by the lens to form a sharp image on the retina. If the object moves further away or closer, the lens changes shape and becomes thinner or thicker so that the image is still focused sharply on the retina. When an image is in focus, a number of light rays converge to form a single dot. The image is clear. When an image is out of focus, a number of dots are formed and the image is fuzzy.

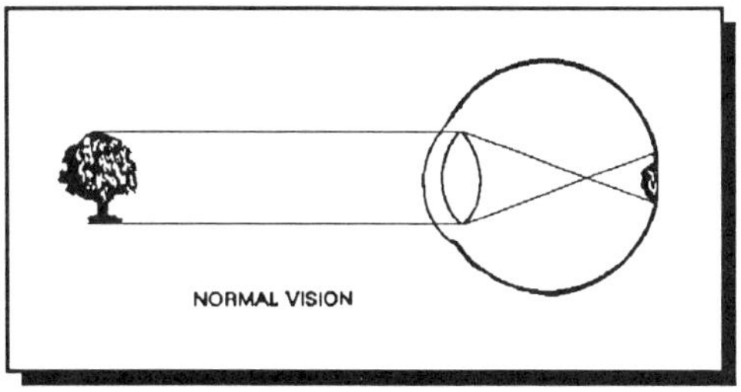

Myopia -- *nearsighted*

In myopia, the eyeball in effect is extra long. The lens focuses the image in front of the retina, so that by the time the image reaches the retina the image is out of focus. Objects that are near remain in focus, butobjects that are distant are out of focus.
A person who can see things that are near is nearsighted or myopic. He or she has difficulty seeing things at a distance. Myopia is the most common eye problem found among school children.

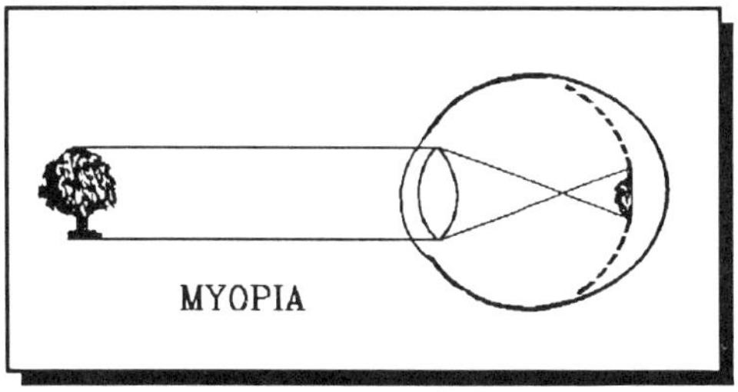

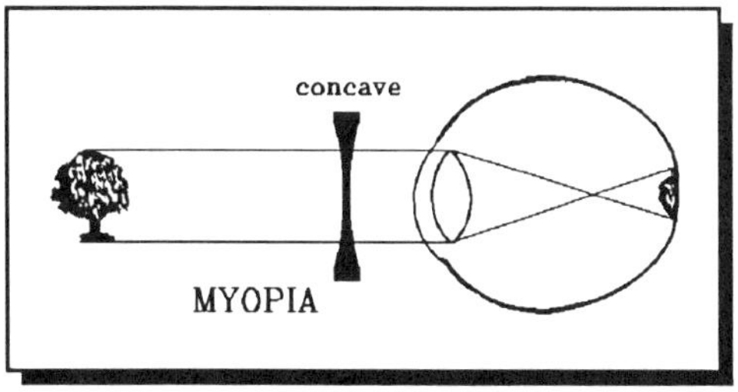

A *snellen* vision screening test can be used to find students who need further examination for possible myopia. A chart is used that has several lines of letters, each line a little larger than the line below it. Each line is marked by the distance from the chart that a person with normal vision can see that line. A person with normal vision can see the 20 foot line (with letters approximately 5/16 of an inch high) at a distance of 20 feet. That is 20/20 vision. However, if a person standing at 20 feet can only see the 50 foot line his vision is 20/50, meaning at 20 feet he can see what a normal person can see at 50 feet. Screening tests for myopia can be con-ducted by a teacher or anyone trained to give them.

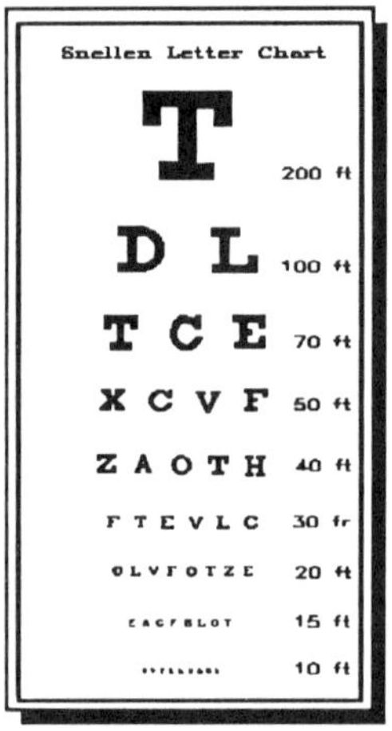

The chart should be placed at average student eye level on a well-illuminated wall without glare. Each student being tested should stand behind a line, perhaps a piece of tape, 20 feet from the chart. One eye is examined at a time, first the right and then the left. Students wearing glasses should be tested with their glasses on. A card is placed over the eye not being tested without pressing against the eyeball. A separate card should be used for each student. The person conducting the test should stand by the chart and reveal only one letter at a time through a card with an appropriate sized hole in the middle. Two or three cards with different sized holes are needed. Start on the 30 foot line and if the student can read the letters on that line move down to the 20 foot line, but if the student cannot read the 30 foot line move up a line at a time until you find the line they can read. A student is considered able to read a line if he or she can read three out of four letters on that line. Record the lowest line the student can read as a fraction with the numerator representing the distance from the chart (20) and the denominator representing the lowest line read correctly. A student who cannot read three of four letters on the 20 foot line should be referred for further evaluation. If a student gets a 20/20 rating, but tilts his head, squints, or shows other signs of eye problem, he or she should still be retested or referred to a vision specialist.

An ophthalmologist or optometrist uses a more sophisticated method, but this same basic idea, to determine the refractive error and prescribe glasses or contact lenses to compensate for the error. The greater the refractive error, the thicker the lenses. Concave lenses are used to correct myopia.

Hyperopia -- *farsighted*

In hyperopia, the eyeball in effect is extra short. The lens projects the image at a point past the retina, but because the eyeball is short, the image does not get that far and the image on the retina is fuzzy. Objects that are far remain in focus, but objects that are near are out of focus. A person who can see things that are distant is farsighted or hyperopic. He or she has difficulty seeing things that are near.

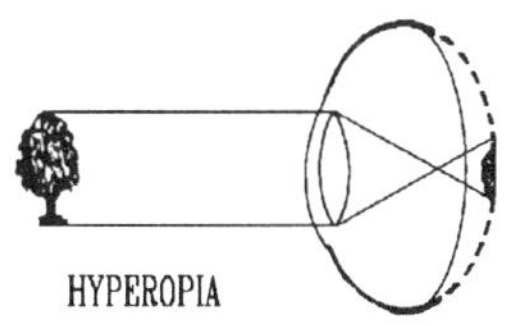

The snellen chart can be used for screening for hyperopia, but it requires that students being tested wear a pair of glasses with +1.75 diopter convex lenses. This test, called the plus sphere test, is given to students who do not wear glasses, who pass the snellen test, but who exhibit other signs of visual difficulty. The test is administered the same as was the test for myopia *except* that if the student can read the 20 foot line he or she has failed the test. The convex lenses blur normal vision, but correct hyperopic vision.

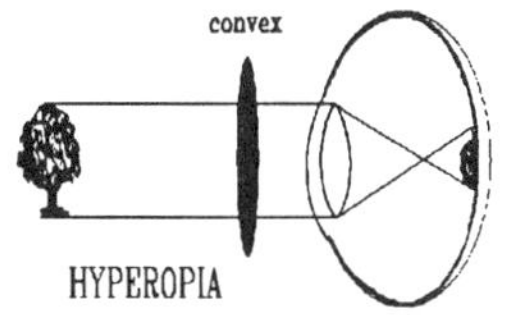

There is another test for the ability to see small objects such as print in a book at close range. It uses a card that contains six paragraphs each written in successively larger print. When the card is held at normal reading distance, 15 inches, the students should be able to see the smallest print clearly. The tester may ask the students if the print seems clear or fuzzy. The tester may also cover the print with a sheet of paper with a hole made by a paper punch and reveal only one letter at a time. The students are then asked to read the letters as they appear. This test is taken with both eyes. A student who can't read the small paragraph is referred.

Astigmatism

Astigmatism is blurred vision due to an irregularity in curvature of cornea. Rays of light passing through the cornea are bent more in one diameter than in another, resulting in some rays being properly focused and others not. This causes distortions such as is produced by a wavy pane of glass. Straight lines and flat surfaces are distorted. It often occurs in connection with myopia or hyperopia. It is probably the second most common vision problem among students. It is usually present at birth and does not grow worse with age.

A large (approximately 14 inch) wheel or clock-like chart is used to screen for astigmatism in the schools. To give this test the examiner covers one of the student's eyes and holds the chart about 15 inches in front of the other eye. The examiner says: "This is

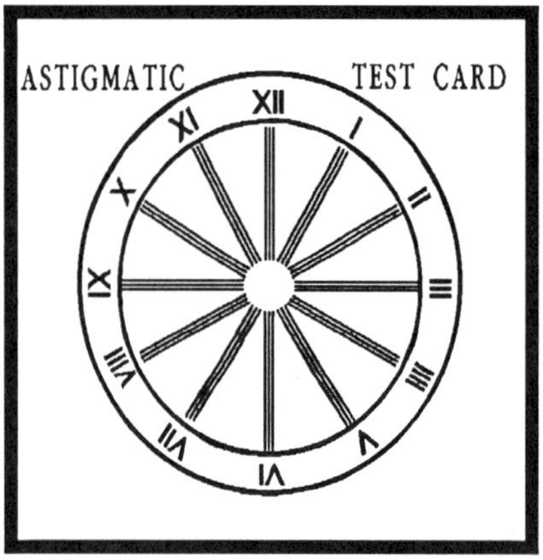

a wheel and the line are spokes which come together at the hub. Look directly at the hub and tell me if any of the spokes are darker than the others." If a student sees a set of lines on one side of the hub as being darker than the corresponding set of lines on the opposite side of the hub, he or she should be referred. A student who is normal for astigmatism will see all of the lines as equally dark. The test is repeated for the other eye. Glasses can be made to correct this problem.

Presbyopia

Presbyopia occurs in some older people starting at about age forty. It occurs when the lens loses its ability to change shapes to accommodate from various near and far points. This is not a problem for students, but it is a problem for teachers who need to see things that are close. People who have never had glasses before may have to be fitted with reading glasses. Those who already have glasses may have to go to bifocals, two lenses in one, and use the upper part for distant vision and the bottom part for near vision.

Alignment dysfunction

Eye alignment refers to how both eyes work together as a pair, so that the image seen with one eye fuses with the image seen with the other eye. *Binocularity* refers to how well the six muscles on each eye work together. Normally, the eyes converge or look inward as they focus on an object close to the eyes, and they become more parallel as they look at a more distant object. They also diverge or look outward. Alignment dysfunction seldom affects clarity of vision, but creates visual stress and fatigue. Students with binocularity problems cannot sustain reading or paper and pencil tasks.

Strabismus -- *cross-eye*

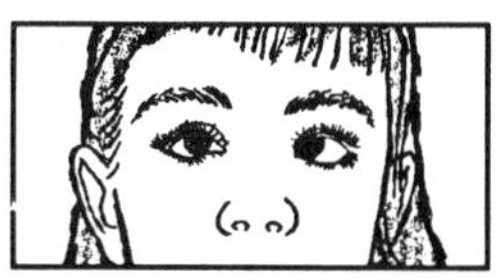

Strabismus refers to a misalignment of the eyes. With *cross-eye*, one eye turns in or converges more than the other normal focused eye. With *wall-eye*, one eye turns out or diverges more than the other normal focused eye. In some children, latent strabismus reveals itself only when they are tired or under emotional stress.

A rough and not very accurate screening test for muscle imbalance is the cover test. The procedure is as follows. Have the student look at an object about 20 feet away. Cover one eye with a card to block its view of the object while the uncovered eye continues to look at the object. Watch the covered eye to see if it maintains its alignment or if it turns in, out, up, or down. As you remove the cover, watch to see if the eye returns to alignment. Repeat the process for the other eye. Then start again having the student look at an object about 10 inches away. If the student's muscle balance is normal, there should be little change in alignment as the eye is covered or uncovered. Students who show noticeable deviations should be retested, and if similar results continue, they should be referred for professional evaluation. A combination of surgery and eye exercises may be used to correct the problem.

Amblyopia -- *lazy-eye*

A preschool child who has an eye muscular imbalance may suppress the use of one eye. This condition is called *amblyopia*, and it will result in the loss of vision in that eye unless treated. Preschool screening tests must be conducted to catch amblyopia before it is too late. Part of the early treatment is to have the child wear a patch over the good eye to force the use of the weaker eye.

Common Eye Infections

The teacher should be alert to the following common eye infections because of the importance of getting them prompt treatment:

Blepharitis is an inflammation of the eyelid producing itching, soreness, and white scales or yellow crusts.

Stye is an infection of a hair follicle on the margin of the eyelid. At first there is pain and sensitivity, and then an abscess forms, ruptures, and discharges pus.

Conjunctivitis is a highly contagious infection of the conjunctiva sometimes called "pink eye." Symptoms include itching, smarting, and burning of the eyelid, and the production of a discharge. Infected students should not attend school.

Trichoma is virus infection that attacks the conjunctiva which eventually leads to blindness, due to scaring of the cornea. It is not common in the United States, except possibly on Indian reservations, but it is still a major problem in the Middle East, Africa, and Asia. Its occurrence is associated with the lack of hygiene.

Other Eye Problems

Ptosis or drooping eyelids is an inherited condition. It may be considered a cosmetic problem, but does not interfere with vision.

Glaucoma means an increased pressure within the eyeball. It occurs when more fluid is formed than can be discharged and this pressure can cause blindness. Since it is most apt to occur among adults over age forty, tests for interoccular pressure should be a part of regular eye exams for adults.

Cataracts occur when the lens of the eye becomes clouded or opaque due to a biological change associated with aging. Treatment includes surgically removing the cataract lens and replacing it with a plastic lens.

Detached retina is a separation of the retina from the wall of the eyeball. A portion of the retina hangs like a torn curtain, and a portion of the person's vision is obstructed. It can be reattached by surgery and requires extended periods of no head movement. It can occur at any age and sometimes occurs to athletes.

HEARING

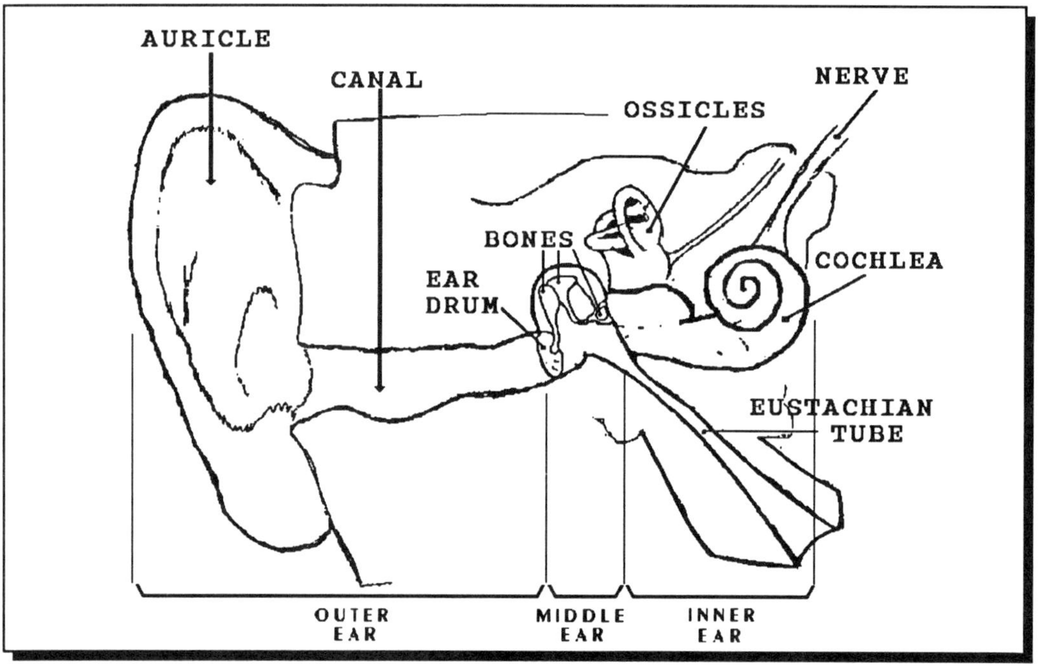

The hearing process begins with airwaves or vibrations created in our environment. Our auditory system is highly sensitive as it picks up and interprets those sounds. It can discriminate among voices and instruments in an orchestra. Its delicate structure is protected within the hard bones of the head. Vibrations can reach the nerves of the ear through the bony structures around the ears as well as by sound waves that come through the ears. Practically everyone is surprised the first time they hear their own recorded voice. When we hear ourselves speak, what we hear comes by both bone and air conduction, but the tape recorder records only what is air conducted.

The ear is divided into three areas: outer ear, middle ear, and inner ear. The external ear (*auricle*) helps direct sound waves into the ear canal which penetrates about an inch into the head. The sound waves cause the ear drum (*tympanic membrane*) at the end of the canal to vibrate. Three little bones (*malleus*, *incus*, and *stapes*) in the middle ear conduct and amplify the vibrations from the ear drum to the cochlea of the inner ear which is filled with fluid. The amplified vibrations pass from the stapes to the oval window of the cochlea and cause the fluid in the cochlea to move in waves. The waves of fluid excite the nerve endings along the cochlea and nerve impulses are sent to the brain.

If the snail-shaped cochlea were rolled out straight, it might be compared to the keys on a piano arranged from low to high notes. However, the inner ear has more than 20,000 "keys," and instead of making sounds, they receive sounds. Tiny hair-like structures along the cochlea are made to oscillate by the waves of fluid. A hair structure called an organ of corti is an auditory nerve receptor. Some of the nerve receptors respond to very low-sounding notes which vibrate as slow as 20 cycles per second; others respond to sounds which vibrate as fast as 20,000 cycles per second; and others respond to every sound in-between. Some types of hearing loss are associated with the destruction to the nerve receptors somewhere along the cochlea.

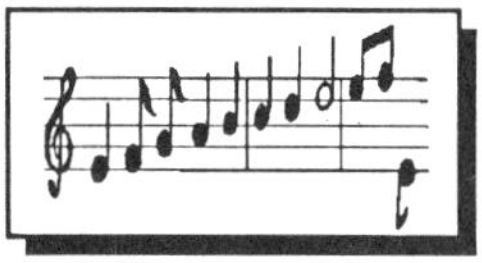

There are two characteristics of sound, frequency and volume. Frequency or pitch has to do with cycles per second and ranges from low to high like the keys on a piano. A piano ranges from 27 to 4,000 cycles per second (cps). Conversational speech ranges from 200 to 3,000 cps. Human capacity ranges from 20 to 20,000 cps. Frequencies below 20 cps can be felt but not heard.

Volume has to do with how loud or soft the sound is, and this can range from as soft as a whisper to as loud as a jet airplane. The volume or intensity of sound is measured in decibels (db) on a logarithm scale where 0 db is the least intensity of sound that a normal ear can hear. (A sound of 10 db transmits *ten* times as much energy as a sound of 0 db. A sound of 20 db transmits *one hundred* times as much energy as a sound of 0 db and *ten* as much as a 10 db sound.) A whisper is about 20 db and conversation is about 60 db. Household appliances and construction equipment may range from 80 to 110 db. A jet airplane takeoff 200 feet away may be 120 db. Sounds in excess of 80 db become annoying. Sustained sounds above 90 db may cause hearing loss, sometimes temporary and sometimes permanent.

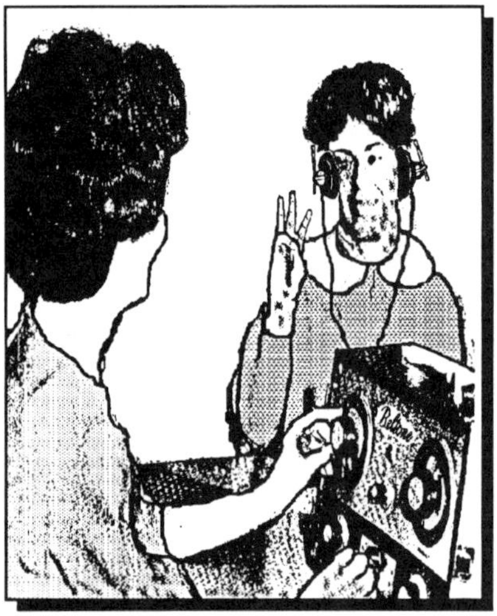

A number of conditions can cause hearing loss: infections, injury, heredity, age, excessive noise, etc. The hearing loss may be limited to a specific frequency. A person may be able to hear sounds at that frequency only if the volume is increased. Since a person may be able to hear some sounds all of the time and all sounds some of the time, he or she may not realize there is a loss. Since they can hear some people speak and not other people, they think those they cannot hear are just mumbling.

Loss of hearing acuity usually occurs so gradually that the individual does not notice it. He unconsciously learns to compensate to some degree by learning to lip read; we all lip read to some extent. A hearing screening test would catch such problems early. Many adults with marked hearing defects could hear better today if the problem had been detected when it first started. Hearing screening should be conducted on a regular basis starting with preschool and periodically throughout the school years. A student with hearing loss may adjust his or her posture or exhibit other behaviors such as inattention, poor pronunciation, or an unnatural voice that a teacher might observe. A student may try to copy other students' work when he or she cannot hear what the teacher says. Poor academic progress may cause a teacher to suspect hearing or vision problems.

There are two types of hearing defects, sensorineural and conductive.

Sensorineural. Impairment of the hairs in the cochlea and the nerves between the ear and the brain. Usually both ears are involved. The hearing loss is complete deafness, and the condition is not serviceable. This condition is obvious.

Conductive. Impairment along the pathway from the outer ear to the cochlea in the inner ear which interferes mechanically with the conduction of sound vibrations. One or both ears may be involved. It is usually a partial hearing loss in the low sounds. It is usually a hard-of-hearing condition which is serviceable.

Hearing screening tests

Hearing screening is important, because good hearing is essential to the child's social and educational development. The following are benefits of a well-planned screening program:

- the prevention of handicapping hearing losses through early detection and treatment.

- the maintenance of adequate hearing for the child in the classroom; many defects go undetected and untreated because of poor screening programs.

- the habilitation for those children with permanent hearing losses which are identified by the screening program.

Some authorities suggest that hearing screening should be conducted for all students in kindergarten and in grades 1, 3, 5, and 7. Tests should also be conducted on all students transferring into the school system (including high school students), students with a history of previous hearing problems, and students whose possible hearing problems may have been detected through teacher observations. There are two types of tests, whisper tests and tests with an audiometer. The Whisper Screening Test is not extremely reliable but can give the teacher some idea as to a student's loss of hearing. The audiometer is usually used by a specialist; however, a teacher could learn to use it.

Whisper Test Procedures

1. Have the student face away from the teacher in a room free from distractions.

2. The teacher should stand 30 feet away and whisper words. The student then will give an indication that he heard the whisper. The teacher should move up five feet at a time if the student can't hear the whisper.

3. Use only one ear at a time, stopping the other with the student's finger.

4. The student should be able to hear the whisper at 30 feet if he has normal hearing. If he can't hear as close as 10 feet away, a man's pocket watch should be used instead of a whisper.

Audiometer Screening Tests

There are several types of audiometer tests that are used to check air conduction and bone conduction factors in hearing loss.

Sweep test. This is the standard screening technique, and it is conducted as follows. Set the hearing level of the screening audiometer at 20 db. Start at the 1000 frequency and sweep up through the 2000 and 4000 frequencies (Hz) and then down through the 500 and 250 frequencies (Hz). Have the students raise their finger or hand when they hear a sound. If a student does not respond at a frequency, increase the intensity to 25 db. A student who still does not respond should be retested after a few weeks, and if there is still no response, the student should be referred.

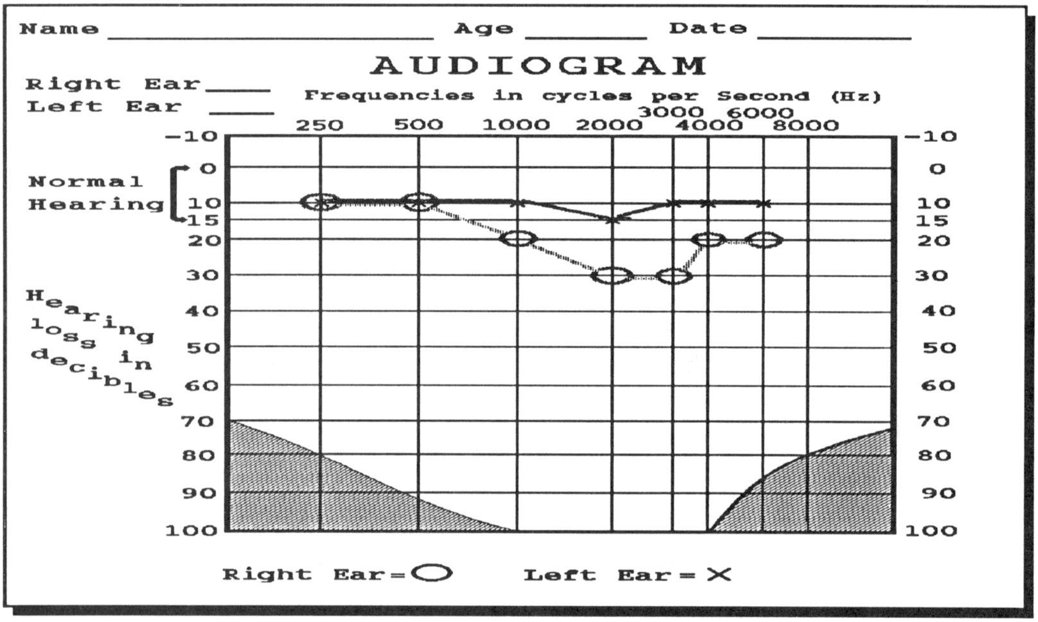

<u>Threshold test</u>. This test determines the exact decibel level at which a tone frequency can be heard. Each ear is tested at 250, 500, 1000, 2000, and 4000 Hz. starting at 0 db and increasing at 5 db intervals until a response is obtained. The child should be referred for further testing if the hearing threshold is 25 db or greater at two frequencies or 35 db or greater at one frequency. More extensive testing would also use a bone conduction device to see if there is a difference in air conduction hearing and bone conduction hearing. This will help isolate the problem and point to the best remedial approach.

Teachers who have hearing-impaired students in the classroom may be able to help by having the student sit in the best location in the classroom. Generally, that place is to the side of the room with the best ear to the classroom, but the best location varies with the individual and the acoustics in the classroom, so it may take some trials to find the best spot. Since the hearing-impaired student generally relies on lip reading, the teacher should avoid anything that might block the student's vision of his or her lips.

The schools should provide further consultation services for children found to have irrem-ediable hearing losses even after medical treatment has been concluded. These services include further audiogram studies that may lead to recommendations for hearing aid use, special seating in the classroom, lip reading or auditory training classes, or referral to special schools or classes.

DENTAL

The dental examination is primarily a preventive measure to detect and correct early dental defects. It can be given by the family dentist or by a school-appointed dentist at his office or at the school. The dentist basically checks for any cavities and other dental abnormalities. Although a teacher's role in observing students' dental problems is limited, if signs or symptoms are detected, the student should be referred. Diseased teeth or gums, misaligned teeth, mouth odors, and student complaints about toothache may indicate a problem. Students should be made aware of the problems associated with poor dental health.

Dental Problems

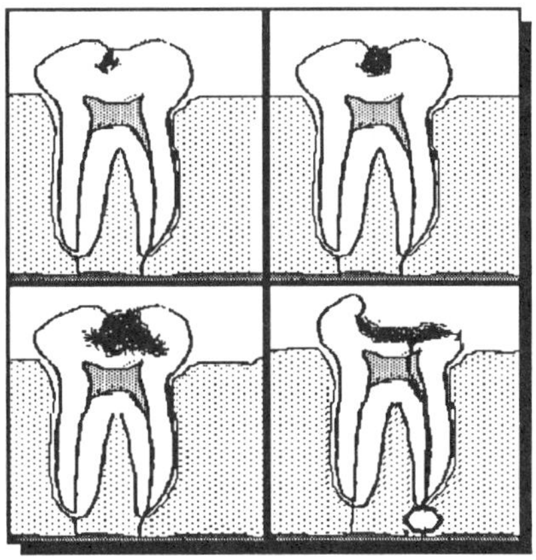

Dental decay (*caries*) are associated with heredity, diet, and neglect. Dental *plaque*--consisting of mucus, food particles, and bacteria--collects between the teeth, in crevices, and on the gum line. Bacteria in the plaque feed on the sugar in the food and generate acid which erodes the tooth enamel and forms tiny cavities. This beginning of dental decay will continue to grow if not treated. When the decay spreads through the dentin and reaches the pulp, inflammation develops. The body responds by increasing blood flow with white cells to the area to combat the infection. This swelling puts pressure on the nerves entering the tooth and causes a toothache. As decay continues, the exposed nerves react to hot or cold and sweets. If there is too much infection, the root containing the nerves will die and an abscess on the root may form. Infection from the abscess is a serious risk to health.

Gingivitis is inflamed and swollen gums. It is also caused by accumulated plaque between the tooth and the gums. The plaque, if not removed, continues to irritate the gums and *periodontitis* develops. If not treated, the gums recede until the tooth is lost. While such problems occur primarily among adults, the pattern of neglect starts during the school age years.

Malocclusions or misaligned teeth may cause a variety of problems ranging from appearance to difficulty eating and speaking. Teeth may be too large for the gums, causing

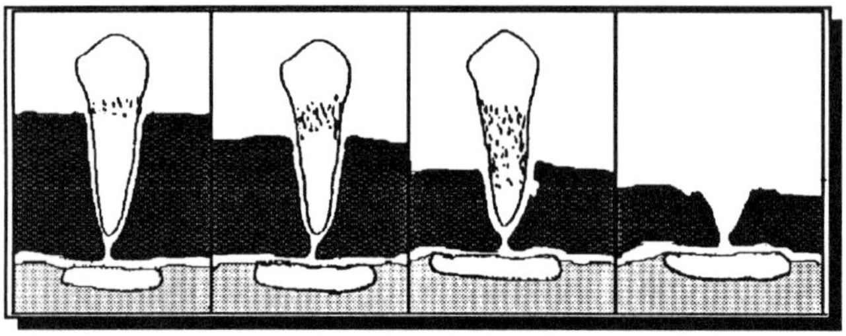

crowding. The bite between the upper and lower teeth may not fit. Teeth may protrude out or be in the wrong place. Dentists specialized in orthodontia use a variety of procedures to correct such problems. Because some malocclusions are associated with speech defects, they should be detected early.

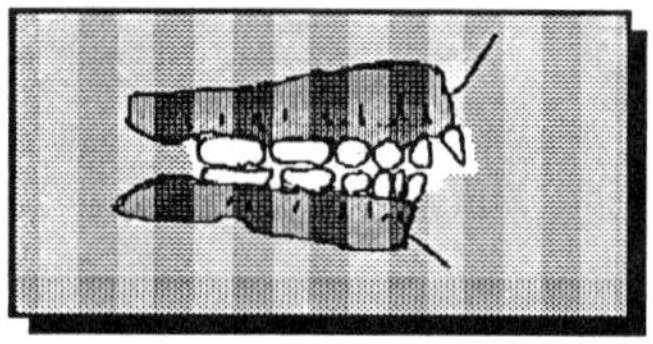

CHILD ABUSE

The role of the teacher in detecting possible child abuse has been gaining attention in recent years. Teachers have been given added instruction on what to look for, and laws have been passed in all 50 states requiring teachers to report such observations. This is a delicate and sensitive area, but one that requires careful attention. There are a number of types of child abuse, but signs of neglect and physical abuse are most apparent. *Physical neglect* involves parents or guardians who fail to provide basic physical needs such as nutrition, hygiene, and safety. *Emotional abuse or neglect* is failure to provide an emotionally stable environment for the child to mature in. *Sexual abuse* is extremely emotionally destructive, but very difficult to detect and deal with. Teachers should work closely with school counselors in all types of suspected child abuse. Teachers generally see the results of *physical abuse* as soft tissue injuries such as bruises, welts, abrasions, lacerations, and burns.

At first, this might seem difficult to distinguish between physical abuse and other circumstances that may cause the injury. But there are some key distinctions. The part of the body that is injured is a clue. For example, the point of the elbow is often injured in accidents, but accidental injuries seldom occur to the inside of the elbow. Persons who abuse children frequently grab and squeeze the child's arm so violently that welts and sores are left. Injuries to protected areas such as the back of the knees, the back of the thighs, the buttocks and genital areas, between the shoulder blades, and to the front of the face are suspicious. Another clue is reoccurring injuries, particularly in the suspicious areas. Children are not likely to admit that the offending person caused the injury, but the way they give explanations is another clue. The explanations may be void of detail, but along lines that challenge the imagination. Failure to concentrate on studies or normal interests and other emotional behavior changes may also be a clue. Put a number of clues together, and you have the basis for a referral. There are a number of agencies which deal with child abuse cases that have been recognized for their expertise and discretion.

OTHER HEALTH PROBLEMS

Head Lice

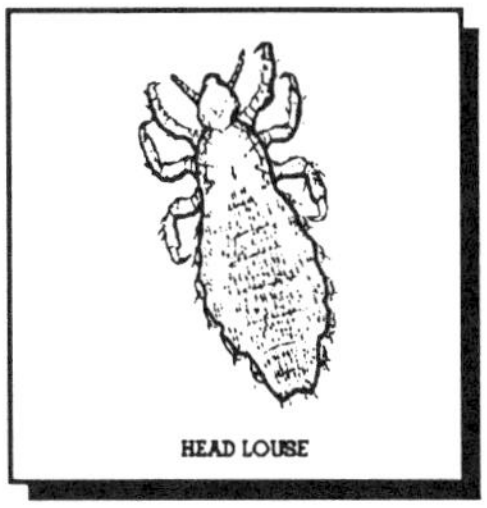

Millions of Americans are infected with head lice, and the number is increasing. The ban on DDT, expanded world travel, and increased social contact has brought screening for head lice back into the schools. An outbreak can quickly reach epidemic proportions. Lice are small, flat, wingless insects with stubby antennae and three pair of legs with sharp curved claws. All three types of lice (head lice, body lice, and pubic lice) need human warmth to survive and live all their life (2 months) on their host's body. Head and pubic lice lay their eggs in the hair; body lice may lay their eggs in the seams of clothing. The eggs take about a week to incubate. They are spread by personal contact or by sharing items like clothing or combs. Head lice are more prevalent among grade school children, pubic lice are more prevalent among young adults, and body lice can infect any age group.

Some schools, particularly elementary schools, conduct periodic screening for head lice; others do not screen unless there has been reported cases in the area. A close examination of the scalp will reveal small, whitish eggs firmly attached to the hair shaft, especially at the nape of the neck and above the ears. Inspection may also reveal hatched lice and irritated red marks. Signs and symptoms of body and pubic lice are severe itching, scratch marks, and local lesions. Once lice infestation has been discovered, all members of the family and all close contacts should be treated. This problem is more prevalent where general hygiene is at a low level; however, lice can spread even where levels of cleanliness are high.

Tuberculosis

Tuberculosis is not the dreaded disease it once was, but some schools still conduct tuberculin screening tests. There are usually no early signs or symptoms, but the tine test identifies individuals who have been exposed to the infection. A little device with needles in it pricks the skin. The nurse will look at the needle mark a few days later. People who have been exposed to TB will develop a red spot at the needle marks. X-ray examinations will be given as a follow up to positive reactions.

Height, Weight, and Posture

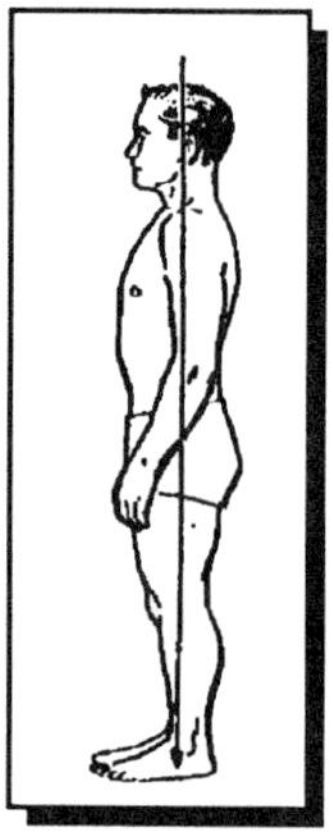

Height and weight measurements interest the students in their own growth and well-being. This can be done by the school nurse or physical education teacher. Students should be measured and weighed with their shoes on and one pound and one inch deducted. Measurements should be taken three times a year and a record should be kept. Various charts are available which can help determine if the child is in the normal, healthy range.

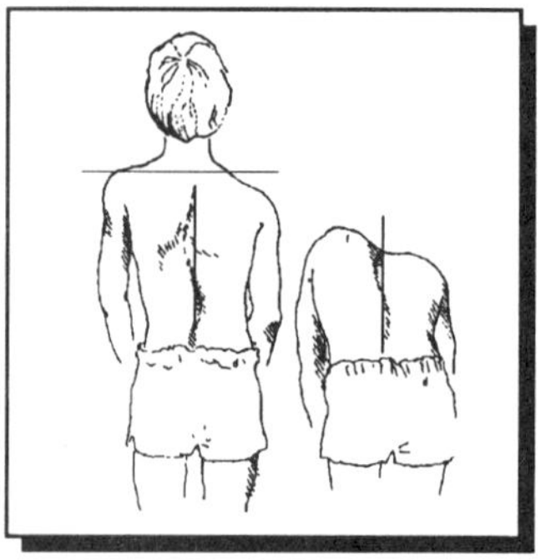

Posture screening is done through visual examination to find any disorders of the spine. There are several types of posture problems, but of most concern is scoliosis or curvature of the spine. The most important factor in ensuring early diagnosis of scoliosis is routine examinations of all growing children and youth at six-month intervals, from early childhood until full maturity. Although a school nurse or physical education teacher are usually best suited to make a thorough exam, other teachers can conduct basic tests. Any teacher can observe marked spinal deviations beneath regular clothing. First, have the students stand against the wall and with a straight line see if each student's shoulders are the same height. Then have the student bend over while you check the spine by running your hand along it to see if it is straight. Such simple tests may reveal minimal scoliosis early so that treatment may correct the problem and prevent it from getting worse.

Speech Defects

About six percent of the people in this country have speech problems. Most common are articulation problems such as the inability to produce certain sounds. Fluency problems such as stuttering are also common. Some have problems with voice disorders, and a few have delayed speech and language development.

Stuttering and stammering are conditions usually related to emotional causes. Anyone acutely embarrassed or terrified is likely to stammer until his emotions are under control. Stammering is usually an expression of self-consciousness, shyness, or fear. In an eager youngster, however, it may be nothing more than failure to keep up with his rapid flow of thought.

One approach to help students with speech problems is to let them know in advance what they will be expected to read in class so they can look it over and gain confidence before actually reading it out loud. When they are speaking, do not hurry them or say it for them. Be patient so they can relax and take the time they need, and they will do much better. People with a possible speech problem should be referred for special help from a speech therapist.

The main adjustment is for parents, teachers, and others--including fellow students--to have patience and try to instill confidence. Do not try to say the words for the student who stutters. Help the student prepare for discussions in advance so that he or she will be under less pressure. Consult with the speech therapist for more specific advice on how to help.

Learning Disorders

The terms "learning disabilities" and "perceptual disorders" are used specifically to indicate the type of learning difficulties encountered by children who are not mentally retarded, but who have a mild central nervous system dysfunction.

In a broader sense, the term "learning disabilities" also applies to children suffering from an educational problem related to minimal motor development, generalized mental retardation, cultural deprivation, and emotional disturbances. Often the nature of the dysfunction is so subtle that it is hard to recognize. We know that the physical and the emotional are often interrelated. The problem operates in a regressive cycle. Poor vision may result in poor reading, which may result in a poor self-concept, which further interferes with learning. From the practical point of view of the normal classroom teacher, we are concerned with any health problem (physical, social, emotional, or intellectual) that interferes with a student's ability to learn.

The basic result of a learning disability is academic crippling and the loss of subsequent opportunities in life. The afflicted individual becomes a burden to his family and society in general. As high as 90 percent of juvenile delinquents are underachievers or nonachievers in school. Many of the problems can be traced back to learning disorders when they were first learning to read and write. Because they did not learn to read and write well, they had learning problems in other areas of education. To this failure, they react emotionally with inappropriate behavior. This results in social rejection, and their self-esteem becomes lower than ever. They become inattentive. They may become antisocial and turn to delinquency and crime. They may become socially dependent. Thus learning disabilities, if not remedied, may place a person in a state of unrealized potential.

Serious emotional reactions can be averted if learning disabilities are detected early. Irreparable damage may take place if a child who has learning disorders is considered to be stupid. Patience is needed until the underlying cause is found and corrected as far as possible. A few signs and symptoms of a learning-disabled child are the following:

- **Associations.** The student has difficulty in being able to categorize, conceptualize, or draw conclusions. The student is easily confused and mixed up and is unable to distinguish right from left or up from down.

- **Short attention span.** The student's attention to a subject lasts only for a short period of time. He or she is distracted by extraneous stimuli. He or she may be in a state of perpetual motion, and he or she may shift moods suddenly and frequently.

- **Visual characteristics.** A student may have difficulty comprehending sequences, discriminating between shapes, or transferring ideas from one situation to another. He frequently confuses letters (p-b-d-g) and reverses words (was-saw).

- **Auditory characteristics.** A student may have difficulty associating the sound of a letter with the appropriate symbol. He or she may not hear the difference between words such as "tree" and "bee" and letters such as t and d.

Dyslexia

One learning disorder that has received a lot of attention in recent years is dyslexia, which means impaired reading or writing. The World Federation of Neurology defines dyslexia as "a disorder manifest by difficulty in learning to read despite conventional instruction, adequate intelligence, and socio-cultural opportunity." Dyslexia is hard to define because every case displays different symptoms. Some of the common problems are on the following page.

- Difficulty in learning and remembering printed words.

- Some letters and numbers are reversed, for example:
(b - d), (p - q), (6-9).

- The order of letters in words are changed, for example:
(tar - rat), (quite - quiet), (12 - 21).

- Confusion of vowel sounds or substitution of consonants.

- Elimination of or insertion of words while reading.

- Persistent spelling errors.

- Difficulty in writing.

There is no known cause of dyslexia, but theories deal with learning sequence and brain dominance. Eighty percent of the cases are among males. Treatment is strongly remedial, focused on the specific needs of the individual. Since students with dyslexia are very slow readers, the use of books recorded on tapes or having someone read for them will help them stay up with their studies. Some dyslexics are successful in college, but have to work extra hard. Teacher encouragement until they gain confidence is important.

The teacher's role in the school health services program includes not only detection but also some areas of remedial work. Sometimes specialists such as speech therapists help in the remedial programs, but often the majority of the adjustments must take place in the normal classroom setting. The handicapped pupil should be treated as nearly like any other pupil as possible. Although there are special provisions that the school may make, to live successfully within their limitations is their challenge.

STUDY HELPS

Match the following.

A. EYES / SEEING
B. HEIGHT/WEIGHT
C. CHILD ABUSE
D. LEARNING DISORDERS
E. EARS / HEARING
F. SPEECH
G. COMMUNICABLE DISEASE
H. TEETH / DENTAL
I. POSTURE
J. OTHER

1. amblyopia
2. astigmatism
3. audiometer
4. auricle
5. blepharitis
6. canal
7. caries
8. cataracts
9. cochlea
10. conductive
11. conjunctiva
12. conjunctivitis
13. cornea
14. detached retina
15. drum
16. dyslexia
17. emotional
18. eyeball
19. gingivitis
20. glaucoma
21. head lice
22. hyperopia
23. incus
24. inner ear
25. iris
26. malleus
27. malocclusions
28. middle ear
29. myopia
30. neglect
31. nerve
32. optical
33. outer ear
34. periodontitis
35. physical
36. plaque
37. presbyopia
38. ptosis
39. pupil
40. retina
41. scoliosis
42. sensorineural
43. sexual
44. snellen
45. stapes
46. strabismus
47. stye
48. trichoma
49. tuberculosis
50. whisper test

1. What is school health appraisal? How does it fit into the School Health Program? How does school health appraisal relate to personal and family-provided health care?

2. What is the basis for school health and dental examinations? What are the various patterns for conducting these examinations?

3. What is the purpose of school-based health screening tests? What type of screening tests are in use in the public schools? Who normally administers the various screening tests?

4. What is the purpose of teacher observation? How do teacher observations fit into school health appraisal? What are the guiding principles for conducting teacher observations?

5. What advantages and disadvantages does teacher observation have as compared with other forms of health appraisal?

6. When a teacher observes a possible departure from normal health, what is the procedure for making a referral? What follow up should a teacher make?

7. When a teacher is in a position to give health counsel, what principles should guide his or her actions?

8. What are some indications of possible problems that a teacher might observe regarding growth, poslture, general appearance, and in the following areas of the body? -- nose, mouth, throat, ears, skin, scalp

9. What is the role of the teacher in detecting and reporting possible child abuse?

Chapter 14

DEALING WITH CHRONIC HEALTH PROBLEMS

Although adolescents as a group are the healthiest segment of society, there are still a few who suffer from a variety of serious chronic conditions. It helps if teachers understand something about these conditions and their impact on students' lives. Chronic refers to those diseases marked by long durations or frequent recurrences of a noninfectious origin. Some of these conditions, such as congenital heart disease, have been affecting the student since birth. Other students may be in the process of adjusting to a recently discovered condition such as diabetes. Some may have conditions that are pretty well under control and others may have conditions that will eventually prove fatal. Some conditions require continual adjustments on the part of the school, teachers, and fellow students; others require only a little understanding, some encouragement, and a chance to try to succeed.

DEALING WITH CHRONIC HEALTH PROBLEMS

When the word disease entered the English language from French, it literally meant "that which makes one uncomfortable or *not at ease*." Its use is associated with a variety of conditions ranging from an indefinable sense of not feeling well or malaise, to specific acute and chronic ailments. Sometimes people are confused by the categories of disease. One way to identify chronic disease is to say they include all the diseases that are not caused by microorganisms. They are sometimes described as stress diseases, functional disorders, degenerative conditions, and noncommunicable diseases. The term "stress" is associated with the body's failure to adapt appropriately to the stress of life. "Functional" describes what happens when parts of the body without pathology fail to function properly. "Degenerative" means that a part of the body simply wears out or breaks down. And "noncommunicable" means that the condition is not due to a disease-producing microorganism that is spread readily from person to person; these will be discussed in the next chapter. "Chronic" means that the unhealthy condition lingers or recurs.

At the turn of the century, communicable diseases were leading the list of causes of death in this country. Today, chronic diseases have replaced communicable diseases at the head of the list. As medical science extends life by combating communicable diseases, people have become vulnerable to the chronic diseases. Heart conditions are the most frequent cause of death and disability among the general population of this country. Cancer is second for the general population and the leading cause of death due to disease among the 15-24 year age group. The most frequent type of cancer among young people is leukemia, a form of cancer in the blood. Several other types of chronic diseases are found occasionally among secondary students. Students are also frequently affected by chronic diseases among members of their families. Teachers need to understand some facts of chronic diseases that may affect their students or the students' families.

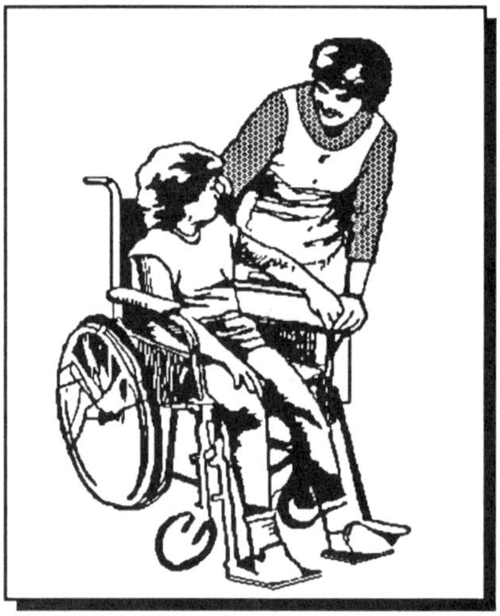

The schools and teachers have two major responsibilities in regard to chronic diseases: (1) to deal with students' current problems, and (2) to help prevent future problems. Medical science is doing much to help with the first, and behavioral science is pointing the way to the second. For example, a few years ago leukemia was always considered fatal, today most young people survive this form of cancer. Schools are also learning better ways of helping students with leukemia through the long recovery period. Schools are in a position to do much more to help students develop lifestyles that will reduce chronic disease risks.

Sometimes teachers go too far in trying to help students with health problems and end up doing psychological damage to the child. The student needs to learn to live with his problems and should not be pampered or receive help beyond his needs. His actual needs are not easily determined; therefore, it is well for a team effort to be employed consisting of students, teachers, and other concerned school personnel. Wise consistency is important. Sometimes parents will request preferential treatment for their child. This may or may not be necessary or advisable. For example, parents may request that a child with a congenital heart condition be kept inside for recess. A check with the physician may indicate that the child needs the fresh air and mild activity such as walking around, but not strenuous activity such as running. The response of the teacher or school should be to the effect that the policy is that whenever a student receives preferential treatment on a continual basis, that treatment must be requested in writing by the student's physician. This provides important guidelines and protection for the student and the teacher. The teacher does not want to pamper and spoil the student, but he does not want to lead him into an activity that may be too difficult or harmful.

Sometimes teachers are too emotionally immature or not professionally qualified to handle the knowledge that a student is somehow different without this knowledge interfering with the normal relationship between the teacher and the student. For example, if a teacher who finds out that a student has a history of epilepsy becomes frightened that the child will have a seizure in class and this fright interferes with the normal teacher-student relationship, it may be better not to have that information. A professionally qualified teacher would be able to handle that information so that he would be prepared in the case of an emergency. The teacher should not let the disease get in the way of seeing the student, yet they still need to be aware of the possible implications of the disease.

While the teacher can encourage his students to follow good sound health practices and this will help prevent some of the chronic diseases, the teacher's role lies more significantly in the area of helping students with such problems adjust to life, particularly in the school setting.

UNDERSTANDING THE CHRONICALLY ILL

Before the teacher can learn to deal with a chronic illness in a student, he must be able to recognize the fears and anxieties of the child and those the child reflects from his parents. A child with a chronic illness is trying to explore life at the same time he is trying to come to terms with the bewilderment of his illness. He may respond to ordinary school experiences in an unordinary way. He may have feelings of failure and doom in looking toward new experiences. The chronically ill adolescent may also exhibit dependency, regression, or uncooperative behavior because of fear felt towards new experiences at school. He may be afraid to join in socially and enjoy the experiences of a new school life because of a fear of rejection or incapability. Also, a fear of death may accompany his illness. This fear may bring out feelings of anger, denial, guilt, and self-doubt. The chronically ill child may also be deprived of normal experiences through frequent hospitalization, medications, etc.

It is important for the teacher to understand the chronically ill student before he can help him. The teacher, instead of reacting with feelings of panic, inadequacy, rejection and fear, should be a source of strength.

COMMON CHRONIC HEALTH PROBLEMS

The following list identifies a number of chronic health problems found among secondary students or conditions that may develop as a result of lifestyles formed during adolescence. Those that occur most frequently among students and will be described in greater detail later in the lesson are marked with an (§).

Acne § — A skin condition common to teenagers caused by blocked pores and resulting in pimples. It affects the face primarily and causes considerable self-consciousness. Serious cases, if untreated, may cause permanent scarring.

Allergy — A distressful or hypersensitive reaction to specific substances which cause no problem in most people. Hay fever, bronchial asthma, bronchitis, and croup are related to allergies affecting the respiratory system. Hives may be an allergic reaction to certain foods resulting in welts on the skin.

Anemia — This condition occurs when either the hemoglobin or red blood cells count is below normal. Since iron is an essential ingredient in hemoglobin, it may be due to insufficient iron in the diet, or it may be due to a shortage of vitamin B^{12}, used in red cell production. Sickle cell anemia, a disease affecting people of African descent only, is an inherited trait which results in the production of abnormal, sickle-shaped, red blood cells. Symptoms include lack of vitality and endurance.

Arthritis — Arthritis is a collection of many crippling diseases. Arthritis is an inflammation of the joints. Rheumatism is a disorder of muscles, tendons, bones, and nerves outside of the joints. The importance of seeking medical advice during the early signs cannot be stressed too much. Even though there is no specific treatment or cure, much can be done to reduce the progress of the disease and avoid disability. Arthritis victims are particularly susceptible to the misleading claims of unproven health practices. The spontaneous but temporary remissions seem to give credibility to the false claims of cure.

Asthma — Bronchial asthma is a condition of spasmatic wheezing or difficult and labored breathing due to the narrowing of the bronchial tubes. It usually has an allergic basis. It is often accompanied by nervousness and inefficiency in functioning because of associated anxieties.

Atherosclerosis
Degeneration of blood vessels in the heart caused by deposits of fatty materials such as cholesterol along the lining of the vessels walls leads to this disease. Although this condition does not show up until later, it may start to develop during the school age years due to improper diet and inadequate exercise.

Bronchitis Inflammation of the air passages. Acute bronchitis is an infection acting at first like the common cold, but settling in the chest. It is common among young people. Chronic bronchitis is a more permanent obstruction and usually occurs among older adults, particularly smokers.

Cancer § Cancer is a large group of diseases characterized by uncontrolled cell growth. Common types of cancer among children and youth include leukemia, or cancer of the blood and bone marrow; lymphomas and Hodgkin's Disease, or cancer of the lymph nodes; and malignancies of the nervous system, kidneys, and other soft tissues.

Cerebral Palsy
A form of paralysis manifested by jerky or spastic movements resulting from damage to the brain center which controls muscles. It also affects speech. It may have several causes including fetal infection and birth injury.

Cystic Fibrosis
A disease of the exocrine glands when secretions are poured into or out of the body instead of into the blood. The accumulated secretions depress the functions of other organs of the body and produce a variety of symptoms including respiratory distress. It is a recessive hereditary trait. It occurs in infancy but may not be recognized until later.

Diabetes § A deficiency in insulin output by the pancreas resulting in fluctuation of blood sugar levels which can bring on insulin shock or diabetic coma.

Emphysema Destruction of the air sacs of the lungs marked by difficulty in exhalation and inadequate oxygen/carbon dioxide exchange. Frequently found among older, long term smokers.

Epilepsy § A neurological disorder marked by periodic recurring convulsions and/or loss of consciousness. The *mal* or seizures are associated with explosive discharges of electrical activity in the brain cells stemming from a variety of causes. There are three types: 1) grand mal, 2) petit mal, and 3) psych-motor mal.

Coronary Artery Disease §

Heart attacks rarely occur among high school students, but they start establishing the lifestyles that will lead to early heart attacks and strokes when they get older. Heart attacks occur when the coronary artery is blocked so that the heart muscles are deprived of oxygen.

Congenital Heart Disease §

Abnormal blood circulation through the heart due to incompetent fetal heart development.

Rheumatic Heart Disease §

Infection of heart during rheumatic fever; usually results in damage to the heart valves. Symptoms: cardiac crisis may sometimes result.

Hemophilia

A person with this problem is known as a "bleeder." This rare disease is associated with a reduced production of blood factors promoting blood clotting. Cuts bleed for a long time. Internal bleeding is caused by bumps and falls, deep bruises occur easily and are slow to heal. Knee joints may become swollen, stiff, and painful. Hemophilia is a sex-linked inherited disease affecting males.

Hypothyroidism

An endocrine gland disorder involving insufficient production of thyroxin hormone by the thyroid gland leading to a slowing down of mental and physical processes. Symptoms include being chronically slow, disinterested, sleepy, and doing poor school work.

Muscular Dystrophy

This rare disease starts among children and is marked by a progressive wasting and weakening of the muscles. It is a sex-linked inheritance affecting boys only. Victims may have to attend schools for the physically handicapped. Treatment is aimed at minimizing deformities. Chest infection and fatal pneumonia usually develop by age twenty.

Ulcers

An ulcer is an open sore with an inflamed base and local disintegration of tissue of the skin or mucous membranes. Canker sores are ulcers of the mouth. Gastric or peptic ulcers affect the stomach, duodenal ulcers affect the first part of the small intestine, and colitis is characterized by ulcers of the colon or rectum. Ulcers are associated with anxieties and stressful situations affecting the patient. Ulcers are showing up with increasing frequency among teenagers and young adults.

ACNE

Although acne is not serious in terms of life and limb, probably no other health problem has caused so much concern for so many people. Young people with acne have put up with all manner of advice from well-meaning parents, teachers, and sympathetic friends. Advertisements and articles in the media have further complicated the matter. For love or profit, it seems that everyone is concerned with clearing adolescent faces. Unfortunately, most time-honored rules for treating acne are irrelevant, and many of the best-selling acne preparations are without effective ingredients. Certainly, teachers do not want to add to the confusion. Well-informed teachers can have more than sympathy for the eight out of ten teenagers who must face the world with a face full of bumps and blotches.

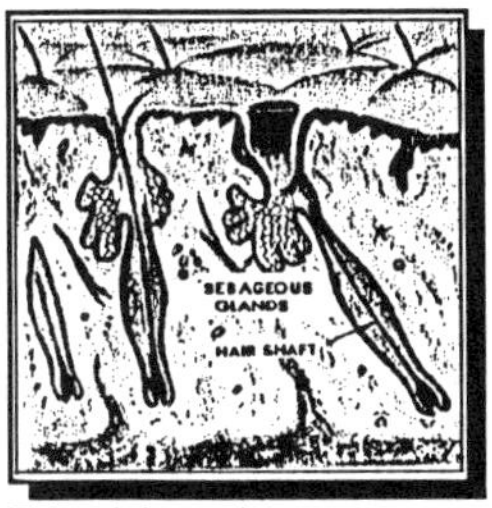

Blackhead

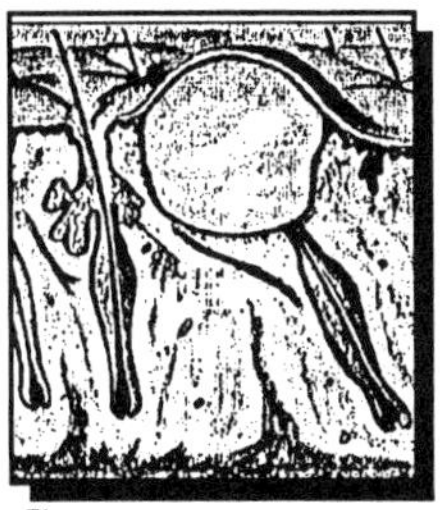
Cyst

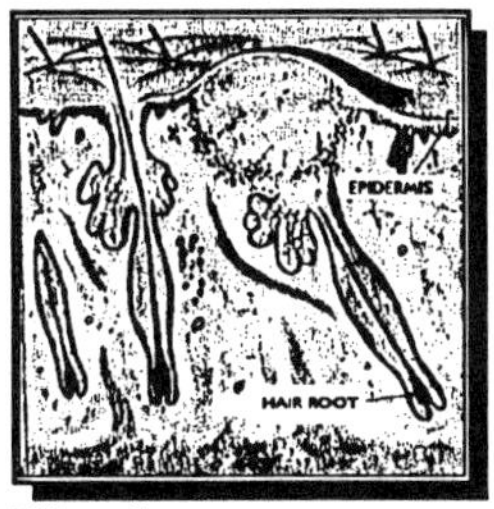

Pimple

What Causes Acne?

To dispel some nasty rumors, acne is nobody's fault. It does not arise from dirtiness or neglect; nor is it a sign of physical, intellectual, or social inferiority. Rather, it is a medical disorder most common in adolescents because of the increase in sexual hormones at puberty. The body mechanisms that lead to acne are imperfectly understood. Among the known culprits are the sebaceous glands, particularly large and numerous on the scalp, face, chest, and back. They secrete sebum, a mixture of fats and waxes, into the hair follicles and through the pores to the skin's surface. In acne patients, the cells that line the hair follicle are abnormal in that dead cells accumulate and block the pores. Sebum accumulates instead of sloughing onto the skin's surface. Combined with oils and bacteria, the cells form comedones or whiteheads (blackheads are comedones open to the air).

But where does the redness and inflammation of acne come from? As oils continue to pour into the stopped-up hair follicles, they are split by bacterial enzymes into free fatty acids, irritants that weaken the follicle walls. Continued irritation causes the walls to rupture, releasing oils, bacteria, and sebum into surrounding tissues and producing inflammation. The result is an acne pimple, medically termed a papule. A pus-filled papule is called a pustule; a larger and more deeply embedded lesion is an acne cyst. Appropriate home care and time will take care of mild cases, but severe cases should have good medical care in order to avert possible scarring and pitting.

What Will Help With Acne?

There are a variety of over-the-counter (OTC) treatments for acne--creams, cleansers, lotions, soaps, powders, gels, cleansing sticks, scrubs, beauty masques, and medicated towelettes. Unfortunately, many of them do not work well, and some add to the problem.

Fortunately, the road to complexion ruin is a two-way street. First stop on the way back: the neighborhood pharmacy. There are many over-the-counter medications that may help clear up mild acne (although doctors can't explain exactly how they work). But there are also some OTC medications that claim to clear up acne but that do not contain the proper ingredients. The four medications commonly used in OTC remedies and believed to be of some value by most dermatologists are benzol peroxide, sulfur, resorcinol, and salicylic acid. They all inflame the skin and cause it to peel. Benzol peroxide is the strongest, creating the most peeling and the most clearing. No single product is ideal for everyone. People's skins differ in sensitivity, and acne problems differ in magnitude.

Teachers can help students develop some consumer skills as they evaluate various acne treatment products. They should disregard most advertisements except to criticize the sales techniques and learn to read the labels. They should suspect the word "antibacterial" in the ads or on the label of acne products. Although bacteria are a part of the problem, they live beneath the skin's surface and cannot be reached by topical antibacterial agents. However, treatment by physicians sometimes includes antibiotics that will get to the bacteria internally. The labels should tell the percent of benzol peroxide (5-10%), sulphur (2-10%), resorcinol (2%), or salicylic acid (2%). Avoid products that do not contain at least one of those four active ingredients or state the percent of the ingredients.

There is abundant misinformation about the cause and treatment for acne. Except perhaps in unique individual cases, there is little evidence to suggest a cause and effect relationship between any of the following and acne:

- Certain food such as fats, fried foods, chocolate, cola beverages, and dairy products. These foods may be associated with other health problems, but probably not acne. However, if an individual sees a connection, it may be prudent to minimize their use. Dermatologists do agree that iodides and bromides can cause skin eruptions that look like acne. Excessive intake should probably be curtailed during acne treatment. Iodides occur in appreciable amounts in certain drugs, foods, and multivitamin/mineral combinations.

- Lack of sleep. "Early to bed" may make you healthy, wealthy, and wise, but it won't make your pimples go away.

- Constipation. Laxatives have fallen out of favor as an acne remedy.

- Sexual behavior. Adolescents were once embarrassed by the notion that masturbation or other sexual activity or inactivity caused or aggravated acne.

- Not washing the face properly. Although washing the face thoroughly is a part of acne treatment, that relationship is controversial. Although there is no scientific proof that not washing causes acne or that washing really helps acne, most dermatologists advise their acne patients to wash several times a day. Scrubbing with a soapy washcloth helps to remove oils, dead skin, and surface bacteria--and produces minor irritation, which may be of some help in very mild acne. For cleansing the skin, ordinary commercial soaps usually do an adequate job. Some heavily advertised cleansing products are no more likely than a nonmedicated bar of soap to fight acne.

Although a teenager's desire to cover up blemishes may be overwhelming, they should be advised not to do it. It's best not to use any cosmetics, particularly oily skin preparations or greasy creams. One should look for water-based products and apply them lightly. If one's hair is naturally very oily, it should be kept off the face and shampooed at least once or twice a week. It is also best to avoid hair dressings with greasy or lanolin bases. Long-term use of those preparations can cause "pomade acne," a clustering of blackheads on the forehead and temples.

One of the prime temptations of acne is to pick and squeeze blackhead and plump pimples. Resist it. Handling acne blemishes can rupture follicle walls, spread inflammation and may eventually lead to deep-pitted scars. If one feels a need to remove blackheads, it may be time to consult a physician. Although a doctor cannot cure acne (only time can do that), he has more weapons at hand to keep it in check. In prescribing medication, he can adjust the dosage and proportion of ingredients to meet the patient's specific needs.

CANCER

Cancer is the leading cause of death due to disease among high school students. Cancer is an uncontrolled malignant cell growth which, if not removed or destroyed, will cause death to the host. Of the various types of cancer, leukemia or cancer of the blood leads the list. Once it was considered always fatal, but recent medical strides usually produce a recovery. Nevertheless, it characteristically tends to sap the patient's strength for some time and makes school participation difficult.

What is Cancer?

Cancer is not a single disease, but a family of diseases all characterized by abnormal cell division. The chromosomes in the cells contain the genetic codes that govern the cell's functions. In the process of normal human cell division, the 23 pairs of chromosomes line up across the axis of the cells. The mother cell divides along a line between the pairs of chromosomes so that one-half of each pair of chromosones goes to each of the two daughter cells. Then a duplicate of each original chromosome is formed so that the chromosomes are again in pairs. The chromosomes in the daughter cells are identical to the chromosomes in the mother cell.

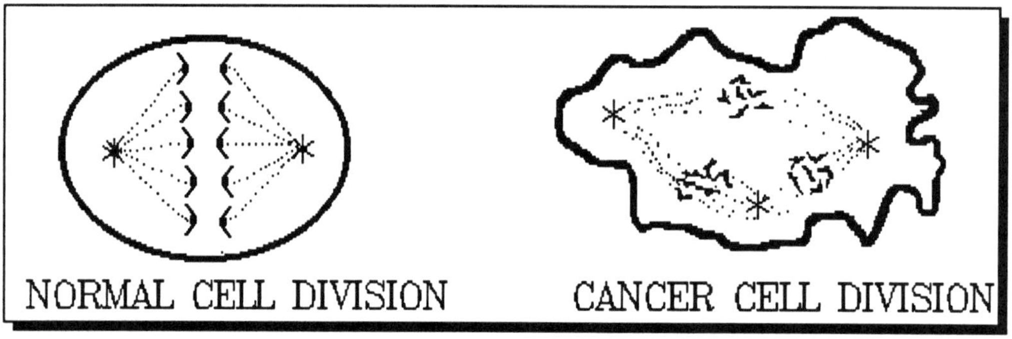

The division is abnormal in cancer cells. The chromosomes do not divide evenly. One cell may divide into several cells, each with a different number of chromosomes. Thus, codes that govern the cell's functions are all mixed up. It is like a cell that has gone *crazy.*

A cancer cell has:

- Abnormal cell division
- Abnormal chromosome configurations
- Abnormal shape, size, and appearance
- No useful function (except to destroy the host)
- A tendency to grow rapidly and spread

A group of abnormal cells is called a *tumor* or *neoplasm.* There are two major types of neoplasms, benign and malignant. A benign neoplasm or tumor is walled off, does not spread, and grows slowly. A malignant neoplasm or cancerous tumor is not walled off; it grows and spreads rapidly. Cancer spreads in two ways. It invades adjacent tissue, crowding and starving normal cells, and it spreads through a process called *metastasis*. Cancer cells leave the original site and travel through the blood and lymph vessels to distant body sites where secondary cancers may develop. If a person has cancer, hopefully it can be discovered and treated before metastasis takes place. After metastasis occurs, cancer treatment is much more complicated and much less successful.

What Causes Cancer?

We do not know for sure how cancer is caused, but the three main theories are:

1. The body for some unknown reason routinely makes cancer cells, but most of the time the immune system destroys the new cancer cells before a cancer develops. However, occasionally an *irritant* may interfere with the immune system and allow a cancer to form.

2. We have a cancer gene (*oncogeny*) in every cell, but it remains inactive most of the time. In some cells, for reasons we do not understand but perhaps it is an *irritant*, the cancer gene becomes activated and a cancer cell results.

3. An *irritant* may cause normal cells to mutate or change and become cancerous. A mutation or abortion is a change in the gene codes on the chromosomes. Somehow an irritant breaks up the chromosomes and changes the gene codes. Most mutations are lethal; the genes have been changed so much that the cell cannot live or divide into new cells. Sometimes a mutation is enough so that it is no longer a normal cell, but not great enough to be lethal. It becomes a cancer cell.

Although the mechanism is not fully understood, somehow an irritant alters the gene codes in the cells. A link has been established between the following irritants and certain types of cancer.

- **Radiation.** Subatomic-sized particles are given off from radioactive material and travel through space at great velocity. This is called radiation, and people are exposed to radiation from a variety of sources such as atomic bomb blasts, uranium mining, X-rays, medical radiation therapy, ultraviolet light from the sun, and cosmic radiation from outer space. The potential for harm as those tiny particles pass through the body depends on the wavelength of the radiation.

  X-rays, for example, pass through the body and expose the film on the other side. Because the X-rays pass through some parts of the body faster than others, the exposed film reveals a pattern of the inner body. If you are in the room when an X-ray is taken, the technician may give you a lead apron to shield the more susceptible parts of your body.

If radiation particles pass through cells during the process of cell division while the chromosomes are lined up across the axis of the cell, they might strike a chromosome, break it up, and change the genetic code. Thus, radiation can be an irritant that might promote the development of cancer. This is most apt to occur among rapidly growing cells such as skin cells, blood cells, and reproductive cells. Since a rapidly growing fetus would be susceptible to radiation, X-rays are generally not taken of pregnant women.

If radiation causes cancer, you may wonder why radiation is used to treat cancer. Since radiation can cause mutations among rapidly growing cells and since cancers are growing very rapidly, cancer patients are sometimes given radiation therapy. Hopefully, it will cause further mutations that will destroy the cancer.

- <u>Chemical agents</u>. Certain chemicals may act as an irritant on certain body cells and somehow promote the mutation of normal cells into cancerous cells. Chemicals that will do this are called carcinogens. A *carcinogen* is a chemical substance that will cause or promote the development of cancer. Cigarette smoke, for example, contains numerous carcinogens along with other chemical substances called *co-carcinogens*. A co-carcinogen is a chemical that increases the effectiveness of carcinogens. Numerous products have been taken off the market, because research has found them to be carcinogenic.

  This poses a dilemma, for some chemicals such as sodium nitrate or nitrite are used to preserve foods. There is a slight chance that they might in some situations promote cancer, so some people believe we ought to stop using them as a food preservative. But other people believe the threat of food contamination, such as botulism, is much greater and we should therefore continue to use them.

- <u>Viruses</u>. Certain viruses invade and become a part of certain body cells. The genetic code of the virus becomes a part of the genetic code of the cell. This is in a sense a mutation that might explain how some cancer gets started. Research is being done to better understand the link between viruses and cancer. If a virus can cause a mutation that results in cancer, viruses may also be used to promote further mutations that will kill the cancer cells.

- <u>Physical irritation</u>. There seems to be a slight link in some cases between constant physical irritation and the development of cancer. For example, a wart or mole that is constantly being irritated by constrictive clothing or frequently being nicked while shaving, might have an increased chance of becoming cancerous.

What Are The Chances Of Getting Cancer?

The chances of a person getting cancer and the chances of recovery after getting cancer depend on the type and location of the cancer. In the United States, an average of one in four people will develop cancer at some point in their lifetime. Ask the students to pick themselves and three other people in the classroom. Then have them identify the one in the group of four who will get cancer. Most people think, "It won't be me." Some groups of people who follow a healthy lifestyle have a much better than average probability, but still the rate is high.

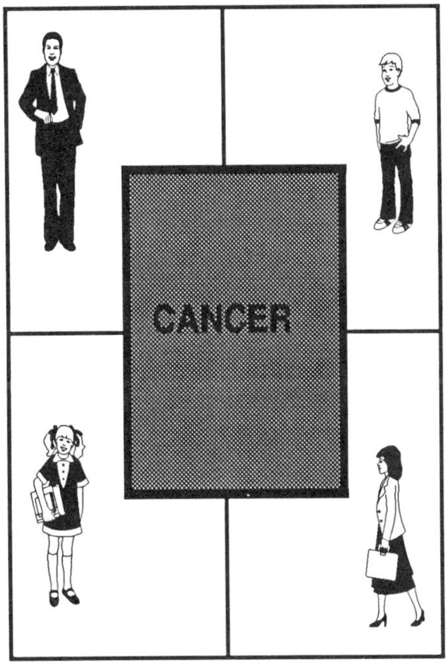

Expressed as a percent, 24 out of every 100 people will get cancer. Of the 24 who get cancer, 12 or about half *could* survive, but only 8 *do* survive. What makes the difference? The gap between technology and application. When we say could survive we mean the location and type of cancer is such that treatment, if started in time, would have a high probability of being effective. Why do four people die who could have been saved? Because of delayed diagnosis and treatment. Of the nearly 500,000 deaths annually in this country from cancer, an additional 170,000 could be saved by earlier diagnosis and treatment. This is a major goal of cancer education.

The chance of recovery from cancer depends on the type of cancer and its location in the body. For comparison, skin cancer has nearly a 90 percent survival rate, lung cancer has only a 5 percent survival rate. Skin cancer can be diagnosed easily and is readily accessible for treatment. Lung cancer has progressed so much that by time it is diagnosed, treatment is very difficult and very ineffective. The chance of recovery decreases with delayed diagnosis and treatment. Breast cancer, for example, now has nearly a 90 percent survival rate if treated in the early stages, but less than a 50 percent survival rate if there is regional involvement before it is treated.

For statistical purposes, the American Cancer Society considers a case as cured when there has been no reoccurrence of cancer after five years. Over the years, the incidence and survival rates for some types of cancer have increased and others have decreased. Lung cancer has shown the most dramatic increase. The overall rate for all cancers as a group has increased, but lung cancer has decreased. In 1987, lung cancer passed up breast cancer as the most common cause of cancer deaths among women.

What Are The Cancer Risk Factors?

Several steps can be taken to help reduce the risk of getting cancer, some are much more significant than others. Not smoking is the most important risk factor. A person should consider all of the factors on the next page.

- Don't smoke or use smokeless tobacco.
- Minimize exposure to environmental tobacco smoke.
- Avoid excessive exposure to the sun, use sunscreens.
- Don't frequent tanning booths and salons.
- Avoid occupational exposure to cancer-causing agents.
- If you drink alcohol, do so in moderation.
- Avoid unnecessary exposure to x-rays.
- Maintain ideal weight; avoid obesity.
- Avoid high fat diets.
- Eat cruciferous vegetables (cabbage, broccoli) regularly.
- Eat foods rich in vitamins A and C.
- Eat foods high in fiber.
- Minimize consumption of smoked and cured foods.
- Minimize consumption of charcoal-broiled foods.
- Eat a wide variety of foods.
- Avoid promiscuity in sexual relationships.

How Can One Improve his Chances of Recovery?

Should cancer strike, a person's chance of recovery is greatly improved if it is detected and treated early. The following steps are important to improve the chance of early detection.

Cancer's seven danger signals. By knowing and observing cancer's seven danger signals, early detection of cancer is more probable. If any of these signals last more than two weeks, a person should consult a physician. Most of the time they do not turn out to be cancer, but sometimes they do. An individual cannot tell.

Regular self-exams. Self-examinations to detect possible early signs of cancer are important. Directions are provided in the textbook. A person may want to consult a personal physician or a competent health counselor for more details. All mature women should conduct a breast self-exam on a monthly basis. Men, particularly those between the age 20 and 35, should regularly conduct a self-exam of the testes.

CANCER'S SEVEN DANGER SIGNALS

- **Hoarseness of Cough**
- **A Sore that Does Not Heal**
- **A Change in a Wart or Mole**
- **Unusual Bleeding or Discharge**
- **A Change in Bowel or Bladder Habits**
- **Indigestion of Difficulty Swallowing**
- **A Lump or Thickening in the Breast of Elsewhere**

Medical examinations. Regular thorough medical examinations are also important. Your physician should tell you how frequent the exams should be, but they should become more frequent with age. It is also important to select a physician who conducts a thorough examination. A doctor cannot detect every type of cancer, but the examination should be thorough enough to discover those that are detectable.

- **The Pap test.** An important part of the pelvic examination for women is the Pap test. This early cancer detection procedure saves over a hundred thousand lives each year. Cells discharged from the cervix and uterus are collected and examined under microscope for pre-cancerous conditions.

- **Prostate exam.** The examination of the prostrate gland is an important examination performed by a physician for men. This exam involves palpating the lower abdomen.

- **Proctoscope exam.** Starting about age fifty both men and women should have a proctoscope examination to detect possible cancerous growths in the lower intestine. Tests to detect blood in the stool should also be conducted.

Special tests are used along with examinations to detect certain types of cancer. A *smear* is a collection of body waste material placed on glass slides and examined under a microscope. A *washing* is a collection of material gathered from the lining of the stomach. A *biopsy* is a very thin slice of tissue that is examined under a microscope. *X-rays* play an important part in diagnosis in some locations.

Avoid cancer quacks. One of the saddest scenes, one that is played over and over, goes as follows. A man suspects he has cancer, but instead of going to a medical doctor he goes to a quack. After months of unorthodox treatments, his condition becomes much worse, so he finally goes to a qualified physician who, after a thorough examination says, "If you had only come to me in time." In spite of the billions of dollars spent in this country each year for cancer fraud, the greatest price for quackery is the loss of time. Time is so very precious in cancer treatment; time equals lives.

Another problem is that many people pay cancer quacks large amounts of money to cure them of cancers they never had in the first place. While some quacks deliberately commit fraud, others are sincere, though ill-informed. Their victims, however, have to pay the same ultimate price, their life.

What is the Treatment for Cancer?

The effectiveness of cancer treatment has improved significantly in the last few years, and people are now being cured from cancers that not long ago were considered incurable. The treatments often have serious physical and emotional side effects, yet new research projects provide some optimism for the future. The three major types of cancer treatment are:

- **Surgery.** Surgery is the oldest and still most preferred type of treatment. It is used whenever the cancer is in a location that surgeons can get to and laser surgery is sometimes used on places not accessible. The patient has to have the physical stamina to withstand the surgery. When surgery cannot be used, other treatments will be employed. Sometimes other treatments are used in addition to surgery when surgery alone is insufficient to remove all of the cancer.

- **Radiation.** Radioactive substances are used to bring about further mutations in cancer cells and thus destroy the cancer. Radiation has undesirable side effects on the rest of the body, but its concentration is focused on the cancer which it hopefully will destroy.

- **Chemotherapy.** Certain chemicals have been developed that tend to poison the cancer. They also have some poisonous effects on the whole body and this produces serious side-effects, but the side effects can be endured in hopes of a cure from the cancer.

It is important to realize that there is a difference between the current rate of survival and the number who could survive *if* the latest technology was employed in time. Of every 100 cancer victims, an additional 16 persons could survive if early diagnosis and proper treatment were obtained.

HEART DISEASE

Heart disease is the leading cause of death in America. For teenagers it ranks second next to cancer as a leading cause of death due to disease. Among secondary students, however, it is not the heart attack, but congenital heart defects that cause so many fatalities. Rheumatic heart disease also occasionally affects adolescents. Students with these problems sometimes need special considerations. For this reason, teachers should understand these conditions. Teachers also need to understand other cardiovascular diseases, so they can help students develop lifestyles that minimize the risk of heart attacks and strokes in later years.

What Is Congenital Heart Disease?

The development of the heart in the embryo is a complex process with numerous opportunities for something to go wrong. It is surprising that there are not more congenital heart defects than there are. Some defects that do occur are so severe that the infant dies within a few minutes of birth. Other defects are so slight that the person is able to live a normal life, in spite of the defect. Some defects are such that they can be surgically corrected, and some are not. The older the child is before surgery has to take place, the better the chances are of success.

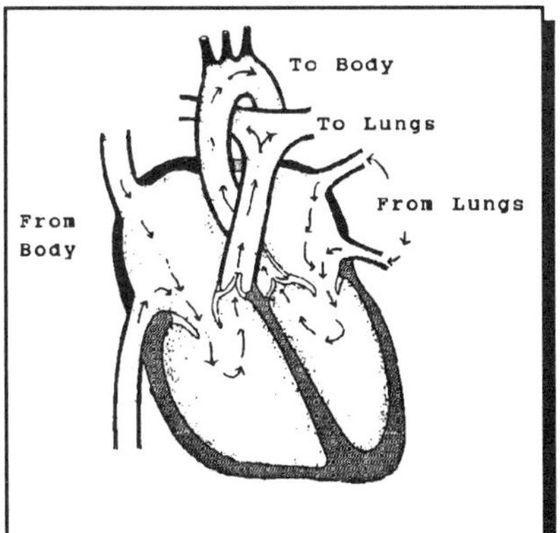

NORMAL CIRCULATION

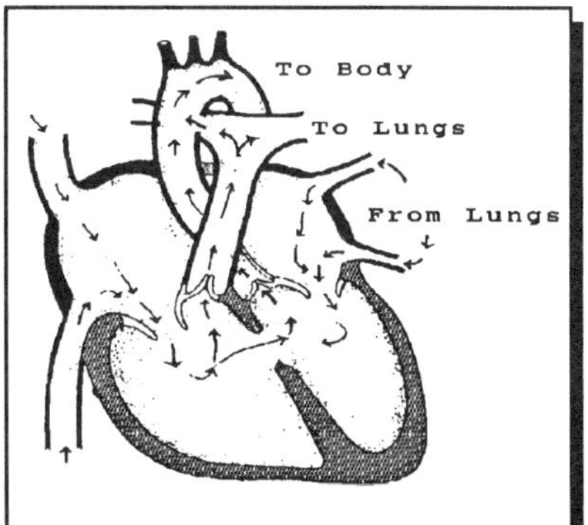

FETAL CIRCULATION

The sequence of blood circulation is different in the fetus at some stages prior to birth than it is in normal circulation after birth. Prior to birth, the infant gets its oxygen supply from its mother through the placenta, but immediately at birth, the infant must get its oxygen from the lungs. Normal blood circulation follows this sequence: (1) blood coming from the body enters the chambers on the right side the heart, (2) the heart muscles contract to pump the blood from the heart to the lungs where the blood picks up oxygen, (3) the blood returns to the chambers on the left side of the heart, and (4) the heart pumps the blood to the body. Months prior to birth, however, since the fetus has no need to pick up oxygen, much of the blood circulation bypasses the lungs. In the fetal heart there is an opening between the right and left chambers of the heart, and there is also an opening between the two major arteries through which the blood leaves the heart. Therefore, in fetal circulation when the heart contracts in step (2) above, much of the blood is pumped directly from the right ventricle to the left ventricle and from the pulmonary artery to the aorta instead of going to the lungs. Before the time of birth, these openings close so that all of the blood must go to the lungs.

In the most common types of congenital heart defects, these openings have not completely sealed off so that some of the blood still bypasses the lungs. Because the blood is not completely oxygenated, the infant may have a blue appearance and may be called a "blue baby." The seriousness of the situation depends on what percent of the blood is not properly oxygenated. If the openings are large the infant may not survive. If the infant lives, surgery may be necessary. But since surgery is risky or may be impossible, it may be delayed or not advised. Many children live normally with congenital heart defects, and some children are limited in the types of activities they can engage in. Some require special understanding and accommodations in their school participation.

Schools should also do their part to help students understand how to avoid those circumstances that increase the risk of congenital defects. Present evidence indicates that although heredity may have something to do with it, events in the life of the mother during early pregnancy are the major factors. These events may include German measles, drugs, and low oxygen environments which can be dangerous to the fetus at critical times.

What is Rheumatic Heart Disease?

Rheumatic heart disease is a chronic disease that results from having rheumatic fever, and rheumatic fever results from having a strep infection. While rheumatic heart disease and rheumatic fever are not communicable, strep infection is. About 10 percent of the children in Utah who get group A hemolytic streptococcal infection develop rheumatic fever. About one-third of the people who have rheumatic fever will recover without damage to the heart, about one-third will show some signs of heart damage but will lead normal lives, and one-third will develop severe heart disease and their life will require special planning.

Rheumatic heart disease is usually more frequent among children living in mountain regions. The exact cause of rheumatic fever is unknown, but it is related to the streptococcal bacteria and may follow sore throats, tonsillitis, and scarlet fever. Initial attacks occur most frequently among children in grade school, but it is not uncommon among college students. It seldom occurs for the first time to people over age 25. Older people who get it usually have had it as children. Unlike most communicable diseases, people who have had rheumatic fever do not develop an immunity to it; they become more susceptible. One who has once had it needs to be more cautious about preventing it and getting immediate medical attention if it starts. Rheumatic fever develops so rapidly that the condition becomes well developed within 24 hours. It usually starts from a few days to a few weeks after a streptococcal sore throat.

Early signs and symptoms of rheumatic fever are the same as for other respiratory infections: a look of pallor, poor appetite, repeated nosebleeds, failure to gain weight, lingering low level fever, and complaints of pain in arms, legs, and abdomen. Definite signs are painful, inflamed joints, irritablity and instability, and possible twitching and jerking of face, arms, and legs. Although rheumatic fever tends to run in families, it is not contagious. The patient will require isolation and bed rest for his own protection. No miracle drugs have been found to cure rheumatic fever; however, a patient may be required to take penicillin to prevent a strep infection. Bed rest is necessary for weeks or months until the fever dies. Failure to do so may cause serious complications, including rheumatic heart disease. Proper living conditions, nutrition, and rest are necessary for recovery and prevention of reoccurrences.

The first attack is over after a few weeks or months. Then the patient must continue to rest in bed until the doctor is sure the active stage is over. This is essential, even though the child may look well and feel fine. Here is where the parents' biggest share of the treatment comes in. It is no easy chore to keep a youngster interested, happy, and quiet when he must lay in bed for months, although he is feeling well. It takes imagination to keep him from boredom. School work should be continued to whatever extent the doctor thinks wise. It is especially important for parents themselves to be as cheerful as possible. If children sense their parents' worry, they worry too.

The real danger of rheumatic fever is rheumatic heart disease, and this is more apt to occur after repeated attacks of rheumatic fever. The infection-causing rheumatic fever will affect the heart by causing inflammation of the heart muscle, the lining of the heart, and the heart valves. Permanent damage is usually due to inflammation, which results in scarring of the valve on the left side of the heart. The scar tissue that is formed restricts the valve from opening and closing properly. This reduces the normal flow of blood through the heart and to the lungs and body. The heart of a person with rheumatic heart disease would have to work much harder than the heart of a normal person to do the same amount of work. This may seriously reduce the amount of exertion the person can safely participate in.

What Is A Heart Attack?

Diseases of the vessels of the heart, brain, and other body organs are the cause of heart attacks, strokes, and other circulatory problems. The coronary arteries supply blood to the heart muscle. A normal coronary artery has a smooth, slick inner surface. Unfortunately, some people as early as the sixth grade start to deposit plaque materials along the coronary arteries. This makes the surface rougher, and this in turn attracts more plaque deposits. Atherosclerosis is the term for this plaque formation. In time, the artery will become so full with plaque that the flow of blood is blocked. A heart attack occurs when the coronary arteries are blocked to the point that the heart muscle cells are deprived of oxygen in the blood.

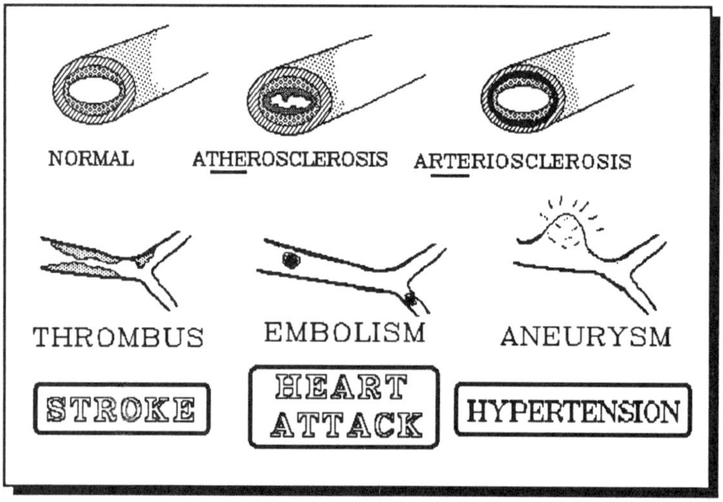

At times, atherosclerosis contributes to the development of two types of clots that can also block the coronary arteries. A *thrombus* is a clot that is attached to the wall of an artery. An *embolism* is a moving clot that may have formed suddenly in the blood vessels or a piece of plaque that has broken loose from a thrombus. Either will flow through the arteries until they reach a narrow point and then block the flow of blood. The seriousness of a heart attack depends on how much of the heart muscle is below the occlusion and is deprived of blood. If a small branch of a coronary artery is blocked, the victim will survive, but if a larger artery is blocked, the attack will be fatal. Muscle cells that do not get oxygen die and are eventually replaced with scar tissue. Obviously, anything that can be done to prevent atherosclerosis will reduce the risk of heart attack.

A stroke is a blockage in a cerebral artery to the brain, also due to atherosclerosis, a thrombus, or an embolism. Aneurysms and tumors also cause strokes. An *aneurysm* is a weak point in an artery wall that balloons and becomes so thin that it breaks and hemorrhages so that the blood does not reach its destination. A tumor growing adjacent to a vessel may squeeze an artery shut and diminish the supply of blood. The severity of a stroke depends on which part and how much of the brain is deprived of blood. The result is unpredictable; it may cause death, paralysis, loss of memory, and many other problems. High school students are extremely unlikely to suffer from a stroke, but they may suffer from a head injury that may impair or destroy brain tissue with results that are similar to a stroke. Many of the same lifestyle factors that will reduce the risk of heart attack will also reduce the risk of stroke.

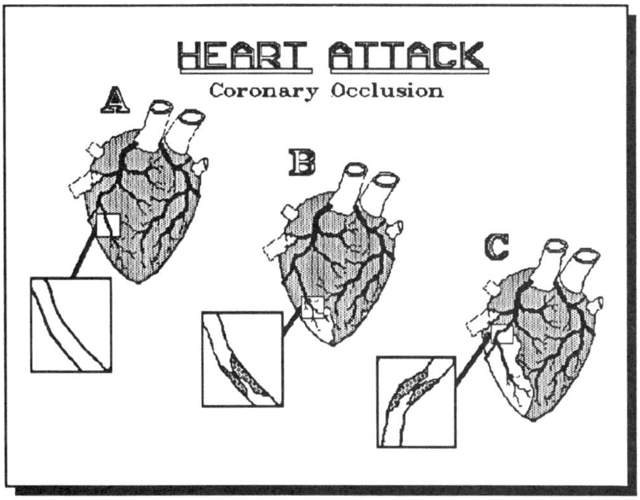

People are asking, "What makes the difference between an attack that can be survived and one that proves fatal?" One difference is artery size. If the arteries are small, a blockage due to a clot will deprive a larger portion of the heart muscle of oxygen-containing blood. Another difference is artery profusion. If there are multiple capillary networks in the heart muscle, the effect of a block in one network will be reduced. Some possible long term benefits of exercise are larger-sized coronary arteries, increased artery perfusion, and reduced plaque formation.

What Are Risk Factors For Heart Attacks?

Some major risk factors such as heredity, sex (male or female), race, age, and diabetes cannot be changed. But some major risk factors that can be changed are smoking, high blood pressure, and cholesterol level. Other contributing factors are obesity, stress, and the lack of exercise.

- **Cigarette Smoking** A man who smokes more than a pack of cigarettes a day has nearly *twice* the risk of heart attack and *five* times the risk of stroke as a nonsmoker.

- **High Blood Pressure** A man whose blood pressure at systole is over 150 has more than *two* times the risk of heart attack and nearly *four* times the risk of stroke as a man whose systole blood pressure is under 120.

- **Cholesterol Level** A man with a blood cholesterol measurement of 250 or above has about *three* times the risk of heart attack and stroke as a man with cholesterol below 194.

What Is High Blood Pressure?

High blood pressure has been called the "silent killer," because it generally has no signs or symptoms. Blood pressure must be measured for a person and his or her physician to know it is high. Fortunately, when it is discovered, there are many things that can be done to keep it under control. The problem with *hypertension*, or high blood pressure, is that it puts too much pressure on the tiny arteries in the various organs of the body.

High blood pressure affects more than 28 percent of the white adults in this country, and among blacks it exceeds 39 percent. Since it is virtually a symptomless disease, people over age forty should have their blood pressure checked periodically, particularly if they have a history of hypertension in their family or if they are overweight. A person whose blood pressure exceeds 140/90 should consult their physician. Depending on other factors such as age, sex, and general health, the physician may suggest some lifestyle changes such as controlling weight, stopping smoking, minimizing alcohol consumption, limiting salt intake, exercising, and in some cases medication.

In recent years, many people have purchased the necessary equipment and have learned how to take their own blood pressure.

How Do You Take Blood Pressure?

A blood pressure cuff and a stethoscope are used to measure blood pressure. The cuff is a long balloon-like device covered with fabric. Connected to the cuff by a tube is a bulb that will inflate the balloon with air when squeezed. A control valve in the neck of the bulb regulates the air flow. Also attached to the cuff by a tube is a meter that measures the air pressure in the cuff.

The person testing your blood pressure wraps the cuff around the upper arm and inflates it by squeezing the bulb. The cuff is inflated too so that air pressure in the cuff exceeds the blood pressure in the artery of the arm. The inflated cuff acts as a tourniquet, and blood flow through the artery is stopped. Now the end of the stethoscope is placed under the cuff, and the tester starts to listen. At the same time, the control valve is lessened and the air in the cuff gradually escapes. At first, no sound can be heard, but when the air pressure in the cuff is equal to the blood pressure in the artery, a sound is heard. As the blood rushes past the constricting cuff, a sound like a heart beat is heard.

The person testing the blood pressure notes the meter reading when this first sound is heard. That is the systolic reading. Two numbers are used to record blood pressure. The higher number is the systolic reading. This is the point when the pressure in the artery and the pressure in the cuff are equal. As the meter shows the air pressure, it also indicates the blood pressure. The tester continues to let the air out as he listens. The thumping sound

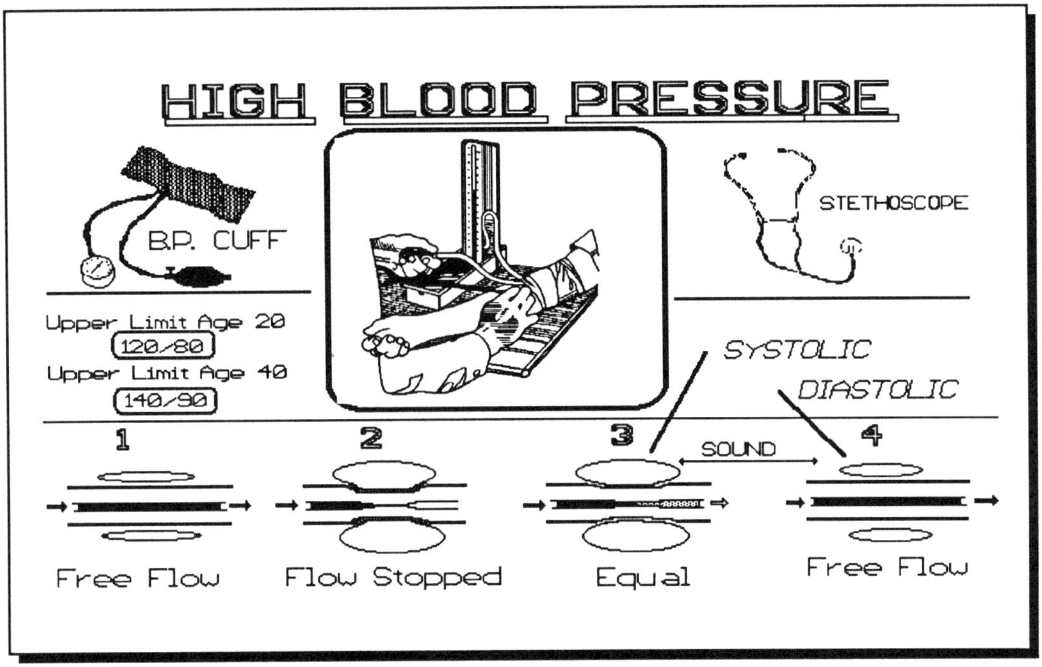

of the pressure in the artery against the pressure in the cuff continues until there is no more resistance. When the sound of the heart beat stops, the number on the meter is noted again. The last sound heard is the diastolic reading. It indicates the amount of blood pressure in the arteries when the heart is at rest.

Both numbers, systolic and diastolic, are important. They would be written as 120/80. They indicate the blood pressure at two points during the heart beat cycle. The systolic--the greatest pressure--occurs as the heart beats. The diastolic--the lowest pressure--occurs between beats when the heart is at rest. Because the earlier methods of measuring blood pressure involved the use of a mercury-filled glass column, the numbers still indicate millimeters of mercury.

If blood pressure gets too high, organs of the body can be damaged and problems such as stroke, kidney disease, and heart disease can occur. But if the pressure gets too low, insufficient blood and oxygen will get to the organs. This is a condition of shock, and it can be fatal. High blood pressure is called *hypertension* and low blood pressure is called *hypotension.* A reading of 120/80 is normal. A reading of 140/90 might suggest the possibility of borderline hypertension. When considering hypertension, the lower or diastolic number is probably the most significant. If that number is consistently above 90, a physician should be consulted. A systolic reading below 100 might indicate borderline hypotension, and a medical evaluation might be suggested.

What About Cholesterol?

A few years ago, researchers found a relationship between high cholesterol levels in the blood and heart disease. People were urged to reduce their consumption of foods containing cholesterol. That suggestion was met with controversy, because cholesterol in the blood comes from varied sources. Some of the food we eat contains cholesterol, and the body also manufactures it. Keeping one's cholesterol level under control is more complicated than simply cutting out a few foods.

It starts with having a special blood test. Since high cholesterol levels are so significantly associated with heart disease, all adults should request their physician to order such a test periodically. The simplest test measures only the total cholesterol (TC). If the results are high, the physician may order a more comprehensive test which shows each of the two types of cholesterol--HDL (high density lipoprotein) and LDL (low density lipoprotein). The LDLs, regarded as the bad kind, are lipoprotein that carry cholesterol, and in large amounts they contribute to the building of plaque in the coronary arteries. HDLs, the good kind, seem to protect against atherosclerosis. If the TC is high but it is made up primarily of HDLs, there may be no problem. The amount of LDL is a better gauge of coronary risk than the amount of TC.

If the level of LDLs are high, the person should take some steps to lower it. The numbers are recorded as milligrams of cholesterol per deciliter of blood. For ages below nineteen, 170 to 185 would be a moderate risk and above 185 a high risk. For ages twenty to twenty-nine, 200 to 220 would be a moderate risk and above 220 would be a high risk. The acceptable level goes up each year so that at age thirty to forty the moderate risk starts at 220 and the high risk at 240. Above age forty the moderate risk starts at 240 and the high risk at 260. At best the TC is a rough estimate of risk. The ratio of TC/HDL is a better estimate. For example: 210 TC divided by 70 HDL = 3. A ratio above 4 is considered undesirable. Among the things a person can do to lower this ratio are the following:

- **Exercise** — Exercise tends to increase HDL and also decrease LDL.
- **Don't Smoke** — Smoking may increase total cholesterol and decrease HDL.
- **Saturated Fat** — Eat more unsaturated and polyunsaturated fats and less saturated fats. Eat more vegetable oils such as corn, soy, safflower, and olive oil and less animal fats, butter, and palm and coconut oil.
- **Fish** — Substituting fish for other meat a few times each week may lower LDLs and increase HDLs. Fish that contain

the omega-3 fatty acids such as salmon, sturgeon, mackerel, whitefish, herring, mullet, and bonito are best. Halibut, swordfish, and fresh water trout are also good.

- **Fiber** — Type I fiber from fruits, vegetables, and oatmeal are high in pectin which decreases the absorption of cholesterol. Taking oat bran daily seems to be one of the most efficient non-drug means of lowering cholesterol.

- **Certain Foods** — Limit consumption of preformed cholesterol in such foods as fatty meat, whole milk, and eggs (1 to 3 per week).

- **Weight Loss** — A benefit of a weight loss diet is that it may also reduce cholesterol consumption.

The danger of heart attack and stroke increases with the number of risk factors present. If a person has a risk factor that cannot be controlled, that increases the importance of reducing those risk factors that can be controlled.

DIABETES

Diabetes is a chronic ailment in which the body loses its ability to metabolize carbohydrates, sugars and starches. To metabolize carbohydrates, we need insulin, a hormone produced by the pancreas. If the pancreas produces too little or no insulin, or if it fails to release needed amounts into the blood, or if other chemicals in the body interfere with the use of insulin, the symptoms of diabetes develop.

Can Diabetes Be Inherited?

Where both parents are diabetic, all children may become diabetic. If one parent is diabetic and the other has a family history of diabetes, there is a 50 percent chance of the children becoming diabetic. If neither parent is diabetic but both have diabetes in the family, the children have a 25 percent chance of getting diabetes. If one parent is normal and has no family history of diabetes, the children should not get the disease.

How Is Diabetes Treated?

Modern treatment is a carefully established balance of diet, physical activity, and where needed, medication--either insulin injections, oral therapy, or a combination of both. If this balance should be disturbed--if the patient overeats or undereats, engages in too much or not enough physical activity, if he skips medication or takes the wrong dose--the complications of diabetes are likely to ensue unless the balance is quickly restored.

How Can Diabetes Be Detected?

In the absence of obvious symptoms, there are a number of very sensitive tests available to the physician. Apart from the ordinary urine and blood tests for abnormal sugar levels--which may not be positive in mild cases--there are such refined tests as the glucose tolerance test and other tests. The glucose tolerance test determines the body's ability to deal with an overload of sugar and takes two to three hours. Tests for urinary sugar show the status of the diabetes and how well it is being controlled. The results of these tests indicate to the doctor whether adjustments in treatment are necessary.

How Does Diabetes Change One's Life?

Diabetes will change a person's life only to the extent necessary to control the disease. The diabetic should be able to do everything he did before the ailment struck, but he will also have to observe the rules of treatment prescribed by the physician. For example, good hygiene is important to everyone and especially to the diabetic. This is because diabetes tends to impair circulation, and any wounds or infections--especially in the feet and legs--become increasingly dangerous and may result in gangrene. Many things--an infection, injury, or some great worry or sorrow--might change the disease to a more severe form. Even a common cold may necessitate a change in treatment. A change of work or physical activity may require a change in diet or medication. Even the normal aging process is a factor for change.

What Are The Complications Of Diabetes?

The two most immediate complications are diabetic coma and insulin shock. Diabetic coma (*hyperglycemia*), or a sugar reaction, is the result of uncontrolled diabetes. It arises from insufficient insulin activity which leads to too much sugar in the blood. Unable to use sugars for energy, the body uses up the fat and protein tissue. In the process, fatty acids accumulate and begin to poison the system. This, if unchecked, may lead to coma and death. This complication develops gradually, and the symptoms are those of diabetes itself. Skin is flushed and dry, there is a fruity breath caused by acetone, and the patient becomes very drowsy. Then breathing becomes deep and labored, there is vomiting, and the diabetic loses consciousness. A coma can result from a number of things: missing medication, too small of a dose relative to food intake or physical activity, illness, or stress. There might even be a change in the nature of the disease. Insulin or injections will help correct the problem. Medical attention may be required.

Insulin shock (*hypoglycemia*), or an insulin reaction, occurs when there is too much insulin and not enough sugar in the blood. It arises when a diabetic takes an overdose of insulin, eats too little, or engages in too much activity. Symptoms usually begin with mild hunger, then comes sweating, dizziness, palpitation, and pale skin. If the reaction is not treated, these symptoms follow: shallow breathing, trembling, blurred vision, mental confusion, and unconsciousness. Insulin reaction can be helped by swallowing some form of concentrated sugar--candy, honey, jam, soda pop, or fruit juice. If the reaction is not treated promptly, recovery becomes more difficult. Immediate medical attention is needed.

Other complications--some of which may be a part of the disease itself--include eye trouble; various circulatory disorders such as arteriosclerosis; and in elderly diabetics, possible gangrene, kidney and bladder ailments, and fungus infections.

<u>What Is The Teacher's Role</u>?

DIABETIC REACTIONS		
CHECK	**DIABETIC COMA**	**INSULIN SHOCK**
ONSET	Gradual	Sudden
SKIN	Flushed, Dry	Pale, Moist
BEHAVIOR	Drowsy	Excited
BREATH	Fruity Odor (*acetone)*	Normal
BREATHING	Deep, Labored	Rapid, Shallow
VOMITING	Present	Absent
TONGUE	Dry	Moist
HUNGER	Absent	Present
THIRST	Present	Absent
URINE SUGAR	Large Amounts	Slight

A teacher should be alert to possible symptoms and see that necessary care is obtained. It may be necessary to adjust curriculum to the child and recognize the pupil's problems. A teacher may also be able to help the pupil adjust to a new pattern of life and adhere to the recommendations of his physician.

EPILEPSY

Perhaps no problem causes more unnecessary concern in a school than a convulsive or epileptic seizure. A teacher may be shocked as he faces a grand mal seizure for the first time. He will feel helpless and perhaps be anxious about the child relaxing and regaining consciousness. Too often a social stigma is attached to it. The disturbed person is ashamed and will not face his problem realistically. The lack of understanding can lead to unhappiness and poor social adjustment of the affected student. The following facts concerning epilepsy are listed so that you may better understand an affliction which too long has been misunderstood.

The word "epilepsy" means seizures. It is not a disease but an outward manifestation of the irregular and overwhelming neurological disturbance of the brain. It is characterized by recurrent or spasmodic attacks of unconsciousness or impaired control. Epilepsy is a neurological disorder usually characterized by some type of "seizure" likened to a temporary electrical storm of the brain. The seizure is caused by a chemical disturbance in the brain cells which results in irregularities in the brain wave pattern. Epilepsy incidents of the general population are 1/200. The likelihood of the appearance of epilepsy in the offspring of an epileptic is 1/40.

An epileptic seizure may be triggered by an acute infection with a high fever or an infection of the nervous system such as meningitis, encephalitis, a mastoid infection, or a brain abscess. Or it may be associated with a profound emotional disturbance, a metabolic disturbance, a brain tumor, brain damage before, or a congenital defect such as cerebral palsy.

The symptoms of epilepsy are the seizures which are caused by brief, recurrent episodes of abnormal energy release by the affected brain cells. Seizures may range in severity from a *petite mal* involving momentary impairment and possible loss of consciousness to a *grand mal* with major convulsions. The severity depends on the spread of the energy discharge. Seizures may vary in frequency from one to two per year to as many as 200 a day. Those under medical control may go for years without a seizure.

Epilepsy does not cause insanity. The intelligence of persons with the disease parallels that of the general population. Epilepsy is not considered hereditary, although the tendency or predisposition may be found in certain types of people. There is no complete cure for epilepsy, but about 80 percent achieve adequate control and lead normal lives. Another 10-15 percent of the cases achieve partial control.

Petit mal seizures or "little sickens" are most common in children and usually disappear after adolescence. They are characterized by momentary lapses of memory, staring into space, slight rolling of the eyes, moving of the lips, twitching of the eyelids or eyebrows, and generalized trembling. The child returns to an awareness of his or her environment rather quickly, and there are no aftereffects. These seizures may occur only occasionally or several times a day. The child seems to be daydreaming. No emergency measure needs to be taken.

Psychomotor seizures affect about one-third of adults with epilepsy. The person's behavior is based on reflexes; it is automatic. The person is unaware of what he or she is doing or what is going on around them. The behavior may appear normal or have varying degrees of complexity. The person may appear restless and move around aimlessly or exhibit repetitive movements such as finger objects. At first, it may be easy to confuse the episodes with emotionally disturbed behavior. People with these type of seizures ignore other people. Little can or should be done about the behavior; it will cease soon.

Grand mal seizures or convulsions are the most common form and may occur at any age. The pattern is varied. Some individuals experience an *aura* or warning. Sometimes the seizure may start with a strange cry or sigh. The person loses consciousness, and the body may stiffen and jerk. Some have violent contractions or muscle spasms. The tongue may be bitten, and the head may be injured against the floor or furniture from the fall or convulsions. The facial color may change; this is because the diaphragm muscles are in spasms and the person is not breathing. This may look bad, but it is not serious. The muscles will relax in a few moments and breathing will be restored. During the seizure, the person will have expended a great amount of energy and may go into a coma for a few minutes, at least he or she will be tired and want to rest a few minutes.

First aid for grand mal seizures is very simple. First, nothing should be done during the seizure except perhaps move away any furniture or other objects the person in seizure might strike his or her head against. When the seizure first starts, it may be possible, in some situations, to ease the person who is having the attack to the ground, but do not try to restrain him or her. After the seizure has subsided, it would be well to turn the person onto his or her side to allow any saliva to escape and avoid choking should vomiting occur. It is also well to loosen tight clothing and make them comfortable. A blanket and pillow may be helpful. Many people who have had a seizure can resume regular activities almost immediately; others will want to rest awhile first.

Occasionally, a person may go into a deep sleep or coma for a few minutes following a seizure. If this occurs, it is important to monitor their breathing and place them on their side. A rule of first aid is to never leave an unconscious person on their back and unattended. If a person in a coma is left on his back, his air passage might close. Note that it is no longer thought appropriate to attempt to insert anything between the teeth.

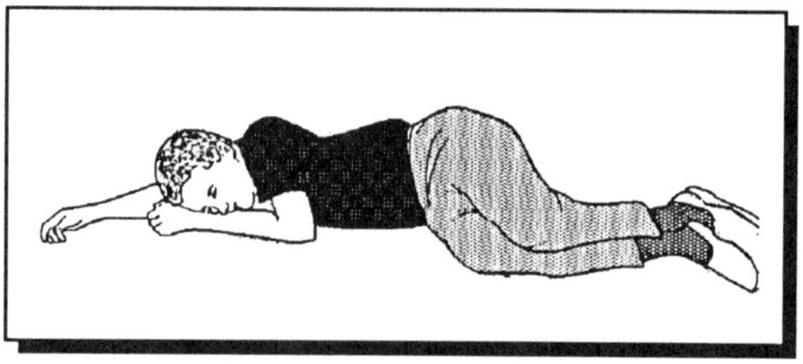

Emotional help is an important part of first aid for people who have gone through a seizure. As they regain consciousness, they will not remember what has happened. It is best if they do not have to deal with a lot of bystanders or with questions. Take steps to help them avoid unnecessary embarrassment. If the bladder or bowels are voided during the seizure, help with clothing or covering may be appropriate. Not only is emotional help important for the person who experiences the seizure, but also for the other students in a school setting. Their fears should be removed, and they should be helped to understand that nothing serious has happened to the person who had the seizure. They should continue to treat that person as though nothing had happened. Although for a few moments occasionally he or she may experience a seizure, the rest of the time he or she is normal. It is particularly important that the teacher show no signs of apprehension.

An epileptic seizure is not a medical emergency, and no medical follow-up is necessary unless it is the first seizure or there are a consecutive seizures. Then, however, emergency medical care should be obtained, and the student's physician should be notified immediately according to school policy. Of course, the parents should be notified also. Observation notes of the seizure should be recorded on the student's health record. Such notes may help the physician and the school officials understand the problem. Restrictions should be placed on the student only as recommended by the physician. For the student's safety should a seizure occur, restrictions might include avoiding hot materials, power tools, swimming, and heights as long as the seizures are not under control. In some cases, the school may be able to help advise the student on career alternatives.

SCHOOL AND TEACHER RESPONSIBILITY

When students are afflicted with the diseases discussed in this lesson, the teacher can do much to help them. Evidence seems to indicate that emotional stress may be a factor in some of these disorders. In some cases, a teacher can help the student adjust to a new mode of life. The teacher should place no limitations on the pupil except those suggested by the child's physician. If a medical crisis should occur, place the student in a comfortable position and call for assistance according to the individual case and the school policies.

It is important that public school systems develop means whereby students with chronic health problems can be accommodated so they can achieve the most from their school environment. The following are general principles that should guide a teacher in directing the activities of a student who has chronic health problems:

- Treat the child as normally as possible.
- Use common sense in excluding him/her from activities which may be harmful to his/her health; i.e. do not let an epileptic swim.
- Help the child understand and correct the correctable problems, but do not make him overly self-conscious.
- Follow any special advice given by the child's physician concerning his/her activities.
- Treat the child as a person, not as a disease.

In addition, if needed, there are special provisions that the school may properly make for handicapped pupils:

- Provide specially constructed chairs and desks for orthopedically disabled pupils.
- Provide appropriate seating arrangements for children with vision or hearing defects.
- Provide hearing aids.
- Provide special educational material and equipment, i.e. books with large type, etc.
- Schedule all classes on one floor for those students confined to wheelchairs.
- Permit rest periods between classes.
- Provide resting facilities.
- Provide permission to attend school only part of the day.
- Adapt physical education requirements.
- Provide transportation to and from school.

Identification of and special provision for handicapped children is an important aspect of school health services. Handicapped pupils are helped to achieve their optimum health and academic potential through the attention given to their physical and mental health. The handicapped pupil should be treated as nearly like any other pupil as possible. To live successfully within his limitations is a lesson to be learned. This is important, even if it means doing things in a different way at different times from other students. Within reason, the child should be protected from feelings of incompetence, frustration, failure, or a sense of being too different.

STUDY HELPS

1. Distinguish between communicable and noncommunicable disease.

2. The schools and teachers have two major responsibilities in regard to chronic diseases. What are they?

3. Explain what is meant by the statements:

    a. "Sometimes teachers go too far in trying to help students with health problems and end up doing psychological damage to the child."

    b. "Sometimes when professionally unprepared teachers learn that a student has a health problem, they allow that information to interfere with the normal teacher-student relationship."

    c. "It may be difficult for teachers to comprehend the complex feelings of students with a chronic health problem, but this insight is needed to help the students through their period of adjustment."

4. Since teachers have a responsibility to help foster among their students a lifestyle that reduces the risk of disease, what is the significance of each of the terms on p. 407?

5. As a teacher looks over his or her class, there may be one or more students with a chronic health problem. If so, the teacher should try to (pick one): (1) see the illness, not the child; (2) see the child, not the illness; (3) see the child first, then the illness; (4) see the illness first, then the child; or (5) all of the above.

6. "It is important that public school systems develop means whereby students with chronic health problems can be accommodated so they can achieve the most from their school environment."

7. What are some common misconceptions about acne?

8. If a student in class asks you, "What is cancer?", how would answer the question?

9. What types of heart disease are most likely to occur among students, what type of problems might this present for the students, and what can a teacher do to facilitate any necessary adjustments?

10. What are the complications of diabetes that a teacher should be aware of?

11. What are the complications of epilepsy that a teacher should be aware of?

12. Some of the health problems listed on pages 376-378 are chronic health problems found among secondary students. Other health problems on the list may develop in the future as a result of the students' current lifestyles. In either case, what should teachers know about the problems, and what should they be prepared to do?

CANCER TERMINOLOGY

The following terms may have special meanings as they apply to this lesson.

benign	biopsy	carcinogen	carcinoma
chromosomes	chemotherapy	chemical agents	co-carcinogens
irritant	leukemia	lymphoma	malignant
melanoma	metastasis	neoplasms	Pap test
proctoscope	prostate	radiation	recovery or cure
sarcoma	self-exam	smear	sunscreen
warning signs	ETS	PABA	SPF

TERMINOLOGY

The following terms may have special meanings as they apply to this lesson.

hypertension	atherosclerosis	arteriosclerosis
thrombus	embolism	coronary occlusion
stroke	myocardial infarction	apoplexy
HDL	LDL	TC
systolic	diastolic	ischemic
pectin	omega-3	cholesterol
blood pressure cuff	stethoscope	saturated fatty acids
coronary risk factors	cerebral artery	

Chapter 15

CONTROLING COMMUNICABLE DISEASE

The prevention or reduction of disease and its attendant suffering has always been a hope of mankind. Perhaps the greatest progress in disease prevention has taken place among the communicable diseases. Some can be prevented primarily through individual knowledge and effort, and some require community action. Schools, teachers, and students have a role to play in this important effort. Buildings must be kept clean and sanitary. Students should be immunized. Students who exhibit signs or symptoms of certain diseases should be excluded from the classroom. Students who have been out of school because of a communicable disease should not be readmitted until certain conditions for that disease are met. The effectiveness of a communicable disease control program is based on appropriate knowledge, attitudes, and practices.

CONTROLLING COMMUNICABLE DISEASE

Disease has been a part of man's existence since the earliest times, but in recent history, major progress has been made in curing and preventing disease. Improved sanitation, waste disposal, water purification, and food processing, and the general upgrading of personal and community standards have greatly decreased the incidence of many diseases in much of the world. Better methods of diagnosis and treatment, required immunizations, and health education in the public schools has contributed to improved health statistics.

The AIDS epidemic has convinced us that the picture is not all good in the fight against communicable diseases. Some diseases that were once pretty much under control are now creeping back in the morbidity reports. Complacency has taken its toll. We must also recognize that as success has moved some diseases out of the public spotlight, others have moved in. A major effort has been directed in recent years toward combating chronic disease. That is good, but we cannot neglect the communicable diseases.

By communicable diseases, we mean those diseases that are caused by certain small and microscopic organisms that are spread from one person to another. The organisms include not only bacteria and viruses, but also fungi, protozoa, and small worms and insects. Efforts to prevent communicable diseases are usually aimed at (1) the person or animal that has the disease; (2) the person in danger of getting the disease; and (3) the means of spreading the disease from one to the other. We are reminded that some diseases are more preventable than others. Some can be prevented primarily through individual knowledge and effort, and some require community action. We all must learn our part and do it.

PATHOGENS

When we hear the word disease, we may think of microorganisms and communicable disease, but this is not always the case. The word disease comes from the French word *disease* which simply means "not at ease." Not all diseases are caused by microorganisms, and not all microorganisms cause disease. In fact, for convenience in studying the cause and prevention of diseases, they have been divided into categories depending on whether or not a microorganism is involved. Diseases not caused by microorganisms were discussed in the previous chapter; this lesson deals with diseases where microorganisms are the cause.

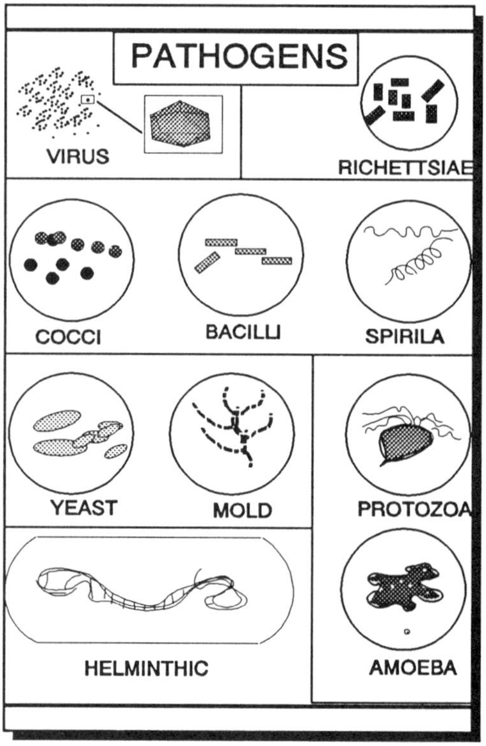

Microorganisms in the human body are classified as *endogenous*, normally present and compatible, or *exogenous*, abnormally present and incompatible. Some microorganisms contribute to the health of the host and are necessary for survival. Conversely, some microorganisms may cause disease if present in the human body in sufficient numbers. *Pathogens*, or germs, are disease-producing microorganisms. They may be a virus, rickettsiae, bacteria, fungi, or protozoa.

An *infectious* disease is any disease caused by a pathogen, whether or not the pathogen is readily spread from one person to another. A *communicable* disease involves a pathogen that is readily spread from one person to another. All communicable diseases are infectious, but not all infectious diseases are communicable. Examples include acne, pyorrhea, and urinary tract infections. Diseases for which we should receive immunizations (mumps, measles, rubella, polio, tetanus, diphtheria, and pertussis) are in this category. There are many communicable diseases for which there are no immunizations--sexually transmitted diseases (STDs), for example.

STAGES OF DISEASE

Most communicable diseases progress through a sequence of stages. The time period for each stage and the period of communicability vary from one disease to another. Some diseases, however, do not follow the pattern. The sexually transmitted diseases (STDs) are noted exceptions--people do not spontaneously recover from most STDs. The chart which follows shows the four main stages in the course of communicable disease. The curved line represents the number of pathogens in the body during each stage.

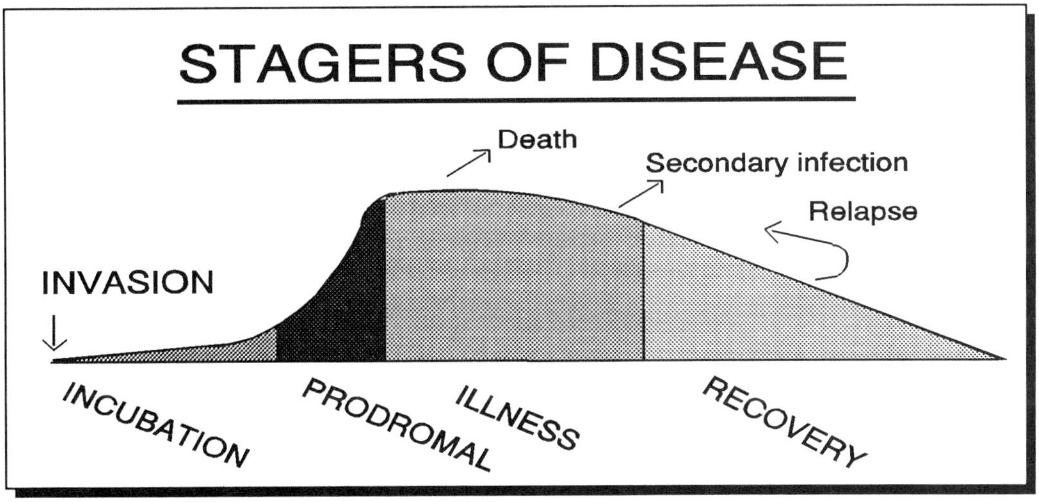

Invasion

This is the point in time and on the anatomy where pathogens enter the body. If the quantity of pathogens present is sufficient, and if the body level of resistance and immunity permits, the pathogens will soon start to multiply.

Incubation

The number of pathogens continue to increase until there are sufficient numbers to cause the early signs and symptoms of the disease. The incubation period may take 48 hours for the common cold, two weeks for chicken pox, or seven days for gonorrhea.

Prodromal

This is the stage of early general symptoms. At this stage, the disease is hard to diagnose, yet very communicable. The number of pathogens rapidly increase.

Illness

The number of pathogens is very high. The symptoms become much more specific. The disease is at its worst. The body's defenses start to combat the pathogens.

Recovery

As the body begins to win the fight, the symptoms begin to subside. However, too rapid resumption of activities may lead to a relapse or a secondary infection. Antibodies are produced to combat that specific antigen (pathogen), and this will confer future immunity. That means that thereafter the disease would be stopped at the invasion stage, but the body does not build antibodies to some disease pathogens. The person does not get over the disease without penicillin or other medical help, and no future immunity occurs. This is the case with STDs.

CHAIN OF INFECTION

For communicable diseases to be spread, the pathogen must somehow get from the old host to the new host--from the person who has the disease to the person who gets the disease. This is called the chain of infection. In between the "old host" link and the "new host" link, there is at least one other link called the "mode of transmission." The goal of communicable disease control is to "break a link in the chain of infection."

Old Host

The body of the person who has a disease acts as a reservoir for growing and storing the pathogens. The pathogen must get out of that person's body through some normal body openings or through infected sores. Since the goal is to keep any of that person's body discharges from coming in contact with another person, isolation is important until recovery or successful treatment.

Mode of Transmission

Direct Some diseases must be transmitted directly from the old host to the new host so there is no intermediate or indirect route. For example, most of the pathogens that cause sexually transmitted diseases (STDs) cannot live outside of human cells, they must be transmitted directly from the infected body tissues of the old host to the susceptible body tissues of the new host.

Indirect. Other pathogens can live for awhile outside of the body. They can be carried by the air, in water, on food and other objects, and by vectors such as flies, mosquitoes, and rats. Public health personnel maintain sanitation control over water supplies and sewage disposal, disinfection control over food supplies and eating utensils, and control over vectors.

New Host

The susceptible host must do his or her job to combat disease. If we maintain a high level of health, we will be more resistant to the disease. We should be careful to protect normal body openings and breaks in the skin, and we should get the immunizations that are available.

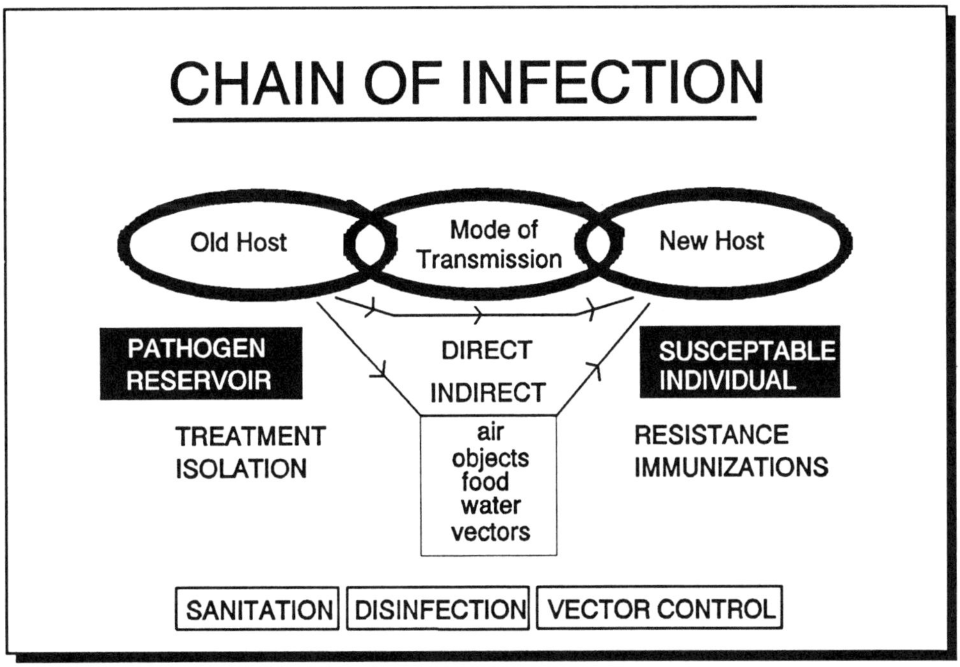

The susceptible host, the person who may get the disease, should take appropriate steps to protect himself or herself from communicable diseases. Parents and guardians have the prime responsibility for insuring that their children are protected. Schools also have an interest in making sure children are protected, since children who are ill and not in school will not be effectively educated. Since the government has a stake in the education and health of its citizens, it should takes steps to combat communicable diseases. Thus the individual, the family, the school, and the government should take the following steps:

- Immunize everyone against the specific diseases for which immunizations are available: polio, measles, rubella (German or 3-day measles), mumps, diphtheria, pertussis (whopping cough), tetanus, and in certain localities, hepatitis, typhoid, yellow fever, etc.

- Follow appropriate personal health practices to maintain a high level of health and disease resistance. This includes proper eating, rest, exercise, and personal cleanliness (this includes clothing and bedding). It also includes avoiding harmful substances and promiscuous sexual relationships.

- Become familiar with the available methods and facilities for prevention, identification, and treatment of disease. People should be motivated to incorporate this information into their daily living patterns.

Some of these things can be done personally or by the family, but some require community action. We should encourage each individual in the community to do his part. We should support the health departments and other community service agencies to carry out their responsibilities such as providing water purification facilities, sewage and garbage disposal systems, and inspecting dairies, restaurants, food handlers, etc. We should do the following to break the "Mode of Transmission" link in the chain of infection.

- Wash your hands thoroughly after using the toilet, changing a baby's diaper, coughing or sneezing into your hand, blowing your nose, or contacting contaminated objects. You should also wash thoroughly before and after caring for the sick and before eating or handling food.

- Prevent the contamination of water and food. This includes thoroughly washing dishes and utensils used in preparing, storing, and eating food.

- Dispose of human waste, sewage, and garbage so that it will not contaminate the water or food supply or otherwise create a health hazard.

- Control insects, rodents, birds, and other animals so that they will not spread disease.

- Maintain a safe and sanitary environment. This includes eliminating dust and dirt from the living, working, and playing areas. It includes keeping one's clothing and bedding clean.

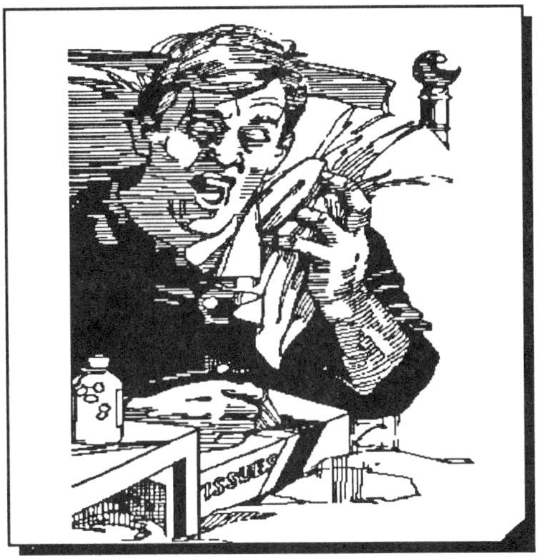

The body has natural lines of defense against communicable disease. *Resistance* is the general ability of the body to ward off pathogens. Several factors are involved in warding off pathogenic organisms. Man's skin serves as a mechanical barrier. Mucous secretions of the respiratory tract serve as a barrier, as well as stomach acidity or intestinal alkalinity. The salinity of the tears prevents infections of the eyes and eyelids. *Fever* is the body's response to pathogens; pathogens become inactive at temperatures above 100 degrees Fahrenheit. *Phagocytosis*, a process by which the white blood cells destroy the pathogens by dissolving and absorbing them, is the body's best defense mechanism. *Immunity* is complete resistance to the disease and is specific for a particular disease through the use of antibodies. *Active* immunity exists when a person's own body produces antibodies to combat the disease either through an attack of the disease or by inoculation to stimulate the body's production of antibodies. *Passive* immunity is attained by injections of serum from other animals or human beings containing high levels of the disease antibody.

SCHOOL PROCEDURES

The following are procedures that may be used by the schools to help control the spread of communicable disease:

- **Sanitation.** In order to insure a clean and healthful environment and prevent the spread of infection, the school must be kept as clean and sanitary as possible. All areas of the school buildings, especially cafeteria, lavatories, and drinking fountains, must be kept sanitary.

- **Immunization.** The school can also require or promote immunization programs to prevent disease.

- **Isolation.** Training teachers to recognize ill students and to exclude them from school will also help to maintain a clean and healthy environment free from infection.

- **Readmission policies.** Sometimes a child is readmitted to school only upon the written approval of a physician. Other times, readmittance only involves allowing the student to come back after he feels better. Caution should be taken about readmitting students that are still contagious.

- <u>Education</u>. A program of health education and public information will help people to maintain a higher level of health in their own lives.

The classroom teacher has a major responsibility in identifying students who may have communicable diseases so that they can be excluded from the classroom and not spread the disease to other students. Since a teacher cannot tell for sure whether a student has a disease or not, the courts have held that it is the teacher's duty to exclude students who merely give the appearance or signs and symptoms of a disease.

<u>Working With Parents</u>

Many communicable diseases are as contagious before the start of signs and symptoms as afterward. For this reason, parents should be instructed to keep their children at home whenever they appear to be ill, even with cold symptoms. The early signs and symptoms of the common cold are the same as some other more serious communicable diseases. Teachers should observe students throughout the day for signs of illness. If a student becomes ill, he or she should be isolated from the other students until a parent can come for them. Students suspected of having a contagious disease should be referred to their family physician by the parents. If a child is diagnosed as having a communicable disease, the parents should not send them back to school until the particular readmission requirements for that disease have been met. When students are exposed to a communicable disease in the classroom, the parents should be notified so that those children who have not had the disease can be observed for symptoms at the end of the incubation period.

CLASSES OF COMMUNICABLE DISEASES

Diseases are classified by mode of transmission, and this table identifies steps that can be taken to prevent the transmission. The following list shows the means of transmission, the pathogens involved, and some examples.

<u>Diseases transmitted to man through the air</u>:

Virus: colds, influenza, polio, measles, mumps, rubella, chicken pox, smallpox

Bacteria: diphtheria, pertussis, meningitis, scarlet fever, rheumatic fever, pneumonia, tuberculosis, leprosy

Fungus: athlete's foot, mycosis

Diseases transmitted to man from fecal materials:

Bacteria: typhoid, paratyphoid, salmonellosis, cholera

Virus: infectious hepatitis

Protozoa: amoebic dysentery

Helminthic: pinworm, roundworms, hookworms, tapeworms, flukes

Diseases transmitted from animals to humans:

Bacteria: tuberculosis, anthrax, brucellosis, tularemia

Arthropods: encephalitis, malaria, spotted fever, typhus, yellow fever

Fungi: ringworm

Virus: psittacosis, foot and mouth disease

Diseases transmitted to man through wounds or bites: (infection)

Bacteria: staphylococcal infection (boils, acne), streptococcal infection (blood poisoning, impetigo), tetanus (lockjaw), gangrene

Virus: rat bite fever, rabies

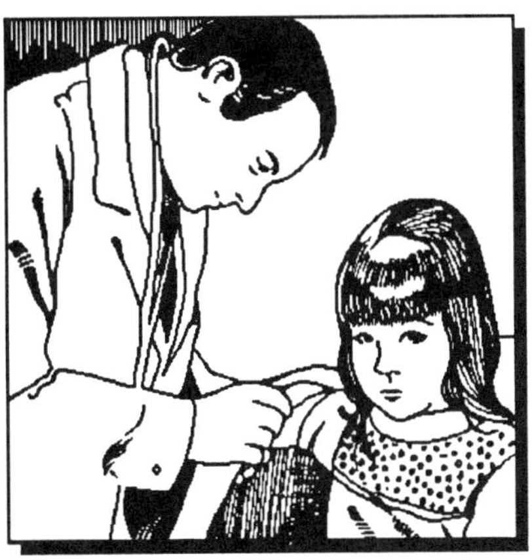

COMMUNICABLE DISEASE CONTROL AT SCHOOLS

The effort of the schools across the nation has done much to combat the communicable diseases across the nation. This has been a part of the worldwide effort that has had success in eliminating smallpox from the earth. Polio has essentially been eliminated from many countries. However, there is concern that the success might lead to apathy. In some cases, diseases that had been significantly reduced are once again appearing on state morbidity reports. Schools must continue their effort to control communicable diseases.

The following information identifies the communicable diseases that may be found among secondary school students and indicates the signs and symptoms and typical exclusion and readmission requirements. The *left* column identifies the disease. The *middle* column lists the symptoms of the disease. And the *right* column lists the control measures the school might follow to control the spread of the disease.

DISEASE	SYMPTOMS	CONTROL MEASURES
CHICKEN POX	Slight fever; few eruptions, mostly on covered surfaces; eruptions in same area at various stages of development.	Readmit after 7 days.
CORYZA	Nasal discharge; watery eyes; mild fever; headache; general aches; irritability; cough.	Readmit after 3 days.
DIPHTHERIA	Early symptoms not striking; temperature not high; throat sore and gray membranes; blood-tinged nasal discharge; illness greater than symptoms indicate.	Readmit after release by health authorities.
GERMAN MEASLES (Rubella) (3-day)	Mild symptoms; slight fever; eruptions varied, but often rose pink and small; lymph nodes on neck behind ear swollen and sensitive.	Readmit after 16 to 18 days.
HEPATITIS	Prodromal signs include fever; hepatitis headache; lassitude, nausea; anorexia; fatigue; marked tenderness and pain in liver; jaundice appears about fifth day and then fever subsides. Not all patients develop jaundice.	Readmit after release by health authorities.
MEASLES (Rubeola) (Red)	Nasal discharge; eyes red and sensitive to light; eyelid irritability; moderate fever; hacking cough; koplik spots on buccal surface of mouth; dusky red rash skin eruptions.	Readmit in not less than 5 days after appearance of rash.

DISEASE	SYMPTOMS	CONTROL
MENINGITIS	Acute onset; intense headache; fever; nausea; stiff neck; irritability.	Readmit after 14 days.
MONO-NUCLEOSIS	Fever; sore throat; headache; fatigue; chilliness; malaise; general involvement of lymph system; white cell count of blood varies between 10,000 and 20,000, excessive agglutinins present in blood.	Readmit after release by physician.
MUMPS	Slight fever; tenderness and swelling over the jaw and in front of the ear, one or both sides; involvement of ovaries and testes may occur in persons with mature reproductive system.	Readmit after swelling is gone.
POLIO	Fever, headache, sore throat, nasal discharge, watery eyes, aches, stiff neck and back, paralysis of muscles.	Readmit after release by health authorities.
RHEUMATIC FEVER	Severe sore throat; then a recovery period of approximately 4 weeks; damage to heart, joints, and other organs.	Readmit after infection is gone.
SCARLET FEVER	Sore throat; fever; nausea; vomiting; flushing of cheeks; pallor about mouth; if rash occurs, it is on the neck and chest and is a fine, scarlet, goose-pimple type rash that blanches when pressure is applied.	Readmit after at least 7 days.
TUBER-CULOSIS	1) Primary type involves infection of the lymph nodes along the windpipe; usually no discernible symptoms, so it is often not detected. 2) Secondary, or reinfection type has a gradual onset; fatigue; fever; cough.	Readmit after release by physician based on periodic chest x-rays.

DISEASE	SYMPTOMS	CONTROL MEASURES
	Skin Infections	
IMPETIGO	Systemic manifestations usually are absent except in infants. Lesions appear as red stains that are first fluid-filled and wet, then filled with pus, and finally form a crust that appears to be pasted on. The face (particularly the mouth) and hands may commonly be affected, particularly the scalp. Pressure generally causes pus to escape from beneath the crusts.	Exclusion from school until pustules have healed.
PEDICULOSIS (louse)	The louse egg (nit), larva or adult louse on the scalp, other parts of the body or in the clothing; nits attached to hair shaft; occasionally a severe secondary infection.	No exclusion if insecticide has been applied.
RINGWORM	Lesions often circular, clear in the center, with fluid like borders; not widely distributed; crusting not present; itching common. Foot ringworm (athlete's foot) is more common in adults; the body, face, and head forms are more common in children, especially in warm weather.	Exclusion if lesions are exposed. Excluded from pool and gymnasium.
SCABIES	Itching of skin often unbearable; frequent locations: the waist, armpit, and crotch; at times lesions on face, scalp, and arms. When infection is mild, systemic symptoms are negligible, but severe infections may result in fever, headache, and discomfort.	Exclusion from school until successfully treated.

RECOMMENDED IMMUNIZATIONS

	STARTING AGE			
VACCINE	2 Months	- 7 yrs.	+ 7 yrs.	BOOSTER
POLIO	2,4,15 Mo.	First Visit 2,4,12 Mo.	First Visit 2, 12 Mo.	4- 6 Years
DIPHTHERIA TETANUS PERTUSSIS	2 Mo. 4 Mo. 6 Mo. 4-6 Yr.	First Visit 2 Mo. 4. Mo. 12 Mo.	First Visit 2 Mo. 8-14 Mo.	4-6 Years [10 Years]
MEASLES MUMPS RUBELLA	15 Mo.	First Visit	First Visit	
HIB	18 Mo.	Up to 5 Years		

Most states require evidence of immunizations before students can be admitted to school, and a record of the immunizations becomes a part of the student's cumulative folder. Some states allow exceptions based on religious grounds, but in the event of an epidemic, students with such exceptions would excluded from school until the epidemic is over. The chart above is a typical immunization schedule; however, everyone should consult their local health department and their personal physician for the local requirements and recommendations. The immunizations should ideally start for an infant at two months; however, children who have not been immunized may start at any age. Some immunizations are given in a single dose, other require a series. The time interval for the series depends on the age of the child when the series was started.

Adults can catch some of these diseases too, and when they do, they are apt to be more serious than when a child is affected. Adults who have not had mumps or have not been immunized against mumps should consult their physician about the advisability of receiving the immunization. Women should have had or have been immunized for German Measles before there is any chance of them becoming pregnant. In addition, people who are traveling to certain parts of the world are required to have specific immunizations; typhoid, yellow fever, and hepatitis, for example. Influenza immunizations are recommended annually for certain health workers, for the elderly, and for people with heart and lung disorders.

The Measles/Mumps/Rubella (MMR) combination is administered in one injection. The Diphtheria/Pertussis/Tetanus (DPT) combination is also administered as a single injection to children under seven years of age. Individuals over age seven are just given the Diphtheria/Tetanus (DT) combination. People should get a DT booster at least every ten years. Physicians may also prescribe the booster following an injury.

The most recent immunization to be added to the recommended list for children is HIB, a bacterial microorganism known as *hemophilus influenza* type B. It does not cause the same type of influenza that we know as the flu. It causes several serious, often life-threatening inflammations. Some of the diseases resulting from HIB are bacterial meningitis or inflammation of the membranes protecting the brain and spinal cord, epiglottitis or inflammation of the trachea, pericarditis which is a dangerous heart condition, otitis media or infection of the ear, cellulitis or inflammation of the skin, septic arthritis or inflammation of the joints, pericarditis which is a dangerous heart condition, and pneumonia. Children under five years are at greatest risk for HIB. One in every 200 children will contract this disease. It is spread easily by coughing, sneezing, and by close facial contact. It can be treated with antibiotics, but immunizations are much more effective. It is given in a single immunization at age 18 months up to 5 years.

SEXUALLY TRANSMITTED DISEASES

Millions of teenagers are exposed to sexually transmitted diseases (STDs) annually in this county. STDs are among the leading communicable diseases in numbers. They are some of the most destructive diseases and some of the most difficult to detect and treat. These are a group of diseases that are transmitted almost exclusively through sexual contact. Until a few years ago this group of diseases were referred to as venereal disease (VD). That name came from Venus, the Roman goddess of love.

There are over twenty-five separate diseases, pathologically quite different each other, but all sharing the same mode of transmission. Their seriousness ranges from some that are extremely irritating to those that are always fatal. Some can be cured, others cannot. Some are on the reportable disease list and others are not. Monthly statistics are maintained by the U.S. Center for Disease Control on the incidence of "reportable diseases." They merely estimate the incidence of nonreportable diseases. For example, the common cold leads the list as the most frequent nonreportable communicable disease, but the STD gonorrhea leads the list as the most frequent reportable communicable disease. Yet another STD, chlamydia (which is not reported), occurs much more frequently than gonorrhea. Even among the reported STDs, there is always a question of the accuracy of the statistics, for many physicians fail to report the number of cases they treat.

Gonorrhea leads the list, and its occurrence is continually increasing despite the fact that the methods of treatment are comparatively easy and inexpensive. This paradox rises from the confusion in our society as to whether to treat venereal disease as a moral or a medical problem. For generations, syphilis was considered to the most serious STD because of its devastating distraction to the body, but that was before the incurable AIDS disease entered the scene. The word panic may be used to describe society's reaction to AIDS. It has certainly caused some school boards to react in panic in trying to decide what to do about a student who may have AIDS. Certainly, schools have to have well thought through policies regarding STDs. Whenever a topic related to sexuality is considered, there are sensitive ethical and moral questions involved that must be handled on a local basis. But the seriousness of AIDS seems to have cut through some of the controversy, so that AIDS education is taking place where traditional STD education was avoided.

Although schools and individual teachers may be limited in what they can do about the STD problem, they cannot turn their back on the problem. They must be a part of the larger community response to the problem. Although there may be a question of what an individual teacher can do, each teacher must be prepared with knowledge about the problem. The school nurse and sometimes teachers, administrators, and counselors will be in a position to counsel individual students who may have a STD. The school, and therefore some teachers, have a responsibility to increase students' knowledge about:

- how STDs are contacted and spread to others.
- the complications of STDs on individuals and unborn children.
- the importance of early medical diagnosis and treatment.
- the importance of assisting health workers in case finding.

Most teachers will not be assigned to teach these topics, but they should be prepared deal appropriately with a discussion should it come up. There is so much misinformation spread about STDs that every teacher should be prepared to correct it when the opportunity occurs. The accurately informed teacher is probably the best source of assistance for most young people. A good teacher will be able to refute the fallacies and provide the intellectual, moral, social, and medical dimensions of the problem. STD education should be systematically integrated within the school curriculum whenever it relates reasonably. Young people need to know about this group of diseases, how they are spread, who may become infected, what are the signs and symptoms, and where are the resources for treatment. Students who will never become infected must be given facts about VD also. They will be adults citizens and parents some day and will have to help combat the problem in their communities and families. Obviously, the schools should play an important role in helping to disseminate this information.

Facts on STDs

For hundreds of years, the venereal diseases, chiefly syphilis and gonorrhea, had no treatment. Then penicillin in the 1950s provided a miraculous treatment. But even with an effective treatment, these diseases go unchecked. Now add to that the even more frightening diseases chlamydia, herpes, and AIDS. The statistics are frightening.

- STDs strike an estimated 20 million Americans a year.
- Within a decade 200,000 Americans will die of AIDS.
- Nearly 85% of all STDs strike the 15- to 30-age group.
- The Center for Disease Control (CDC) estimates that 20 percent of all college students in America are afflicted with chlamydia.
- The medical costs for STDs are more than $2 billion a year. By 1991, the total cost of AIDS alone will be $55 billion.
- Approximately 16,000 people have developed AIDS in this country; more than half have died. By 1991, 270,000 will have been diagnosed; 179,000 will have died.
- The CDC estimates the new cases of STDs each year to be:

chlamydia	--------	$4,000,000
gonorrhea	--------	$2,000,000
genital warts	--------	$1,000,000
herpes	--------	$ 500,000
syphilis	--------	$ 90,000
AIDS	--------	$ 15,000

Who Is At Risk?

A lot of people who did not think they were at risk ended up with an STD, sometimes tragically, because they were what might be called "an innocent party." Since there is virtually no sure way of eliminating all risks, a better way to phrase the question is, "Who is least at risk?"

- **Least at risk.** Those who abstain from sexual relations prior to marriage and maintain a mutually monogamous relationship after marriage.

- **At greater risk.** The more sexual partners one has, and the more partners they in turn have, the greater the risk. A STD could come from any one of those partners.

- **Innocent infants**. Unfortunately, at particular risk are babies born to women who have active STDs. The effects vary from one disease to another, but this often results in death or serious deformity.

Signs and Symptoms

There are now over twenty-five separate sexually transmitted diseases, and each has specific signs and symptoms. More specific information on several STDs is found later in this lesson, but here are a few general signs and symptoms.

- Sores on or near the sex organs.
- Pain in the genitals.
- A burning sensation in the genitals.
- An unusual discharge.
- Abdominal pain.
- Itching around the genitals.
- Growths or warts in the genital area.

Some other important points about signs and symptoms are the following:

- A symptomless person can still be communicable.
- If the symptoms go away, it does not mean you are cured.
- Sometimes the symptoms are confusing; they frequently mimic signs and symptoms of other conditions.
- Sometimes the signs and symptoms seem to come and go.
- Men are much more likely than women to notice the signs and symptoms of STDs.

SYPHILIS

In the United States, there are over 90,000 cases of syphilis and approximately 3,000 persons die from it each year. Hundreds of others suffer blindness, heart disease, and insanity caused by syphilis, and many babies are stillborn or have congenital defects due to syphilis in the mother. The cost to the taxpayer for taking care of these problems exceeds 100 million dollars annually.

History

Syphilis has a fascinating history. It is generally believed that this disease was brought back to the Old World from the New World by the sailors of Columbus in 1493. This new disease devastated Europe for the next several centuries. Syphilis caused so many deaths, resulted in such striking disfigurements, and aroused such fears that it made a profound impression on all aspects of the society of that time.

The disease received its name from a poem by Fracastoro in 1530, "Syphilis Sive Morbus Gallicus." (In those days physicians were frequently poets). The poem described the afflictions of a Greek shepherd boy, Syphilis, who had the misfortune of contacting the disease through intimate contact with sheep when he offended the sun god.

From 1500 to about 1900, little progress was made in controlling it. As the public image of morality became more puritanical, the manner in which syphilis was transmitted from person to person assumed more importance. It became a disease that no one liked to talk about. It frequently was named after peoples' enemies, the English called it the French disease, etc. Epidemics of syphilis frequently followed the trail of invading armies and the women who followed their camps. Syphilis has truly changed the history of the world, for many kings and rulers were afflicted with this disease. Frequently, in its later stages, syphilis caused paresis (insanity due to syphilis), and this affected their decisions.

In 1905, the causative bacteria was identified. In 1907, Wassermann established the first reliable diagnostic blood test. In 1910, Ehrlich developed the first somewhat effective drug, Salversan 606, for treatment of syphilis. It was nicknamed the "Magic Bullet." Finally, in the 1940s penicillin provided medicine with an effective, rapid treatment necessary for control of this major disease. It was called the "New Magic Bullet."

<u>Cause</u>

Syphilis is a communicable disease caused by a corkscrew-shaped micro-organism called *Treponema pallium*, a member of the family of spirochetes, (literally, "spirally curved hairs"). The spirochete of syphilis outside the human body is an extremely delicate organism that dies in seconds when exposed to light and air. Introduced into the body, however, it is an exceedingly tough and invasive microbe which circulates rapidly in the blood stream, multiplies with ease, and comes to inhabit every tissue of its human host.

<u>Transmission</u>

Syphilis is passed from person to person by sexual relations. Since the organism cannot live outside of the human body, this has to be a direct transmission where the infected tissue of the old host comes into direct contact with the susceptible tissue of the new host. This is usually through sexual intercourse, but the organism has been transmitted by oral\genital contact, and even from prolonged intimate kissing when the old host had a lesion in the mouth. Dentists have contacted syphilis when their fingers have come in contact with a lesion in the mouth of their patient. It can be spread in homosexual relationships. Babies of mothers with syphilis are often aborted or are born with syphilis and congenital malformation. Premarital blood tests were instituted to prevent this tragedy.

Following the original entrance of the spirochete into the human body, an incubation period of between 10 to 90 days--usually 2 to 6 weeks--elapses before the appearance of the first signs and symptoms. A person may be infected and yet show no signs of the disease for as long as three months. During this time, in the absence of lesions, a person will not be infectious.

Symptoms

Primary stage. The spirochete enters a new victim through mucous membranes or a tiny break in the skin, generally in the region of the reproductive organs. The first visible effect of the infection is found at the site of entry about two to six weeks later. A small open lesion sore called a *chancre* develops and may become the size of a dime. Being small, painless, and temporary; it often escapes detection. This is particularly true in females, for the lesion frequently occurs within the recesses of the body.

The chancre is moist like any other localized injury in which a spot of skin has been completely destroyed. The fluid obtained from a chancre and viewed under a darkfield microscope displays an abundance of slightly quivering spirochetes. This makes possible an immediate, certain diagnosis of infection. The chancre is dangerously infectious and easily transmits syphilis through intimate contact with another person.

Even without treatment the chancre disappears within several weeks, leaving behind a small, flat, unobtrusive scar or no mark at all. This has misled people into thinking that they are well and have no problem. The disappearance of the chancre means only that the spirochetes have entered the bloodstream and are spreading throughout the body.

Secondary stage. The secondary stage of syphilis begins usually from two to six months after the appearance of the chancre. For the most part, its manifestations involve the skin and mucous membranes. The secondary lesions contain spirochetes; the moist lesions are highly infectious. The disease is very insidious because the signs and symptoms resemble so many other diseases; syphilis has been called "The Great Imitator." Signs and symptoms of secondary syphilis may include the following:

- Skin rashes covering all or part of the body. The rash may be fine and grainy similar to measles. It may consist of flat, sharply marked off areas like ringworm or pustules like chicken pox.

- The condyloma--a small, flat lesion, usually multiple, that occurs when the skin is moist as in the perineal area, between the toes, and at the corners of the mouth.

- Apoecia--a spotty, irregular, temporary baldness.

- Mucous patches--whitish lesions on mucous membranes in the mouth and throat.

- Constitutional symptoms--malaise, the feeling of not being well; low fevers; headaches; swelling of lymph glands all over the body.

The secondary stage is variable. Three-fourths of all persons with syphilis escape this stage. It may be delayed for as long as a year after the initial infection. Its symptoms may be severe and disabling--or so mild that they escape attention. They often persist for only a few days, but sometimes for several months. There may be little damage to the surrounding tissues. The lesions heal without scarring--and like the chancre, without treatment of any kind--thereby ushering in the latent stage. Again, the individual erroneously believes he is over a temporary condition.

Latent stage. The latent stage of syphilis may last for a few months or a few years. While it lasts, the infected person is apparently disease-free except for positive reactions to blood tests. There may be relapses with development of lesions characteristic of the secondary stage. But except at these times, the man or woman (for all practical purposes) is noninfectious (except from mother to unborn child). The latent stage marks a point of near equilibrium in the war between the body and the disease.

Late stage. In the late stage, the equilibrium turns in favor of the spirochetes as they concentrate their attack on a particular area of the body. After the passage of time, maybe twenty years, the disease becomes active again. This produces the last and most destructive stage of syphilis which again plays the role of the "Great Imitator," since it can successfully simulate almost any disease. Progression may cause a chronic inflammation of almost any tissue of the body. It is possible, however, to distinguish three major categories:

- **Central nervous system syphilis.** CNS involvement is slowly progressive, eventually causing disasters such as blindness, crippling, or total disability from syphilitic insanity (general paresis).

- **Cardiovascular syphilis.** It involves the heart and large blood vessels and may cause death from syphilitic heart disease or rupture of a major artery.

- **Gumma formation.** It is growing tumors or ulcerations which destroy the tissues around them. A gumma may develop in almost any part or organ of the body. When a syphilitic gumma involves external parts of the body, the effects may resemble leprosy in appearance.

Congenital Syphilis

This is a special form of the disease, transmitted from an infected mother to her unborn child. The disease is modified by the special circumstances of the baby's development at the times of infection, the duration and stage of the mother's disease, and the treatment she has received. The fetus cannot be infected before the fourth month of intrauterine life. Infection occurring at about the fourth month is likely to result in death of the baby before delivery (a stillbirth) or in the birth of an obviously disease-deformed child.

Infection occurring late in pregnancy may result in delivery of an apparently normal baby who in future months or years develops signs of syphilis. The syphilitic baby may grow and develop poorly, or develop various syphilitic "stigmata," such as malformed teeth, blindness, deafness, or defective bones. While it may take an adult two decades to reach the latent stage, a child may reach that stage in a few months. The child may suffer any of the late stages seen in the adult. If a pregnant woman is treated for syphilis, the infections of unborn children will also be treated. The baby will be born without syphilis, but will still have any physical damage which occurred before the treatment.

Diagnosis

Before one can treat a disease, it is necessary to recognize its presence. Syphilis is particularly difficult to recognize. Its causative organism cannot be seen with an ordinary microscope or grown on culture media. The course of the disease is marked by periods in which the spirochete is not found in blood or other body fluids, and its symptoms may imitate many other diseases.

Three laboratory tests help physicians detect syphilis, particularly the laboratory test of the blood.

The darkfield microscope. The watery fluid exuded from a syphilitic chancre, secondary skin lesion, or mucous patch is examined under the microscope with a particular kind of indirect illumination. By darkfield lighting, the spirochetes are "silhouetted" as pale white spirals against a black background. A "positive darkfield" furnishes positive proof of infection at the time the disease is most infectious.

The serologic test for syphilis. In about four to five weeks following infection with syphilis, a chemical substance called "reagin" appears in the blood. The presence of reagin in the blood can be recognized by different biochemical methods. These tests are not perfect, and occasionally they may fail to detect the reagin or may even produce a false positive result.

The spinal fluid test. When syphilis invades the tissues of the brain, it produces biochemical changes in the spinal fluid long before any mental symptoms occur. These changes can be recognized by appropriate laboratory tests. A spinal fluid test may detect syphilis that was not identifiable through a blood test.

Treatment

Fortunately, it is no longer necessary for anyone to experience the forbidding course of untreated syphilis. Treatment is readily available and inexpensive. Adequate treatment will bring about a true cure. Progress of the disease is permanently stopped, lesions are healed, and transmission is no longer possible. The symptoms of the illness are abated and disappear, except destruction of tissue. Destroyed tissue heals by scar formation which does not contribute to physiologic function. The badly damaged brain of syphilitic insanity cannot be restored, nor can total blindness. However, treatment given the partially blind syphilitic usually stops further progress.

Penicillin became available in 1943. Penicillin is safe, quick, effective, and inexpensive. Today, injections of penicillin will cure most cases of the disease in 10 days and also render them noninfectious. However,it takes a series of very large doses of a special type of penicillin. It takes more penicillin to cure syphilis than any other disease for which penicillin is given. Alternative modern antibiotics are available to the small but growing number of persons sensitive to penicillin.

Immunity

There is no known natural immunity to syphilis. In other words, any person in the world who does not have the disease can acquire it when exposed. There is no known artificial immunity to syphilis. As yet, we have no vaccines, serums, antitoxins, or other biological medicines that will prevent infection. Unlike many other communicable diseases, having syphilis once does not confer immunity to succeeding infections. One can be infected with syphilis again and again; in fact, a person could have both primary and latent syphilis at the same time.

GONORRHEA

History

Gonorrhea is one of the oldest diseases known to man. There are written references to gonorrhea dating back about 3,000 years. It was known to Hippocrates in 460 BC and was named by Galen, a Greek physician of 200 AD. It was sometimes confused with syphilis. A famous English surgeon, John Hunter, intentionally infected himself experimentally with what he thought was gonorrhea, but it turned out to be syphilis and eventually resulted in his death.

Cause

In 1879 the causative organism was identified by the German bacteriologist Neisser, and the organism was scientifically named *Neisseria gonorrhoea.* They stain easily and are plainly visible under any ordinary microscope. These bacteria are found in the discharge from mucous membranes lining the genitourinary tract. They will produce the disease when transferred to susceptible membranes of another person.

Transmission

Gonorrhea is transmitted principally by sexual relations, including homosexual practices, and occasionally from an infected mother to the eyes of her new baby as the baby passes through the birth canal.

Symptoms

Gonorrhea affects men and women in quite different ways because of differences in anatomical structure.

Gonorrhea in the male. Within one to nine days after exposure (usually two to six days), the disease begins with a painful inflammation of the urethral canal in the center of the penis. The inflammation causes a copious discharge from the penis that in the beginning is thick and purulent. Later it becomes thinner and watery. The inflammation of the urethral canal results in a sharp, burning pain when urine is passed. These symptoms usually subside after two or three weeks. When the infection reaches the prostate gland and the testicles, the symptoms are extremely painful and distressing to the patient and impel him to seek medical assistance. If involvement of the testicles is not treated, it causes sterility by blocking the production of sperm. A small percentage of men have no symptoms; however, they are still infectious and may subsequently suffer some bodily damage.

Gonorrhea in the female. Most women aren't aware of infection. Within a few days after exposure, symptoms may begin with a mild burning or smarting in the genital area, and there may be a slight discharge, but these are easy to confuse with some other female characteristics and ignore. An examination at this time could reveal a mild inflammation of the vagina and cervix. Somewhat later, after the occurrence of one or more menstrual periods, the infection ascends the reproductive tract. It may involve the fallopian tubes and ovaries, or spill purulent material into the abdomen, giving rise to peritonitis. At this time, pain and fever may be severe, or be mild enough to be passed off as a stomach upset. This could be followed by a chronic infection, lasting for years, that may cause extensive damage to the reproductive tract. The most frequent serious damage is sterility resulting from damage to the ovaries and the fallopian tubes. Tubal pregnancy sometimes occurs when a tiny sperm gets past the blocked fallopian tubes, but the larger fertilized egg is unable to descend. Meningitis, arthritis, septicemia, and damage to any organ of the body may also occur. In the majority of cases, the symptoms of infection are slight or mild, arousing little or no apprehension. Consequently, there is little impulse to consult a physician. Gonorrhea usually goes undetected in females until the person is named as a contact.

Homosexuals. Rectal and pharyngeal gonorrhea infection is found in males and females, heterosexuals and homosexuals. Rectal infection, like infection of the vagina and cervix, often has no symptoms. If infection persists for many months, rectal discharge and pain sometimes develop. Pharyngeal (throat) infection may involve a sore throat, pus pockets, and swollen cervical lymph nodes; however, absence of noticeable symptoms is not uncommon.

Laboratory Tests

Blood tests are not useful in the diagnosis of gonorrhea as they are for syphilis. However, two laboratory procedures are useful. (1) Microscopic examination of a stained discharge from the genital infection in men. (2) A culture, or growing the organisms on isolation media in the laboratory, is used for vaginal or rectal infection. Cultures may be negative even with infection, especially in the chronic phases when the offending bacteria are few in number. They are also expensive; therefore, it is cheaper to treat suspected females than it is to run the culture.

Treatment

The gonococcus is susceptible to a variety of therapeutic agents, but the preferred treatment is a single massive dose of penicillin. It will cure most cases of acute gonorrhea in men. Chronic cases may require repeated doses over a considerable period of time. The female is more difficult to treat and cure. Penicillin is not always useful with gonorrhea patients. First of all, some patients are sensitive to penicillin. Secondly, certain strains of gonococci develop resistance to penicillin. With these patients, other modern antibiotics can be used effectively. In late or serious cases, therapy may continue for as long as thirty days or more.

Gonorrhea in the Eyes of Newborn Babies

This condition is properly called *gonorrheal ophthalmia neonatorum*. It has probably made more people blind than any other disease, with the exception of trachoma. The bacteria are passed to the baby's eyes while passing through the birth canal. Within a few days an extraordinarily severe inflammation and a copious purulent discharge develop. When symptoms subside, the baby may be completely blind from scarring of the transparent portion of the eyeball. In 1884, Crede, a German physician, discovered that infection in the eyes of newborn babies would not occur if a few drops of silver nitrate were put in the baby's eyes. Today penicillin drops and other antibiotics are also widely used. This treatment, known as Crede prophylaxis, is so effective that it is required by law in most states and countries. As a result, blindness from gonorrhea is now rare when infants are delivered in modern hospitals.

Immunity

With gonorrhea, immunity does not seem to exist. One infection does not protect against a subsequent one. There are no biological materials that will confer a passive immunity.

AIDS

Acquired Immune Deficiency Syndrome (AIDS) first appeared in the United States in 1981. The way that the number of AIDS cases increased and the fact that it is almost always fatal produced a panic among many people throughout the world. The disease has been covered so widely and so thoroughly by the media that it is hard to imagine anyone who does not know the basic facts. The Surgeon General mailed a pamphlet, *Understanding Aids*, to every address in the country. The President of the United States called AIDS "Public Enemy Number One." With a few years of medical and epidemiological research, the AIDS hysteria has given way to a more intelligent approach to the problem--not that the problem is any less, but the parameters have been better defined. The knowledge that has been gained should have focused some fears and removed others, but should not have reduced the resolve to fight this menace called AIDS.

AIDS Statistics

A report issued by the Public Health Service, *Facts About AIDS*, Winter 1986, said that since 1981 there have been 15,000 reported cases, 52 percent of which have resulted in death. It was estimated that between 1/2 and 1 million people had been infected by the virus that causes AIDS, but as of that date had no symptoms. It is estimated that at least one-fourth to one-half of those infected with the virus but without symptoms will develop AIDS within four to ten years. Approximately 45 percent of all AIDS patients will be dead one year after being diagnosed, 85 percent will be dead after three years. The Center of Disease Control (CDC) estimates that by 1992, as many as 365,000 cases of AIDS will have been reported. People who engage in high risk activities are more apt to get AIDS. Homosexual and bisexual men account for 73 percent of the reported cases. Intravenous drug users account for another 17 percent. About 4 percent of the cases were heterosexual contacts. About 3 percent got AIDS through contaminated blood and blood products, 1 percent of the cases were infants who got it from their infected mother, and 3 percent cannot be classified.

What Is AIDS?

Two STDs are caused by a virus, genital herpes and AIDS, and there is no cure for either. Before continuing with the discussion, it may be interesting to look at virology, the study of viruses. Virology is at the frontiers of medical science and philosophy. We still do not understand the nature of the virus. It appears to be living in that it can reproduce itself; yet it appears to be a chemical in that it can crystallize into a lifeless form. Viruses are the smallest organisms that infect man. They are large molecules similar to the DNA molecules in the genes of the human cells. Once inside the body, a virus can invade and take control of a cell's functions and instruct the cell to produce more virus molecules. The newly formed viruses escape and take over neighboring cells. The possibility of a virus mutating is a concern of some health workers, and a report of another new form of the AIDS virus has already emerged.

A virus that causes AIDS is called the Human T-lymphotropic, type III (HTLV-III). It is also called the AIDS Related Virus or ARV. In AIDS it is not the virus that kills; however, the AIDS patients become vulnerable to a variety of illnesses that are not serious for normal people but are fatal to people with AIDS. The virus affects the immune system so people are unable to defend themselves against other *opportunistic* diseases.

The time between infection with the HTLV-III virus and the onset of symptoms may range from 6 months to 5 years or longer. Diagnosis is usually made in connection with care for an opportunistic disease. There are no clear-cut symptoms to indicate the loss of immunity. Early symptoms may include fatigue, weight loss, persistent low-grade fever, swollen glands, sore throat, loss of appetite, and diarrhea. Night sweats and deterioration of the mucous membrane and skin may come later. Then a number of conditions called AIDS-related complexes develop such as infection of the brain and lung, parasite infection, pneumonia, and cancer (Kaposi's sarcoma).

What Is the Risk of Getting AIDS?

The AIDS virus can be transmitted from one person to another through blood and semen. It may be present in other body fluids such as tears and saliva, but not in a strong enough concentrations to be transmitted. There is no risk of a child getting the AIDS virus at school or for an adult getting it at work. Virtually all cases are the result of direct sexual contact, the sharing of intravenous (IV) drug needles, or from an infected mother before or during birth. One does not get AIDS by being in a swimming pool with an AIDS patient, from casual contact, through a kiss, or from a mosquito or other insect bite. One won't get AIDS from saliva, tears, sweat, or urine (some authorities question the safety of feces and vomitus and say when in doubt wear latex gloves). One will not get AIDS from peoples' clothes, a telephone, from a toilet seat, or even from sharing eating utensils. There is no danger in donating blood. The danger of getting AIDS by receiving blood transfusions has been greatly reduced since new protective measures have been introduced.

A person may get AIDS by having vaginal, anal, or oral sex. A person can get AIDS by sharing drug needles and syringes. The risk goes up if a person has any type of sex with a person who shoots drugs or who also has sex with pickups, prostitutes, or a variety of partners. While using a condom provides some protection, it does not make the situation fully safe. The safety of a condom is improved if it is used properly, if a water-based lubricant is used, and if a spermicide is also used. Safe behavior is not shooting drugs, not having sex, or having sex only with a mutually faithful partner.

AIDS in Education

Surveys of high school students reveal that for the most part they know the basic facts about AIDS. This sounds positive, but when asked if this knowledge has altered their behavior in a way that would help prevent AIDS, the response was largely in the negative. It appears that the work that needs to be accomplished is in the area of attitudes. The information provided above contains most of the basic facts about AIDS. Appropriate behavioral change techniques can help young people adjust their attitudes. Some proponents of more extensive AIDS education have seized upon a unfortunate situation to try to introduce information into the classroom that tends to vindicate and invoke empathy for the homosexual community.

Another problem for schools is to deal with a student who has AIDS or to deal with a student who has a parent with AIDS. A teacher's role in the life of such children is primarily that of support. These students face the possibility of being ostracized by other children. The teacher can minimize the situation by educating the class about AIDS. The classroom may not be the best place for the child since it would be a fertile ground for transmitting the opportunistic diseases. The need for protection must be weighed against the need to live a normal life, and this question is best dealt with on an individual basis.

HERPES

Herpes is a disease of the genital organs caused by the herpes simplex virus (also called the herpes virus hominis - HVH). There are two closely related kinds of herpes virus, type 1 and type 2. Herpes infection of the genitals is usually caused by the type 2 virus, while infection of other parts of the body such as "cold sores" and "fever blisters" are usually caused by the type 1 virus. The herpes virus has an excellent relationship with the human body. Once the virus invades, it causes symptoms for just a few days. It then becomes dormant and continues to live in the cells of the body without causing symptoms for the rest of the person's life.

Transmission

The manner in which the herpes virus type 2 reaches the genital organs is not completely understood. It is currently thought that the virus is usually transmitted by vaginal, anal, or oral-genital sexual intercourse; however, there are cases of herpes genitalis in people whose only sexual partner has no evidence of herpetic infection. Herpes genitalis is more common in women than in men.

Symptoms

After an unknown incubation period following infecting sexual intercourse, one or several groups of small and painful bumps or blisters appear on the sexual organs. In women, the areas most often affected are the vaginal lips; but the clitoris, outer part of the vagina, anal area, and cervix can be involved as well. In heterosexual men, the glands or shaft of the penis are the most commonly affected areas. Homosexual men can have blisters in or around the anus. The blisters soon rupture to form soft, extremely painful open sores on a reddish base. On the cervix, sores are painless and usually not noticed. The sores are covered by a yellow-gray secretion. In women, sores can spread and involve the entire surface of the vaginal lips. If bacteria infect the exposed tissues, the sores discharge pus or blood, and the lymph glands in the groin may become tender and enlarged.

After 4 to 5 days, the sores become less painful and begin to heal by themselves. The skin is gradually replaced, starting from the edges of each sore. The sores usually heal completely, with little if any scarring, by the end of 10 to 20 days.

Complications

Recurrent infection. In most cases of herpes genitalis, the sores on the vulva or penis disappear and never return, even though the virus continues to live in the cells of the genital organs; however, in some cases the sores keep reappearing and the whole 10 to 20 day process of healing has to occur again. The herpes virus is most likely to become reactivated when the body is weakened by such things as fever, cold, emotional upset, fatigue, and sunburn. The best defense against reoccurrences of herpes genitalis is to maintain the body in a state of good health by sufficient good food, rest, and exercise.

Cancer. Although the relationship is not completely understood, an infection by the herpes virus makes women more susceptible to cervical cancer. Fortunately, cervical cancer can be detected at an early stage by the simple Pap test. If detected early, cervical cancer has a 100% cure rate. It has been known for many years that cervical cancer is far less common in women who have sexual intercourse only with men who are circumcised. It is known that the herpes virus can be carried in the secretion produced under the foreskin in uncircumcised men, and that such men are more likely to transmit the herpes virus to their sexual partners.

Infection of the newborn. An infant may become infected during birth with herpes virus type 2 while passing through its mother's infected cervix or vagina. It is also possible that some infants become infected while still in the uterus. Premature babies are particularly susceptible to such infections. The results of herpes infection of the newborn are extremely variable. In some cases, the child recovers completely; while in others, it develops a severe brain infection which rapidly becomes fatal. It has been suggested that some stillbirths and miscarriages are actually the result of herpes infection.

Diagnosis

Diagnosis of herpes genitalis is often missed because many doctors fail to suspect the virus as the cause of genital sores. Herpes genitalis is often misdiagnosed as syphilis or chancroid. Therefore, the disease is probably more common than is generally realized. It has been estimated that as many as six percent of women and three percent of men attending VD clinics in some areas have herpes genitalis. In all cases of multiple sores on the genitals, herpes infection should be suspected.

To test for herpes genitalis, a cotton swab is passed gently over the genital sores and the secretions and cells picked up are smeared on a microscopic slide and stained. Secretions from the cervix should also be tested, even if no sores appear on its surface. Attempts should also be made to culture the virus. But this can only be accomplished by a well-equipped hospital or research virology lab.

Treatment and Follow-Up

There is no antibiotic yet available that can kill the virus. Sulfa cream should be placed on the herpes sores to kill bacteria that can infect the exposed tissues. A set dressing of cool water and the use of a surface anesthetic such as Pontocaine may be useful in relieving pain. Oral pain killers such as aspirin with codeine should be prescribed.

Experiments are being performed with chemicals which appear to interfere with the reproduction of the virus, but results have been inconsistent.

People who have herpes genitalis should be examined once or twice a week until the sores disappear to ensure that secondary bacterial infection does not develop. Women who have herpes genitalis and women who have regular sexual intercourse with a man who develops herpes genitalis must have a Pap test for cervical cancer every six months for the rest of their lives.

OTHER STD'S AND GENITAL INFECTIONS

Chlamydia

Chlamydia is probably the fastest growing STD epidemic in this country with more than five million new cases a year. It is caused by a bacteria that acts very much like a virus. It can do staggering damage to the reproductive system without giving any warning signs or symptoms. Over 60 percent of the women and 10 percent of the men who have it have no symptoms. Many of the people, both men and women, who have it become permanently sterile. It increases the chance of ectopic (tubal) pregnancies, and babies that are born are at higher risk for other diseases. Women who have had chlamydia are apt to pelvic inflammatory disease and suffer chronic pain the rest of their life. A problem with chlamydia is that it is hard to diagnose. Its signs and symptoms match other STDs. Tests are expensive and unreliable. A twenty-one day regime of oral antibiotics is an effective treatment.

Genital Warts

Genital warts are so tiny that they may be hard to see, but they can grow large enough to obstruct the urethra, vagina, or anus. Genital warts have been known to cause cancer of the cervix. An infant born to a mother with genital warts may develop warts all over the body. Usually, they do not cause any symptoms at first and may be located where they are difficult to see on the cervix, vagina, vulva, penis, anus, rectum, mouth, or throat. They may be successfully treated, particularly while they are small. Several types of treatment are optimal, freezing with liquid nitrogen, dissolving with chemicals, electrosurgery, or laser surgery. Unfortunately, if a tiny wart is left, the condition will soon reoccur.

Chancroid

Chancroid, meaning chancre-like, is sometimes called "hair cut." Somewhat like syphilis, chancroid produces a small, but painful ulcer at the place where the causative bacteria (*Hemophilus ducreil*) enter the body and there are painful, swollen lymph nodes in the groin. Microscopic examination of material from the initial ulcer or from infected lymph nodes shows the small bacteria and assists in diagnosis. Treatment takes one to two weeks with "sulfa" drugs or other modern antibiotics.

Lymphogranuloma Venereum

This infection is usually transmitted during sexual relations and occasionally by contact with infectious discharges on clothing and bedding. Lymphogranuloma venereum is a disease that may cause much personal suffering. Sometimes starting with very tiny pimples, the organism causes an extensive inflammation of the lymphatic circulation in the region of the genital organs, particularly the lymph nodes of the groin in men. As a result of the interference with lymph drainage, elephantiasis of the genital organs may occur. In women, the disease may cause stricture of the rectum and necessitate extensive surgical alterations and repairs. Modern antibiotics and sulfonamide are effective in treatment.

Granuloma Inguinale

This is a mildly communicable disease transmitted by direct contact during sexual relations. It is caused by a tiny bacterium-like organism. The initial lesion is a small ulcer which may be mistaken for syphilis or chancroid. The surrounding tissues are invaded, damaged, and replaced by scar tissue. If not treated, the disease may cause extensive destruction of the genitals and surrounding structures. Diagnosis is made from the appearance of the lesions and by laboratory demonstration of Donovan bodies. A number of modern antibiotics are effective in treatment.

Other Genital Infections

There are a total of about twenty-five sexually transmissible conditions. Some of these are also transmitted through nonsexual contact. *Pediculus pubis* is a small parasitic insect about the size of the head of a pin which causes itching. *Morilias* (yeast) is the overgrowth of fungus which is indigenous to the female vagina. It may cause a whitish mucous which causes itching and inflammation. *Trichomonas viginalis* (Tric) is a protozoan that seems to cause no problem to the male except that he can pass it on to sex partners; however, in the female it causes a profuse watery, frothy, clear discharge that causes an extreme amount of itching. Other than crabs, these problems can be diagnosed and treated only by a physician.

CONTROLLING STD'S

Education

STDs, in most instances, are medically hidden as well as socially hidden. Socially, persons with venereal diseases ordinarily do not inform their friends or relatives about their infection, and they resist having their disease reported to the health department. The following are two measures paramount to success in controlling STDs which are particularly significant in teaching:

- Whenever anyone has any vague signs or any reason to suspect he or she may have contracted an STD, he or she should immediately go to a physician or a public clinic for an examination. They should not wait for definite signs or symptoms.

- Contacts to all cases must be obtained quickly in order to remove the reservoirs of infection in the community and to prevent further spread. Most patients who come to STD clinics have been named as a contact. They do not usually have symptoms and very frequently laboratory tests provide the only sign that they may be infected.

The role of physicians in treating patients and the role of epidemiologist in tracking people who need to be treated has become more complex because:

- New STDs are developing
- Organisms have increased resistance to treatment
- People develop allergic reaction to treatment
- Other diseases are now transmitted by sex contact
- Many people have more than one STD
- People are becoming more internationally mobile

Although the characteristics of each of the STDs are quite different, the principle process of infection is the same for all STDs--intimate sexual contact, usually of a questionable or promiscuous nature. The number one preventive measure is being selective in sexual activity. Abstinence from sexual activity is the option that is most secure. Abstinence prior to marriage and a mutually monogamous relationship after marriage is essentially safe. Knowing one's partner is extremely important.

Other precautions that provide considerably less protection are the use of condoms and washing the genitals with soap and water before and after sexual activity. A source of reliable information in the classroom is important to offset the unreliable information that is often passed by word of mouth from one student to another.

STUDY HELPS

1. Understand the stages of disease and the chain of infection.

2. Understand the procedures that may be employed in the schools to help control the spread of communicable disease.

3. Identify the causative agent and understand the mechanism of transmission for each of the diseases most likely to be found among young people of secondary school age.

4. Identify the symptoms a teacher might possibly observe for each of the diseases most likely to be found among young people of secondary school age.

5. List the typical exclusion and readmission procedures schools might employ to control the spread of the communicable diseases.

6. Indicate the diseases for which immunizations are typically required by state or local school administrations.

7. State and defend your personal policy in regards to your attendance as a teacher at school when you have or might have a communicable disease.

8. Distinguish between basic facts and fallacies in regards to the common sexually transmitted diseases.

9. What precautions are taken by health workers to increase the likelihood that young people with STDs will receive prompt and proper treatment?

10. What special problems and considerations does the AIDS disease present to the schools?

11. What special precautions should a teacher take if they have a student with AIDS attending class on either an elementary or secondary level?

12. What can schools and teachers do to help reduce the incidence of sexually transmitted diseases?

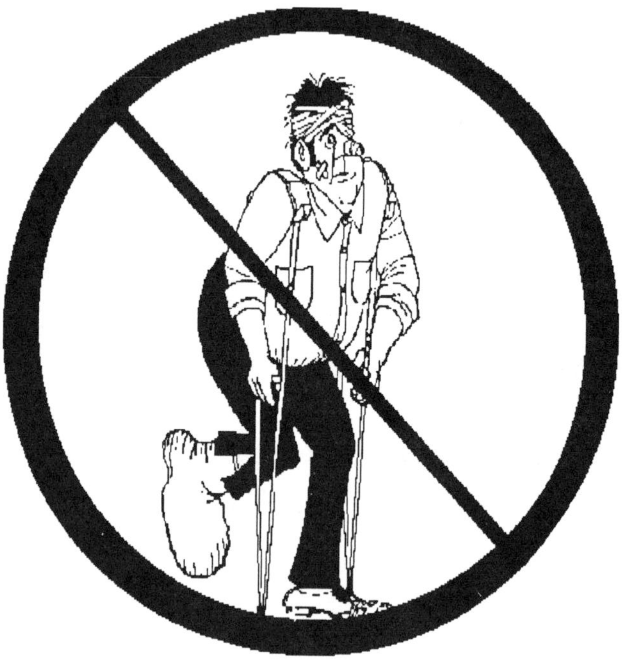

UNIT 4

SAFETY AND EMERGENCY CARE CONSIDERATIONS

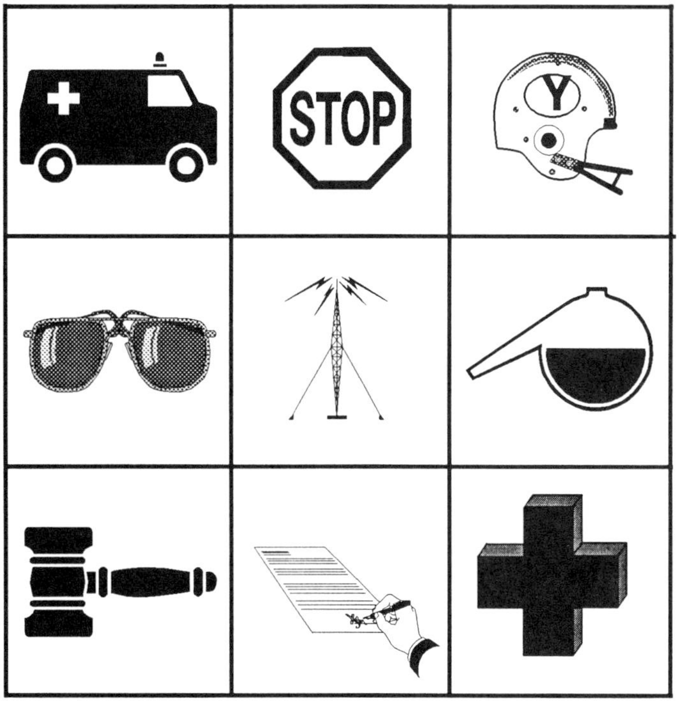

Most accidents do not just happen, they are caused.

Effective safety programs deal with things that never happen.

SAFETY AND EMERGENCY CARE

A teenager's world is one of intense activity and risk, and because of this, accidental injury is the leading health-related problem of this group. This is true when students are in school as well as when they are not. Nearly half of the accidental deaths among school-aged children are connected with school life. Because of this, safety and emergency care are important considerations for secondary school teachers.

Prevention has become the key word in dealing with accidents and sudden illness. Schools have a legal and moral responsibility to maintain an effective safety program and to provide for appropriate care in an emergency. Each teacher needs to intelligently and enthusiastically support the school's safety program and be able to give first aid when it is called for.

The schools need to have official policies pertaining to emergencies, and teachers need to be familiar with the policies and be prepared to carry them out. These policies should cover safety, emergency care for injuries and sudden illness, and contingency plans for major emergencies.

The teacher and the school may face disastrous legal implications if the policies are not well conceived and thoroughly carried out. Civil court action against negligent teachers is becoming a great threat. These considerations cause many prospective teachers to believe that this unit is the most important one in the course.

OBJECTIVES

At the conclusion of this unit, you should be able to meet the following objectives.

1. ACCIDENTS IN THE SECONDARY SCHOOLS

BE FAMILIAR WITH THE ACCIDENT PATTERNS IN THE SCHOOL SETTING AND TAKE APPROPRIATE STEPS TO HELP ALLEVIATE THE PROBLEM.

- Discuss the significance of accidents as a teenage health problem.
- List the school areas and activities where accidents occur most frequently.
- Explain the purposes and procedures for filling out accident report forms.
- Explain the meaning of various terms used to analyze accidents.

2. POLICIES AND EMERGENCY PROCEDURES

EXPLAIN THE NEED FOR AND BE ABLE TO FOLLOW SCHOOL POLICIES AND PROCEDURES FOR EMERGENCY SITUATIONS.

- Explain the purpose for school health policies for emergency situations.
- List the guidelines for establishing emergency policies.
- Discuss the importance of disaster contingency plans.

3. ORGANIZATION FOR SAFETY

IDENTIFY THE ORGANIZATIONS THAT MAY BE ESTABLISHED WITHIN THE SCHOOL SETTING TO HELP PROMOTE SAFETY.

- List some criteria for effective safety education.
- Identify the organizations which may be involved in school safety.

4. LEGAL IMPLICATIONS OF SAFETY AND EMERGENCY CARE

BE AWARE OF THE LEGAL RESPONSIBILITIES FOR PREVENTING INJURY AND DEALING WITH EMERGENCY SITUATIONS.

- Define the legal terms involved in school safety and emergency care.
- List the teacher's responsibilities for safety and emergency care.
- List ways to avoid negligence and liability for student injuries.

5. FIRST AID AND EMERGENCY CARE

RECOGNIZE APPROPRIATE FIRST AID PROCEDURES THAT MAY BE EMPLOYED IN THE SCHOOL SETTING.

- Outline the general directions for first aid in the school setting.
- Describe the procedures for giving life-saving first aid.
- Describe first aid for common injuries.
- Describe first aid for the common cases of sudden illnesses.
- List appropriate first aid supplies for school and classroom.

Chapter 16

LEGAL IMPLICATIONS

One of the questions most frequently asked by prospective teachers is, "What are my legal responsibilities in an accident or other emergency situation?" With the attention given in the media to legal suits of various kinds, this is an expected concern. The material which follows should help answer questions about liability.

LEGAL IMPLICATIONS FOR SAFETY AND EMERGENCY CARE

In this country, every person has the right to be free from bodily harm or personal injury caused intentionally or carelessly by acts of others. If a person believes that his or her injuries were caused by the negligent acts of others, he or she has the right to initiate legal proceedings in order to recover financial compensation for the damages. If a student or his parents believe that a teacher has caused the student harm, they have the right to sue the teacher for sufficient money to pay for the costs associated with the injury.

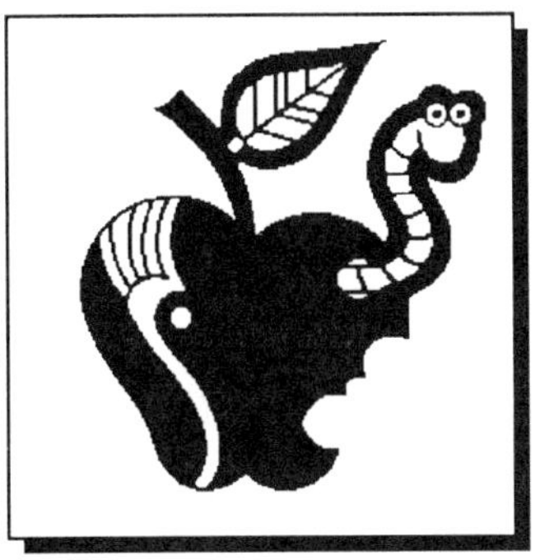

Liability suits of this type are becoming more frequent, particularly in certain states. The threat of liability may be a worm in the apple of education. Teachers are becoming very concerned by this threat. Court actions can devastate a person's life emotionally and economically. Having to go to court, even if not found liable, is very inconvenient and emotionally taxing. Yet such legal recourse is necessary to protect people's rights. The threat of being sued may also help prevent wrongdoing. We don't like to think of teachers being sued, but one court case may send a message that helps prevent many students from being injured. While students need to be protected from teacher negligence, occasionally teachers also need to be protected from unjustified accusations. The legal system exists to protect the rights of both. Teachers need to understand our legal system.

Suits against teachers occur much more frequently today than they did a few years ago. Peoples' attitudes are changing. Years ago fewer people felt inclined to sue a school teacher, and the courts also had a tendency to protect teachers. The traditional doctrine that the "king could do no wrong" provided governmental immunity to suit, and this included the schools. Schools could not be sued unless they agreed to be sued. At the same time, teachers were considered "judgment proof," because they didn't have enough money to be worth suing. While this protected the schools and teachers, it meant that some people who deserved compensation for medical expenses were unable to get it.

As the cost of medical care escalated, the only recourse for injured parties, since the schools could not be sued, was to sue the teachers or other school personnel. Because it was basically unfair to deny the injured party needed compensation and because it was also unfair to force them to sue the teachers, a few school districts started waiving their right to immunity. Some courts also started to overthrow the traditional governmental immunity. At approximately the same time, liability insurance was becoming available to teachers. Today most teachers have liability insurance that can partially pay the judgments if they are found liable.

Consequently, because it is becoming easier to sue and because the amount of the judgments are becoming larger, more and more teachers and schools are being sued. Teachers need to understand the operations of our legal system. This knowledge may reduce their chance of being sued. It will reduce their chance of being successfully sued, but perhaps more importantly it will reduce the chance of a student being injured at the hands of a teacher.

TORT LIABILITY

Under our legal system, every person has the right to be free from bodily harm or personal injury caused intentionally or carelessly by others. If anyone by his actions or neglect causes injury to another person, he or she may be legally responsible to pay for any damages suffered. The branch of law that deals with such offenses is called tort law. Teachers are not immune; they too must suffer the consequences the law affords when they are responsible for injury to their students.

A *tort* is a harmful act against a person which gives the person the right to collect money to pay for damages suffered. Tort law is mainly concerned with injuries to one's person, one's reputation, or one's property. A tort may include not only physical injury, but also the threat of injury which interferes with peace of mind, privacy, or reputation. A tort is a wrongdoing against an individual. Liability is a determination by the court as to the responsibility for paying for the damages. Court action may be initiated by the individual or by someone in behalf of the individual, such as a parent in behalf of their child. Tort cases are heard in *civil court.*

A *crime* is a wrongdoing against society and court action is initiated by the state in *criminal court.* Any fines collected go to the state. *Contract law* is another branch of law which deals with damages resulting from failure to keep a promise or fulfill a contract.

A tort may also be a crime. For example, if someone hits you in the face with his fist and breaks your nose you can sue him in civil court to collect money to pay for the medical expenses. The state can also take him to criminal court to punish him for breaking the law. In the civil court, you collect the money; in the criminal court, the state collects any fine.

Because of their exposure to students and potentially libelous situations, educators must understand their legal rights and responsibilities. While a knowledge of school law in general is important, an understanding of the tort law is imperative. Although physical educators and shop teachers are particularly vulnerable to accident situations, all people who supervise youth activities on either a professional or voluntary basis may encounter civil court action. This discussion will help teachers, youth activity leaders, and others serving the public to better understand our legal system.

Tort law is based on the fundamental premise that all individuals are liable for the consequences of their conduct. If a person feels that he or she has been injured due to the irresponsible actions, or inactions, of another person, he or she can initiate civil court procedures in order to try to force the other person to pay for the damages. In the court proceedings, the injured person becomes the *plaintiff,* and the person who was allegedly responsible becomes the *defendant.* If the court finds that the defendant was liable, the court will order the defendant to pay the plaintiff the monetary value of the damages awarded by the court. Regardless of the court decision, both the plaintiff and the defendant must pay the cost of their own legal fees. Many people feel it important to have insurance that will help pay the legal fees as well as any damages.

Although tort laws vary slightly from state to state, teachers and school districts are not immune from liability. The doctrine of government immunity that once applied to school districts, but not to teachers, has been changed by state legislatures as well as the courts. Some states under the concept of *in loco parentis* (in place of parents) have provided partial immunity for teachers in strictly educational activities unless willful or wanton misconduct is established. Some courts have protected school districts while conducting normal educational functions, but have ruled that extracurricular activities are outside of the school's education mission and not protected by immunity. A distinction has also been made between the school building and equipment within the building. Schools may not be granted immunity if it is found that they have maintained an *attractive nuisance* that has resulted in harm to an individual.

People who have been injured, or parents acting in behalf of a child who has been injured, may consult a lawyer to help them determine whether there is a strong enough case and whether the rewards may be sufficient to warrant the effort of a suit. They may consider the case strong enough if they believe they can prove all three of the following:

- The plaintiff was injured.
- The defendant contributed to the injury.
- The defendant acted in a negligent manner.

Even if a teacher may be negligent in maintaining classroom order, he or she will escape liability if no provable injuries occur. People have tried to fake injuries in order to collect insurance benefits or receive an award in court; therefore, to establish liability, the plaintiff must be able to prove that an injury occurred. Next, it must be shown that the defendant's actions or inactions caused or substantially contributed to the injury. But that is not enough, it must also be shown that the defendant was acting in a negligent manner as he or she contributed to the injury. This is not easy, because sometimes the actions that contributed to the injury were the proper thing to do under the circumstances. For example, moving a person with a broken leg from a burning building may contribute to the severity of the fracture, but that action would be preferable to leaving the person in the building. In a case where it is contended that a teacher was negligent because a *failure to act* contributed to the injury, it must also be proven that the teacher had a duty to act. It is not always easy to prove breach of duty. For example, spontaneous "horseplay" by a student may result in an injury that was not foreseeable.

In addition to having a strong case, the plaintiff must also decide whether any financial awards will be worth the effort. They may ask, "Can we collect enough money to pay the court costs and attorneys fees and still have enough money left to cover the damages or losses?" Sometimes teachers have not been sued because of the "deep pockets" principle; that is, teachers may not have enough money to pay any substantial liability awarded by the court.

Attorney fees and court costs are expensive, and usually the plaintiff must be able to pay these costs before an attorney will take the case. The fee may be based on a flat rate for that type of case plus expenses. Sometimes, lawyers are willing to take a case with the agreement that they will take a percentage of what ever is recovered. If they lose the case, they make nothing. If they win the case and are able to use legal maneuvers to increase the

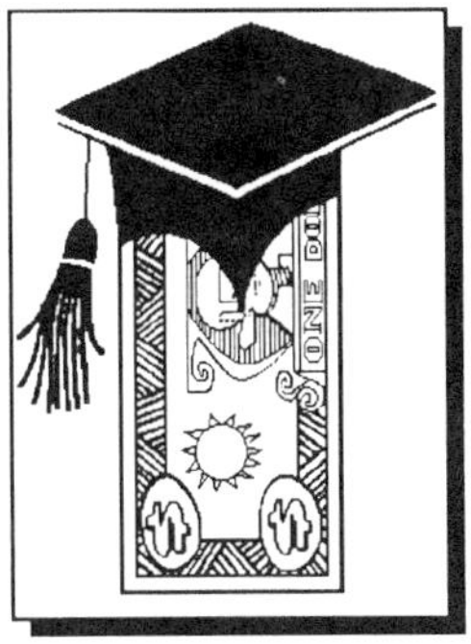

amount of the awards, they will make substantial fees that will offset losses on other cases. Sometimes, the court will award excessively high damages in order to make a statement that it hopes will reduce the incidence of that particular type of negligence.

The plaintiff has a choice of whether or not to take the case to court. The defendants, on the other hand, have no choice. The defendants must pay their attorney fees and their portion of the court costs whether they win or lose. If it looks like people are going to be sued, they should consult a lawyer and notify their insurance carrier, if they have liability insurance. However, if a case is decided in favor of the defendant, the defendant may countersue on the grounds of malicious process and attempt to recover the costs of defense. In the countersuit, the defendant in the original case must prove that the plaintiff in the original case had no grounds for probable cause, that the proceedings involved malicious abuse of due process, and that the original suit was motivated by malice.

The suit begins when the lawyer for the plaintiff prepares and has a summons and complaint served upon the defendant. The summons says that the defendant must appear in court to answer charges. The defendant engages an attorney to draw up an answer to the complaint. The answer may be a denial that the alleged wrong doing occurred or that it constituted a tort. Often pretrial proceedings will be held in which the lawyers for both sides meet to clarify the issues. If there appears to be insufficient evidence or a strong defense, the plaintiff may withdraw the suit. Or if there is an inadequate defense, the case may be settled without going to trial. A compromise may be reached that would save both time and money for both sides. Sometimes arbitration may be agreed upon. An impartial expert acting as an arbitrator listens to all sides and submits an award that he or she thinks is fair. Arbitration is quicker, costs less, remains private, and can deal better with technical information. If a pretrial settlement, compromise, or arbitration is not agreed upon, the case will go to court.

Today many litigations are being settled out of court. The insurance companies are afraid that the courts will award large settlements that may set new precedents. If the case goes to court the defendant might be cleared, but the defendant might also be found liable. Attorneys and insurance companies may feel it is wiser to settle one case out of court than to allow the court to render a decision that might affect the outcome of hundreds of future cases. Also, a large financial award may be used as basis for determining future awards.

If the case goes to civil court, the decision can be determined either by a judge or a jury. Cases involving simple questions of law will be determined by a judge. Cases involving questions of fact are decided by a jury. The plaintiff's lawyer has the burden of proof, he or she must present a preponderance of evidence that is more convincing than the

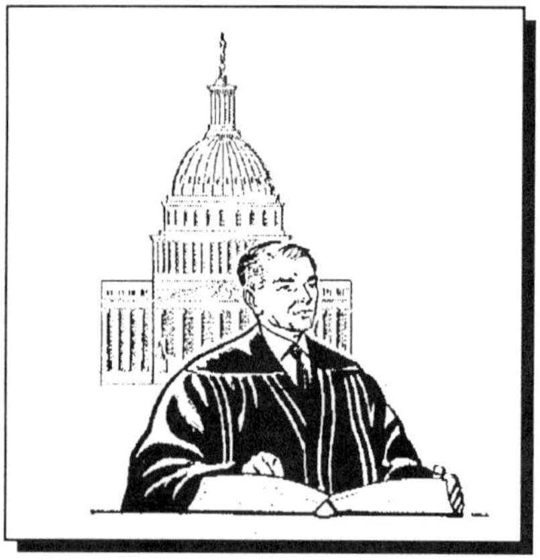

defendant's. As the trial begins, the lawyers for each side make brief opening statements outlining their client's version of the facts so that the court may understand the significance of the evidence that will be presented. Then the case for the plaintiff is presented as witnesses for the plaintiff give their testimony under direct examination by the plaintiff's lawyer. Then each witness for the plaintiff is cross-examined by the lawyer for the defense. When all evidence for the plaintiff has been presented, the plaintiff rests his or her case. At this point, the lawyer for the defense may ask the judge to dismiss the case, because the plaintiff has failed to prove a *cause for action.* If the motion is denied, the lawyer for the defense brings forth his evidence. Witnesses for the defense give their testimony, first under direct examination and then under cross-examination. When the defense rests its case, the lawyers for each side summarize their case. If the case is heard by a judge, he or she renders the decision. If the case is herd by a jury, the judge instructs the jury regarding the law, and the jury retires to consider the case and make a decision before returning to announce the decision.

The jury verdict or the judge's decision may be to dismiss if the defendant has won or to order the defendant to do something if the defendant has lost. The judge can reverse the decision of the jury if he deems the decision erroneous. In some cases, the court order may simply be an injunction to stop the defendant from doing something. In other cases, the court order may direct the defendant to pay the plaintiff a certain amount of money to cover damages or to compensate for the injuries.

In order to recover damages, the plaintiff must prove to the satisfaction of the court that he or she was actually injured, that the defendant committed an act that caused or contributed to the injury, and that the defendant committed the act with deliberate intent or that the act was the result of negligence. A tort involving physical injury may take place even when there is no intention to harm anyone. In torts involving libel or trespassing, the element of intent is essential. The courts award the plaintiff financial compensation for actual and anticipated medical costs, custodial care, and potential loss of income. The courts also now the reward the plaintiff financially as compensation for suffering, distress, and anguish. Punitive damages may be awarded for untrue statements which result in defamation of character by slander of libel. Slander is oral or statements made in the presence of others, and libel is statements written or broadcast by radio or television that can be seen or heard by others.

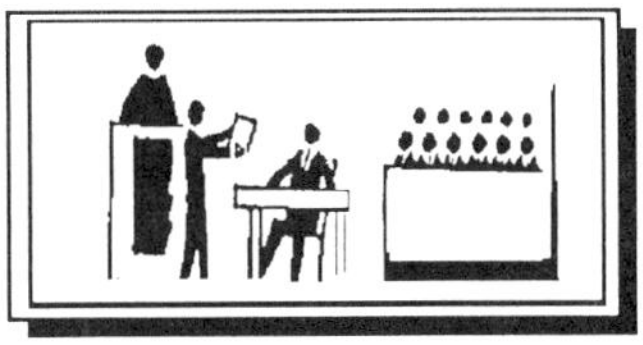

Sometimes a tort involves assault and battery. Assault is a threat to bodily contact without permission, and battery is actual contact without permission. A person waving a fist or ruler and making a hitting gesture may be committing an assault. Any contact with a part of the body such as a hand or foot or any object attached to the body such as a ruler in the hand may be battery. Even a touch without permission may be considered battery. In some circumstances, the courts may hold that the defendant who caused injury to the plaintiff acted with *privilege*. Acting in self-defense, in defense of others, or to protect one's property may be covered by privilege. However, in such circumstances a person should not use greater force than he is defending against. Cases of assault and battery may be tried in both civil and criminal courts. The plaintiff, the police, or other citizens may prefer criminal charges if they believe the law has been broken. Any fines levied in the criminal court will be paid to the state. The plaintiff may also wish to take the case to civil court in order to try to recover damages and to collect compensation.

Sometimes the courts will determine that both the defendant and the plaintiff contributed to some extent to the injuries, and the defendant will have to pay only his portion of the damages. A form of defense a teacher may use is that of *comparative negligence*. He may try to show that the student performed in a way that was negligent, and this caused or contributed to the injury. Another consideration is *assumption of risk*. If an individual knows of the dangers involved in a certain activity and voluntarily assumes those risks, he may not have a basis for charging another person with negligence. This is why it is important for teachers to adequately warn students about risks. Even then, due to the assumption of natural immunity of judgment by adolescents sometimes held by the courts, the teacher may be found negligent. If the court finds that the student assumed the risk or that the student's negligence contributed to the injury, the recovery of damages from the teacher may be denied or reduced.

Sometimes a suit will name several defendants. For example, an injury to a student in a physical education class activity or a city park playground followed by alleged incompetent medical care at a hospital may result in the teacher, the school district, the city, the hospital, and the doctor all being named as defendants. The court may find all, some, or none liable and proportion out the judgment. The proportion assignments may be based on degree of responsibility and/or ability to pay.

Almost all employers are liable for the torts committed by their employees during the course of their employment. However, the government, including the public schools, is an exception based on the doctrine of sovereign immunity. Furthermore, public officials such as police officers in the course of their duty are not liable unless it can be proven that they used excessive force. Parents generally cannot be held liable for torts committed by their children nor can husbands or wives be held liable for the acts of their spouse. One exception would be if the parents or spouse encouraged the acts of the child or spouse. Another exception would be if a child had established a propensity for viscous behavior and the parents failed to try to control the child.

There are three categories of tort action. Strict liability deals with injuries resulting from the creation of unusual hazards. Intentional liability deals with injuries resulting from a desire to inflict harm. Negligence deals with injuries resulting from conduct which falls below an accepted standard. Most tort cases involving school personnel are in the negligence category.

NEGLIGENCE

Negligence is the breach of one's duty to protect others from unnecessary risk of harm. It may involve careless or irresponsible acts of commission and acts of omission. Negligence is the violation of an obligation to take proper care and caution, especially when such acts or inactions result in injury to another person. There are three types of negligence.

- **Nonfeasance**. Failure to perform a legally required duty. Usually an act of omission. If the plaintiff was injured because the defendant had a duty to act but failed to perform his or her duty, the defendant may be found negligent due to nonfeasance.

- **Misfeasance**. Performing a legally required duty improperly. If the plaintiff was injured because the defendant performed a lawful act in an unlawful or improper manner, the defendant may be found negligent due to misfeasance.

- **Malfeasance**. Performing an act without permission or wrongdoing and misconduct in office. If the plaintiff (usually an organization) was harmed because the defendant (usually an employee or elected or appointed official) misused his or her authority to commit an act that was unlawful, the defendant may be found negligent due to malfeasance.

A teacher is more likely to be charged with nonfeasance or misfeasance than malfeasance. A teacher is not apt to misuse his or her authority or perform acts without proper consent. An example of malfeasance might be when a person rendered first aid without first gaining consent. But in the case of a teacher, because the courts have consistently held that teachers stand *in loco parentis*, they have the right to give first aid to students. The teacher has the parents' duties and responsibilities while the child is in school or is engaged in school activities and does not need to gain consent.

In order for the plaintiff to prove negligence, or for the defendant to establish a defense, the following legal questions must be dealt with.

- <u>**The reasonable man test**</u>. To prove negligence it must be established that the defendant's behavior was unusual, unreasonable, and imprudent. The question is, "Would a normal, reasonable, and prudent person with the same background and training as the defendant have acted as the defendant acted in the same circumstances?" The reasonable man test compares a teacher with other teachers, not with a man on the street. The courts consistently hold teachers to a higher standard of care than they do ordinary citizens. Evidence that the defendant's behavior was notably unusual and beyond reason would strengthen the case for the plaintiff.

- <u>**Proximate cause**</u>. To prove negligence, it must be established that there was a causal or contributory relationship between the alleged negligent behavior and the injury sustained. In other words, it must be proven that the plaintiff's injury would not have occurred if the defendant had not performed as he or she did.

- <u>**Foreseeability**</u>. The ability to foresee harm is an important factor in determining negligence. The question is whether or not in that set of circumstances a reasonable and prudent person would have anticipated or foreseen the possibility of harmful consequences and have taken steps to avoid them. There is an important difference between foreseen and foreseeable.

- <u>**Comparative negligence**</u>. The plaintiff's behavior must also be examined. If the plaintiff's own behavior falls below the standard required for personal protection, the plaintiff may have contributed to the injury. If so, the defendant may only have to pay a certain percent of the total liability awarded. The judgment is reduced by the percent the court feels the plaintiff contributed to his or her own injury.

- <u>**Assumption of risk**</u>. Another question of importance to the defense has to do with whether or not the plaintiff knowingly assumed certain risks. The responsibility of the defendant may be significantly reduced if it can be established that despite a knowledge of the hazards, a plaintiff voluntarily entered the area of risks.

- <u>**Pure accident**</u>. In spite of the fact that most accidents are caused, occasionally injuries result without anyone being at fault. When injuries are the result of some uncontrollable force, they may be described as "a freak of nature," "acts of God," or pure accidents. A pure accident was not caused by negligence nor was it avoidable; therefore, no one should be found liable.

- <u>**Duty**</u>. Duty is an existing responsibility relationship between two individuals such as a teacher to a student. In cases of nonfeasance, the question of duty is very important. If a person has no legal duty to act, he or she cannot be found negligent for failing to act. Therefore, in order to establish negligence through nonfeasance, a duty relationship must be established between the defendant and the plaintiff.

Courts today are demanding a greater degree of responsibility. They are less tolerant of mistakes committed by teachers. The courts are demanding more accountability and a higher standard of performance. They expect the teacher to exhibit customary care based on the circumstances. If a case goes to court, the attorney for the plaintiff will try to establish that the teacher was guilty of one or more of the following:

- Was not providing proper supervision.
- Did not give sufficient warnings about inherent dangers.
- Did not give the proper instruction in the proper sequence.
- Did not provide proper safety equipment.
- Did not maintain the equipment properly.
- Did not administer proper emergency first aid.
- Did not perform his assigned duties.
- Did not follow the rules and regulations.

SUPERVISION

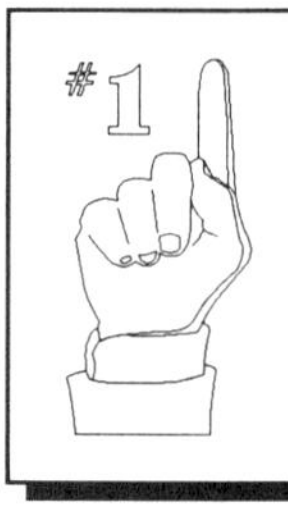

A key question in teacher negligence cases is, "Was adequate supervision provided?" Because the question of supervision shows up most frequently in court cases, it is very important. If an accident occurs and the teacher is not present, the courts are likely to hold that if a supervisor had been present the injury might not have occurred or would have been minimized. There are two types of supervision, and the type required depends on the situation. *General supervision* is when a teacher is present in the classroom or area, but not directly involved in the students' activities. For example, before school starts in the morning the teacher may be working at his desk while students are lounging around the classroom waiting for class to start. In this situation, the teacher can be providing general supervision. *Specific*

supervision is when the teacher is directly involved in an activity. For example, during a physical education class, the students are learning a gymnastics skill and the teacher is acting as a spotter thus providing specific supervision.

To avoid the problem of supervision, a teacher should never leave a class unsupervised at any time, including before and after school. When an emergency occurs and the teacher must leave, a certified person should be left in charge of the class. A teacher in an adjacent room may be able to provide general supervision for two classrooms. A teacher should never release a class early or late. A teacher is liable for what may happen to the students during that time. A teacher should provide the type of supervision required for the particular situation. Younger children, inexperienced students, and dangerous activities require a higher degree of supervision. Recent court decisions have placed greater rather than less emphasis on the teacher's role in providing classroom supervision.

WARNINGS

Another key question in teacher negligence cases is, "Was adequate warning given?" Warnings are particularly important in situations with inherent risks such as in sports and with the operation of equipment. Rules, regulations, and routines should be followed precisely every time without exception. If a shop teacher gives the proper instructions in proper sequence most of the time, but not always, it may be difficult to prove that adequate warning was given the particular time an accident occurred. It may be advisable to keep a record when warnings are given. A check sheet, such as a pilot and co-pilot use before take-off, may be helpful. A student-completed form to verify that the student received and understood the warnings is sometimes used. A teacher should establish reasonable classroom rules that include safety regulations.

PRECAUTIONS

The question of reasonable caution is also important. For example, in sports activities, it is important to make sure the players are in proper physical condition. Also in contact sports, the mismatching of size and strength should be considered. Do not allow student access to potentially dangerous equipment, chemicals, apparatus, or hazards. Periodically inspect classrooms, furnishings, and equipment to insure a safe environment for students. Record the inspections and, if any deficiencies are found, notify the school administrator in writing. A teacher must exercise caution in regards to students in the classroom who exhibit the signs of what might possibly be a communicable disease. The Supreme Court has backed teachers in their responsibility to exclude students from the classroom who merely exhibit the signs of a communicable disease. The potential is there for a suit if a teacher fails to exclude such a student and another student suffers serious consequences because he or she contacted the disease in the classroom.

CHARACTER DEFAMATION

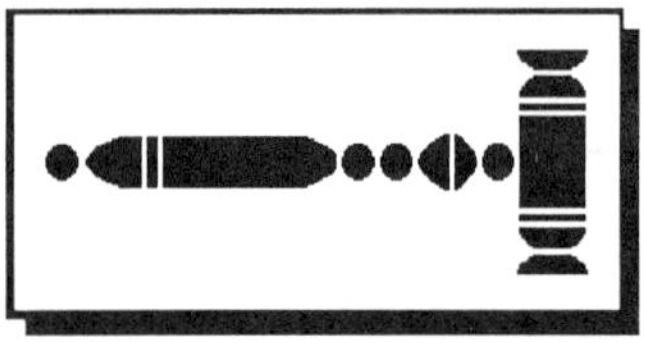

Punitive damages may be awarded for untrue statements which result in defamation of character by slander or libel. *Slander* is oral or written statements made in the presence of others, and *libel* is statements written or broadcast by radio or television that can be seen or heard by others. Teachers must be careful to safeguard information that comes to them that might, if "spread about," tend to damage a student's reputation. A teacher must be careful about anything potentially damaging to a student that the teacher puts into writing or shares orally with others. If it can't be backed up with objective evidence, state it as an opinion, not a fact. Even then don't say it unless there is substantial merit in doing so. Don't make defamatory statements about a student in front of a class or to other members of the faculty. Don't call a student any inappropriate names or attach any derogatory labels. To do so might cause embarrassment and harm to the student and invite a suit for defamation of character.

Any information of a personal nature disclosed by a secondary school student who is receiving counseling is confidential. Such information should not become part of the student's record without the written consent of the student. It should only be revealed and discussed in the following situations:

- For the purpose of medical or psychiatric treatment, but only after the student has signed a waiver of confidence.
- Reporting child abuse and neglect as specified by law.
- To avert a clear and present danger to health, safety, or welfare of the student members of the school community.
- When a crime has been or may be committed involving personal injury or substantial property loss.
- As ordered to do so by law enforcement agencies to aid in investigating a crime or in any judicial proceedings.

A teacher is not generally entitled to *privileged communication.* In some situations, teachers must reveal certain types of information to certain individuals, even when it was shared in confidence, but they should not share confidential information in other circumstances. Doctors, lawyers, and the clergy are entitled to privileged communication, but school teachers, counselors, and administrators are not. Yet there seems to be a trend to allow school administrators, teachers, and especially counselors to have *qualified privileges* in information about students. Under court order, however, teachers must reveal confidential information. If a teacher has information brought to his attention that may be incriminating for a student, in most districts, his or her first duty is to share that information with the principal or another authority who will determine if it should go any further and if so, make the appropriate contact. If he does not do so, he may be liable for withholding information. It is well for the teacher to discuss any questionable situations with the principal. If any legal problems come up, it is important that the principal was aware of the situation and concerned in any actions taken by the teacher. It may create a big problem for a teacher to try to operate in questionable areas on his or her own. For example, information relating to illegal drug use or distribution must be given to appropriate police officers. The child is a minor and the school is acting in the place of the parents while he is still in school. Parents are entitled to most information about their children.

Information about possible child abuse must also be revealed to appropriate state social workers. Generally, anyone making a nonmalicious report of child abuse or taking part in legal proceedings to remedy child abuse will be made immune from liability. On the other hand, willful failure to report child abuse to proper authorities may be cause for civil liability. In a case of suspected child abuse, the school nurse should be contacted to make a preliminary appraisal. If there is a basis for a complaint, the civil authorities should be informed and a complaint filed against the parents.

Written or oral communication which may result in defamation of character is another sensitive legal question. Written communication (*libel*) or oral communication (*slander*) to one other person, other than the defamed, may be grounds for tort liability even when the communication is to the parents of the defamed. This is particularly true when the information is disseminated with lack of good will or with intent to harm. While there is a move toward the legal protection of the rights of privacy, there is also a move toward disclosure of information on school records. Parents, guardians, and students over 18 years of age have the right to inspect and challenge the accuracy of school records. This has significant implications upon what is recorded in the student's health record.

TEACHER MALPRACTICE

Teachers today are joining the ranks of doctors, lawyers, and architects in having to defend themselves against charges of negligence in malpractice suits before a civil court. Malpractice suits in education recognize a new type of injury to students. Psychological, emotional, and educational damage results from the schools' and teachers' failure to provide appropriate teaching, testing, placement, and reporting. Students have a statutory right to receive an education, and students and parents have the right to receive accurate feedback regarding academic progress. Teachers today are being held more accountable for the quality of classroom instruction, and they must develop the potential of all students under their care.

A teacher malpractice tort occurs when 1) the teacher had a duty towards a student, 2) a breach of that duty occurred, 3) an injury occurred, and 4) there was a causal relationship between the breach of duty and the resulting injury. The teacher has a duty to ensure that the students receive competent instruction. Teachers may violate that duty when they intentionally or unintentionally do any of the following:

- Consistently enter the classroom unprepared to teach.
- Exclude basic skills and concepts from the curriculum.
- Improperly advise students on progress requirements.
- Use inappropriate testing and evaluation procedures.
- Use improper student placement procedures.
- Promote or graduate students without minimal skills.
- Do not provide parents feedback on student lack of progress.
- Deny students access to remedial programs in basic skills.

Foreseeability is a critical issue in liability cases. If a teacher can predict that the continuation of certain practices may result in students' academic failure and nevertheless continues without effort to change the outcome, he or she may be inviting a malpractice lawsuit.

DISCIPLINE AND PUNISHMENT

Teachers are responsible for maintaining classroom order, and this occasionally requires some type of disciplinary measures. The *Legal Reference for California School Administrators* states, "Every teacher in the public schools shall hold pupils to a strict account for their conduct." It further indicates that teachers shall not be subject to criminal prosecution for exerting the "same degree of physical control over a pupil that a parent would be legally privileged to exercise but which in no event shall exceed the amount of physical control reasonably necessary to maintain proper and appropriate conditions conducive to learning."

Years ago *corporal punishment* was a common disciplinary measure, but today its use in schools has declined even in states where it is still legal. Corporal punishment is the willful infliction of, or willfully causing the infliction of, physical pain on a pupil. Some states have banned it. Even in states where it is legal, districts may have a policy against its use.

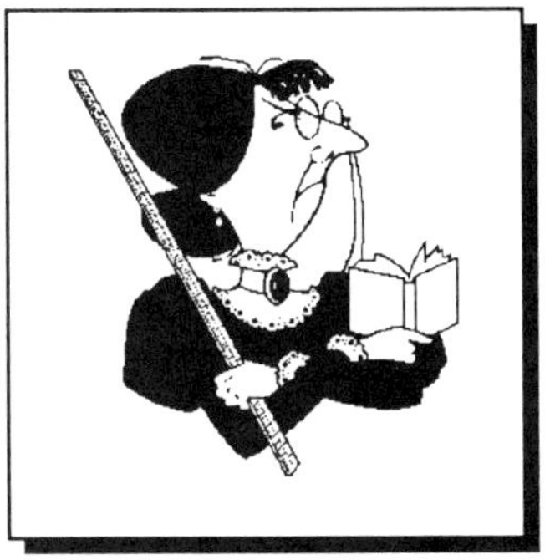

Its efficacy in the teaching situation is seriously questioned. A teacher should be aware of the state laws and local policies in regard to corporal punishment. Yet in some part of the country students are still getting the paddle.

Where it is lawful, within policy, and deemed appropriate, certain conditions should be met. If corporal punishment is to be administered, care should be taken so that it cannot be interpreted as a spontaneous act motivated by anger or vengeance. It would be wise to delay the punishment until it is clear that a cool head prevails and malice is not intended. When corporal punishment is administered, there should be another adult, preferably a school administrator, in attendance as a witness. The student should understand the reason for the punishment and see the relationship between his or her behavior and the punishment. The type of punishment used should not be excessive or malicious, the penalty should fit the violation.

If necessary a teacher may act in self-defense, but his actions should be strictly defensive. There may be legal problems if the teacher badgers the student to incite an attack. A teacher may not provoke an attack in order to exercise force in what appears to be self-defense. Teachers may use physical force to quell a disturbance that threatens physical injury to another person or threatens to damage property. They may also use force to obtain possession of a weapon or other dangerous object, but they should only use the amount of force that is reasonable and necessary.

LEGAL ASPECTS OF FIRST AID

Before considering first aid in the school setting, we will explore the legal implications when members of the general public administer first aid. Sometimes people refuse to give first aid, because they are afraid they might get sued. This fear is very unfortunate and rarely justified. The courts traditionally have been conscientious about supporting and protecting the concept of voluntary assistance in time of emergency. Doctors have been sued for malpractice and teachers have been sued for nonfeasance when they failed to give needed care to an injured student, but the courts have allowed volunteer first aid providers a wide margin of error. Volunteer first aid providers, trained and untrained, have rarely if ever been successfully sued unless they grossly exceeded their limitations or had malicious intent.

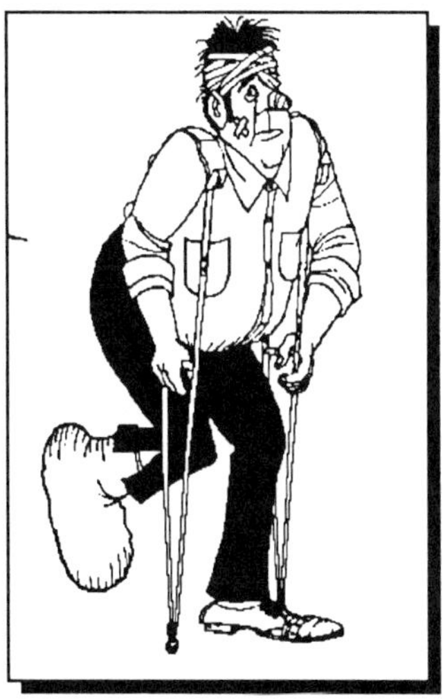

Who is Legally Required to Give First Aid?

In this country, a bystander is not legally required to give first aid. Hopefully, if you are a bystander you will feel a moral obligation to help an injured person, but unless there is a duty relationship between you and the injured person, you are not legally obligated to give first aid. If there is a duty relationship, however, you are legally obligated to give the best care you are capable of giving.

Who has a Duty Relationship?

The following are examples of duty relationships and therefore are legally required to give first aid and other needed care to the best of their ability:

- Police officers or firemen to members of the general public.
- Park or forest rangers to people in the park or forest.
- Proprietors to customers in their place of business.
- Home owners and tenants to guests in their home.
- Drivers or car owners to passengers in their car.
- Group of hikers to members of their group.
- Parents and guardians to their children.
- Adult children to their elderly parents.
- Voluntary youth leaders to the youth in their charge.
- **Teachers to their students.**

If a person who does not have a duty starts to give first aid or other assistance, he or she voluntarily assumes a duty relationship. To abandon the injured person later would be a violation of duty. Also, to fail to send help after volunteering to do so would be a violation of duty.

What is the Duty?

If you have a duty or assume a duty, your duty is to do the best you can under the circumstances. You cannot be expected to exceed your ability. Your ability may be limited by your training, strength, the availability of supplies and equipment, and environmental conditions. Anyone should be able to at least call for help, provide general aid and comfort, prevent further injury, and take charge of the situation until relieved by someone with training and authority. You should not attempt to go beyond your level of first aid training. Stay with the standard first aid procedures taught in a recognized first aid course. To fail to do your duty may constitute nonfeasance and to do your duty improperly may constitute misfeasance.

What about School Teachers?

The policy governing the administration of first aid varies from one school district to another, and each teacher should know and follow the policy in his or her district. In general, however, the courts have ruled that an educator can administer first aid and that a coach has a duty to administer first aid, but in all cases it must be done properly. The courts hold teachers to a higher standard of performance in administering first aid than they do the general public. A teacher may face charges of nonfeasance if they fail to respond to a duty to give first aid. A teacher may also face charges of misfeasance if they give first aid improperly.

First aid providers should not attempt to go beyond their ability. A teacher should render the best first aid he can within his ability and within school policy. A first aid provider should stay with the standard first aid procedures taught in a recognized first aid course. When school policy allows or requires a teacher to give first aid, the teacher should take the responsibility to become adequately trained. The expected standard of performance is comparable to what is provided in an American Red Cross standard first aid course.

A teacher may wonder about giving first aid outside of his school-related responsibilities. Although it is hoped that they would assume a moral duty to help others in distress, the common law of this country (unlike some European and Asian countries) has not made it a legal duty. Unless there is an existing responsibility relationship between two individuals (duty), having received first aid training does not legally obligate a person, including teachers, to give first aid. However, in volunteering to give first aid there are a couple of legal implications to keep in mind. First, once a person voluntarily starts to render assistance, he has voluntarily assumed a duty and can be held liable for failure to provide reasonable care and protection. When people have a higher level of training, a higher standard of performance is expected. Second, occasionally a first aid provider may be charged with malfeasance and/or battery because he or she allegedly performed first aid without first gaining consent. An individual has the right to choose whether or not he wants emergency care. If a victim is unconscious, irrational, or unable to communicate and emergency care is needed, consent can be "implied."

What about Good Samaritan Laws?

Because people sometimes have felt it better to do nothing rather than to run the risk of liability, Good Samaritan laws have been passed in most states to provide protection for professional volunteers such as doctors and nurses and perhaps others who are acting in good faith and are providing care as a reasonable prudent individual would. Protection for the volunteer first aid provider has been provided traditionally by the courts. The Good Samaritan laws, however, are generally not an issue in the school setting because the teacher is not a volunteer. The teacher has a legal duty relationship with the student. The teacher has a duty to act *in loco parentis* to function as a surrogate parent. For this same reason, there is usually no question of consent.

PERMISSION SLIPS

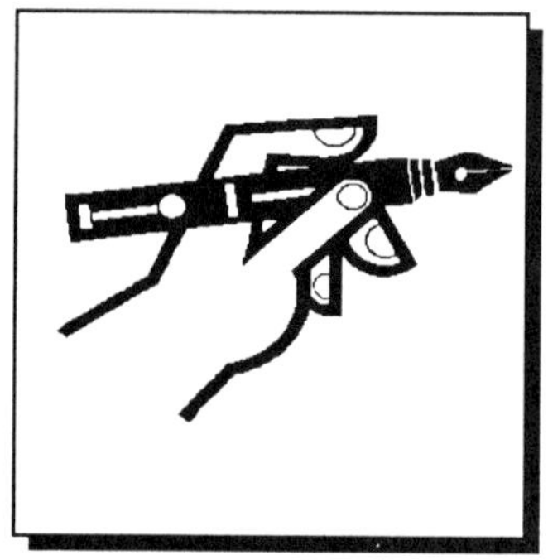

Frequently, schools and youth groups have the students' parents sign permission slips and waiver forms before students participate on field trips and other special activities. Such forms are valuable, but not for the reason commonly believed. They may not protect the teacher or school from liability. Even though they sign the form that says, "I hereby voluntarily waive any claim against the teacher and school," it may not hold up in court. A parent or guardian might be able to waive their right to sue, but they cannot waive their right to sue in behalf of a child. A waiver form will not stand up in the event of gross negligence or malicious conduct on the part of a teacher or other youth leader.

The chief value of a permission slip is that it shows that the parents or guardian were aware of the activity and gave their permission for their child to participate. That fact may be important in case there is an injury and court action. If a teacher took a student on a field trip without the parents being aware of it and the student was injured, the teacher could be in serious legal trouble. The form should contain the pertinent details about the trip or activity such as:

- When they will leave and return.
- Where they will be going.
- What they will be doing.
- Who will be in charge.
- Who they might contact in case of an emergency.

Another important value of the form is the part which authorizes medical care in case of an emergency. It may say, "In the event that I cannot be reached in an emergency, I hereby give my permission to the physician, selected by the adult leader in charge, to hospitalize, secure proper anesthesia, or order injections or surgery for my child." Not only is it important to have this item signed by a parent or guardian, it is also important to have it in hand when the child is taken to the medical care facility. There should also be space available for the parents to comment if the child has any medical needs such as required medications, allergies, or special restrictions. The form may also have a space for recording health and accident insurance data. Finally, the form may solicit the parents' help in encouraging the student to obey the rules of safety while on the trip or activity.

CONCLUSION

To summarize, a teacher can become involved in a precarious legal position. It may be impossible to completely protect oneself from a lawsuit, but a knowledge of the laws and responsible action will help a great deal. The information in this lesson will not keep you from being sued--a person can be sued for anything; however, the success of the suit or the defense rests on well-established legal principles. The information in this lesson discusses those principles and, if followed, should keep you from being successfully sued. Actually, comparatively few teachers are either sued or found liable. Foreseeability, or the ability to anticipate hazardous situations or potential accident causes, is usually accepted as the first test of negligence. If a teacher fails to foresee a foreseeable hazardous situation and fails to remove or diminish the risks, he may be found liable. This will be tested by what is considered to be normal, reasonable, and prudent judgment by a competent teacher in that situation. The teacher's responsibilities are the following:

- To anticipate foreseeable risks.
- To remove all *removable* risks.
- To warn students about unremovable risks.
- To provide care for the injured.
- To not increase the severity of an injury.

Questions of liability are complex; the jargon may be complicated, and the issues confusing to many people. While the information presented here may be oversimplified to a lawyer, hopefully it will be of some help to school teachers. At least it should open their eyes to questions that may have to have more definitive answers at the local level.

STUDY HELPS

Understand the following terms as they relate to this lesson.

1. assumption of risk
2. attractive nuisance
3. cause for action
4. character defamation
5. civil court
6. comparative negligence
7. corporal punishment
8. deep pockets
9. defendant
10. duty
11. foreseeability
12. foreseeable risks
13. general supervision
14. governmental immunity
15. gross negligence
16. *in loco parentis*
17. legal jargon
18. liability
19. liability insurance
20. malfeasance
21. malicious conduct
22. medical care authorization
23. misfeasance
24. negligent
25. nonfeasance
26. nontributory negligence
27. permission slips
28. plaintiff
29. precaution
30. privilege
31. privileged communication
32. proximate cause
33. punitive damages
34. qualified privileges
35. reasonable man test
36. removable risks
37. self-defense
38. specific supervision
39. supervision
40. teacher malpractice
41. tort
42. unremovable risks
43. warning

Chapter 17

SCHOOL SAFETY

A teenager's world is one of intense activity and risk. Because of this, accidents are the greatest threat to life and health for the adolescents. Over half of all deaths to teenagers are due to accidents. It is tragic when deaths and disabling injuries interrupt the life of a young person, but it seems even more pathetic when those accidents occur within the protection of the schools. The schools need to provide safety education at all levels, but accident prevention is a particular concern of teachers.

ACCIDENT STATISTICS

Accidents are the leading cause of death for all ages between one and thirty-eight. In America, accidents are the fourth leading cause of death overall. Each year almost one-third of all Americans will be sufficiently injured to see a doctor or be disabled for a day or more. Among young people age 15 to 24, accidents cause more deaths than all other causes put together.

For men, the accidental death rate is 67 per 100,000; for women, it is 27 per 100,000. The age group that has the highest accidental death rate are those aged 75 or older, most of these are due to falls. Next highest is the age group 15 to 24 with a rate of 97 per 100,000 and most of these are due to motor vehicle accidents. The National Safety Council, *Accident Facts*, lists the leading causes of death due to accidents for the year 1983. The number of deaths per year for each cause is listed as follows.

- Motor Vehicle 44,600
- Falls 11,700
- Drowning 6,600
- Fires & Burns 4,600
- Choking, suffocation 3,200
- Oral Poisoning 3,000
- Firearms 1,900
- Gas Poisoning 1,300
- All Others 14,100

TOTAL 91,000

In addition to being a major cause of death, accidents are a major cause of disability. For example, each year more than 80,000 people are permanently disabled due to back and spinal injuries. Accidental injuries also cost this country approximately $100 billion each year. Approximately one hospital bed in eight are occupied by patients suffering from accidental injury. The number of accidents are on the increase, about one percent per year over the last few years.

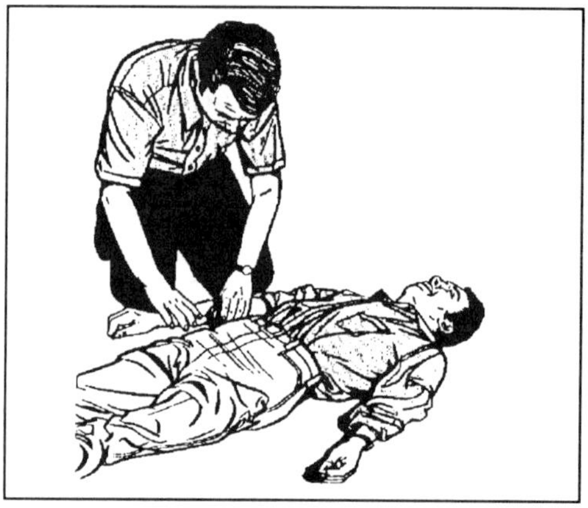

- Motor Vehicle 58%
- Drowning 15%
- Fire & Burns 7%
- Firearms 5%
- Railroad 1%
- Other 14%

As youngsters reach the teenage years, there is a dramatic increase in accident rates. Forty-five percent of the deaths in the ten to fifteen age group and fifty-seven percent of the fifteen to nineteen age group are due to accidents. On the next page is a list of the most common causes of death among young people ranging in age from five to nineteen.

The National Safety Council reports that each year nearly 2 million school age children receive injuries requiring the attention of a doctor or causing absence of more than half a day from school. Many of these accidents occur within the schools, and some of them result in deaths. Forty-three percent (43%) of accidental deaths among school age children are connected with school life. The following list shows the most frequent places where the school related fatalities occur.

GREEN CROSS FOR SAFETY ® **National Safety Council**

- SCHOOL BUILDINGS -- 20%
  - **1st** gym
  - **2nd** stairs and hallways
  - **3rd** shops and labs

- SCHOOL GROUNDS -- 17%
  - **1st** organized sports (the majority are from football)
  - **2nd** activities involving playground apparatus

- TRAVEL TO OR FROM SCHOOL -- 6%

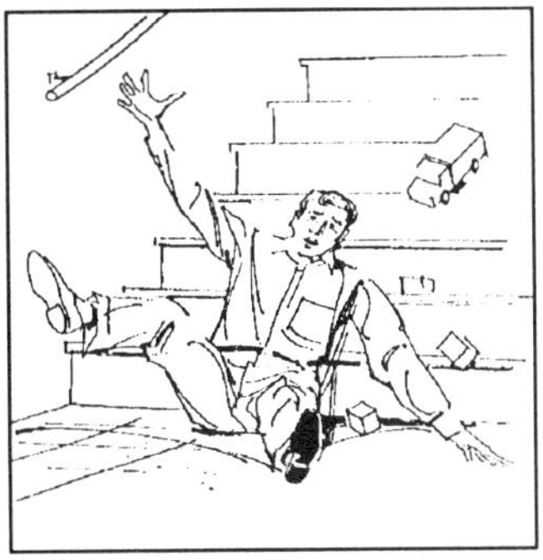

Accident statistics are not just numbers, each case involves human suffering. There are thousands of cuts, fractures, burns, poisonings, and even drownings that take place within the schools each year. Most of the accidents result only in minor injuries that can be taken care of by the teacher, but some are much more serious. There is the girl who falls on a sharp pencil and puts her eye out, the boy who sees his fingers in the sawdust beside the table saw in his shop class, and the boy who spends weeks in a coma and suffers brain damage when he is hit in the head by another student who threw the baseball bat. Then there is the girl who is pushed on a crowded stairway at school and suffers a crushed vertebrae. The pain does not stop after a few weeks in a body cast, it recurs periodically throughout her life. But she is lucky, the boy who broke his neck in a football accident remains a paraplegic for the rest of his life.

A part of the tragedy is that most of these accidents could have been prevented. Accidents are sometimes called "the forgotten epidemic" or "the neglected killer." In spite of the fact that accidents cost this country nearly 100 thousand lives and one billion dollars each year. A 1985 report showed that only two cents of every dollar spent for health problem research goes to accident research.

UNDERSTANDING ACCIDENTS

The fatalistic connotation often associated with the word accidents may be an obstacle to accident prevention efforts. What does the word *accident* mean? It obviously means different things to different people and at different times. It does not have a clear definition. The word *accident* stands for a makeshift or hodgepodge concept that is neither legally, medically, or statistical useful.

The various definitions of the word *accident* are in agreement on the first two points, but insofar as accident prevention is concerned,the third and fourth points are mutually exclusive.

1. Accidents are unintended and unplanned events.

2. Accidents usually have undesirable or unfortunate consequences.

3. Accidents occur by chance or coincidence. They are without cause.

4. Accidents are contingent upon predisposing events or conditions. They are preceded by unsafe acts, they are controllable.

The distinction between points (3) and (4) is central to the safety movement. Point (3), the historical and fatalistic concept of accidents, stands in the way of accident prevention. Point (4), the modern and positive approach, believes that accidents are usually proceeded by acts and/or conditions that cause the accident. The acts or conditions are variables that if altered could have prevented the accident.

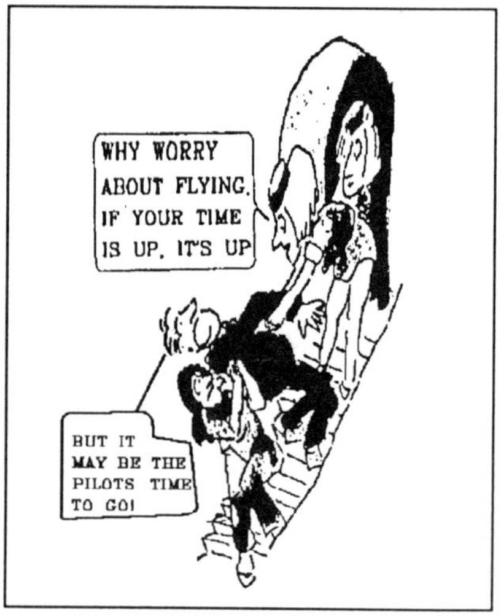
WHY WORRY ABOUT FLYING. IF YOUR TIME IS UP, IT'S UP
BUT IT MAY BE THE PILOTS TIME TO GO!

The word *accident*, as in point (3), is frequently attached to an unfortunate occurrence in order to remove blame and responsibility. All too frequently people say, "It could not be helped. It was an accident!" People are not apt to take steps to prevent accidents when they believe that accidents are:

- unforeseen
- uncontrollable
- inevitable

Some people believe that death or injury is due entirely to fate or some unseen power and that, "When your number is up -- it is up," or that, "If it is not your time to go, you won't go," and, "If it is your time to go, you can't change it." When people believe that they can't do anything to prevent an accident, they are not likely to try. This fatalistic approach may absolve some people of guilt, and that might be good; however, it often leads people to reckless behavior, and that is not good. While we must acknowledge that some conditions are outside of human control, insurance policies sometimes refer to them as *acts of God* or *freaks of nature*, we should not allow this to keep us from exercising the fundamental steps of safety.

<u>Accidents can be:</u>

- understood
- identified
- predicted
- controlled
- prevented

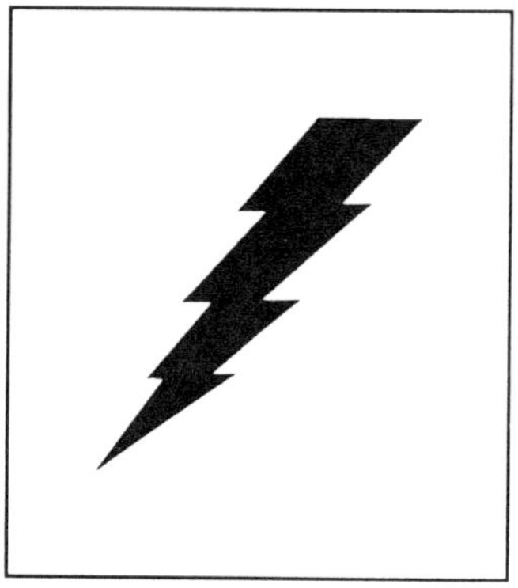

A key concept associated with accidents, as in point (4), is *foreseeability*. Events causing an accident are frequently unforeseen, but not unforeseeable. The modern scientific approach to accident prevention has helped us understand and avoid accidents today that once were considered unavoidable. If the causes of accidents can be identified, understood, and controlled, they can be predicted, and if they can be predicted they can be prevented.

REPORTS

A teacher must fill out and turn in an accident report form on any school-related accident which occurs within his jurisdiction. The analysis of data gathered from past accidents may help indicate steps that can be taken to eliminate or reduce further accidents. The accident report may become a legal document if legal action takes place regarding the accident. The report could contain objective statements about what was observed, but should not contain conclusions as to who was at fault. The report should be complete, correct, and accurate so that those who are responsible for making judgment can be fair.

- The accident report form may be needed for future reference. The data gathered from reports may be useful in developing preventive measures for the future. To prevent future accidents is the most important reason for filling out accident reports.

- Another reason for teachers to fill out accident reports is because it is a legal requirement. Failure to fill out the accident report form could cause legal trouble for the teacher.

- Because court action may follow an accident, the report is needed to make justice possible. The reports should be factual; hearsay discussions should be avoided.

ACCIDENT ANALYSIS

When filling out accident reports, familiarity with the following terms may be helpful. They may help you better understand the process of accident analysis.

Factor

An accident factor is *any condition accompanying an accident.* There are host factors or characteristics of the victim, agent factors or objects associated with the injury, and environmental factors or conditions and locations. Several factors may have contributed to an accident, but frequently only the final factor gets blamed.

Cause

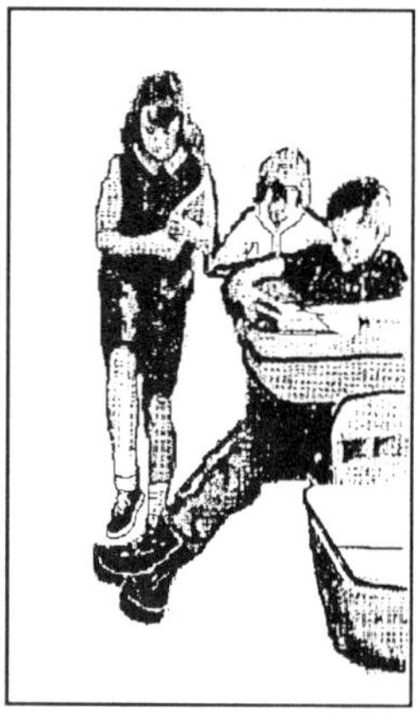

The cause is *any factors contributing to the accident.* All causes are factors, but not all factors are causes. The cause is probably a combination of factors, but the event immediately preceding an accident, the *final factor*, is often inappropriately labeled as the cause. The accident was probably a result of *multiple factors* and probably could have been avoided by removing any one of the factors. A person can probably keep several factors under control, but add the final factor and the situation gets out of control. Accident investigations attempt to look at all of the contributing factors. It is like a police investigation--they collect every detail they can about the crime and the crime scene, and some of them may turn out to be clues. Likewise, an accident report should contain all of the factors. Later analysis by the experts may determine which factors are causes.

Phases

There are three phases of an accident. The pre-event phase includes the factors which determine whether or not an accident will take place. The event phase involves the contact of the forces which cause the damage to people or property. The post-event phase involves the attempts to save or salvage the people or property after the damage has been done. The chart below gives some examples of possible causal factors and countermeasures.

PRE-EVENT	**EVENT**	**POST-EVENT**
	CAUSAL FACTORS	
habits	steering wheel	fire
fatigue	dashboard	delay
ignorance	window glass	improper first aid
inattention	swing seat	improper EMT care
alcohol and drugs	ground	second event
weather conditions	tree	explosion
mechanical defects	weapon	cold
	COUNTERMEASURES	
laws	safety belts	first aid training
enforcement	padded dashboard	ambulance service
inspections	safety locks	flares
education	engineering	flashers

ACCIDENT REPORTS

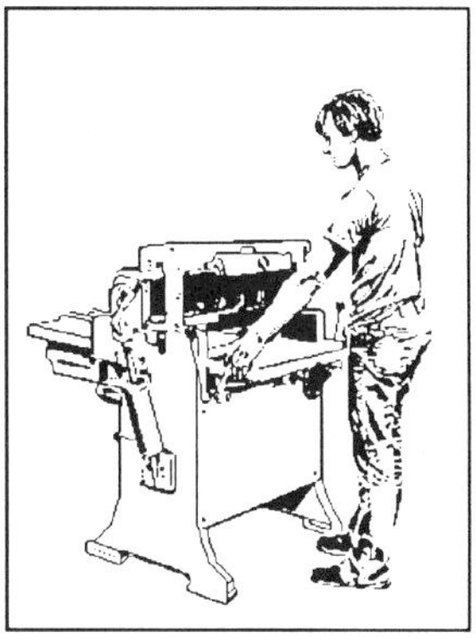

Accident reports should be made out as soon as possible after an accident has occurred. Copies of the reports should be retained in the instructor's file. Additional copies should be filed in appropriate administrative offices. In addition to the accident report form, a teacher would be wise to take detailed personal notes about the accident. These notes may prove very helpful in the event the teacher is called on to give testimony in court or for an insurance investigation.

A variety of accident report forms are available, each district may have their own; however, they should all contain the basic information. William A. Williams wrote an article, *Accident Prevention Manual for Shop Teachers*, published in Chicago in 1963 for the American Technical Society. It outlined the following information that should be found in an accident report.

- **What** was the nature of the accident? What were the circumstances leading up to the accident? What was the nature of the injury or damage? What were the persons involved doing? What unsafe act or acts were committed? What were the direct or indirect causes? What machine, tool, substance, or object was most closely connected with the accident? What corrective action is indicated?

- **Who** was injured or nearly injured? Who were the participants in the accident? Who committed the unsafe act? Who were the witnesses? Who administered first aid to the injured? Who completed the accident report?

- **Where** did the accident occur? Where was the instructor at the time of the accident? Where was the injured person with respect to the machine, tool, substance, object, or person most closely associated with the accident?

- **When** did the accident occur? When was the accident investigation made? When was the accident report completed?

- **Why** was the unsafe act or the hazardous condition permitted? Why did the person act unsafely? Why did the accident occur?

- **How** did the accident happen? How did the physical environment contribute to the accident? How can similar future accidents be prevented?

STUDENT INJURY REPORT FORM

1. Child's Name ________________ 2. [ ] Male [ ] Female 3. Grade _______

4. Parent's Name ________________ 5. Date of Birth ___/___/___

6. District ______________ # ___ 7. Date of Accident ___/___/___ 8. Fatal [ ]Yes

9. School ______________ # ___ 10. Time of Accident _________ [ ] am [ ] pm

11. Days Absent From School [ ] 1/2, [ ] 1, [ ] 1-1/2, [ ] 2, [ ] 2-1/2 [ ] More (Specify) ___

12. Action Taken BY SCHOOL (Check)
 a. [ ] First Aid Administered
 b. [ ] Parent or Guardian Notified
 c. [ ] Remained in or Returned to Class
 d. [ ] Sent Home [ ] Taken Home
 e. [ ] Checked by School Nurse
 f. [ ] Checked by Paramedics / EMTs
 g. [ ] Taken to Physician
 h. [ ] Taken to Hospital
 i. [ ] Other (specify) ______________________________

 Action taken BY PARENTS
 a. [ ] Parents deemed no medical action necessary
 b. [ ] Taken to Hospital or Emergency Care Facility. Diagnosis: ______________
 c. [ ] Other (specify) ______________________________

13. Hospitalized (Specify length of hospital stay.) ______________________

14. Restricted School Activity (Specify number of days) ______________________

15. **NATURE OF INJURY / SYMPTOM:** (Specify in descending order of severity.)
*Abrasion, Contusion, Burn, Concussion *, Laceration, Dislocation *, Fracture *, Loss of Consciousness, Nosebleed, No Pulse, Not Breathing, Pain/Tenderness, Puncture, Shortness of Breath, Sprain/Strain, Swelling/Inflammation, Other.*
*(* = Possible)*

16. **AREA AFFECTED:** (Specify area of body affected by corresponding injury/symptom.)
HEAD: Chin/Cheek, Eye, Ear, Forehead, Mouth/Lip/Tongue, Neck/Throat, Nose, Scalp/Skull, Tooth/Teeth.
TRUNK: Stomach, Back, Buttocks, Chest, Collarbone, Genitalia, Internal, Pelvis/Hips, Shoulder.
EXTREMITIES: Ankle, Arm, Elbow, Finger/Thumb, Foot, Hand/Wrist, Knee, Leg, Toe.

17. **CONTRIBUTING FACTORS:** (List factors that may have contributed to the injury.)
PERIOD: Before School, After School, Class, Assembly, Field Trip, Lunch, Recess, Athletic Competition, Other (specify).
LOCATION: Athletic Field, Gymnasiums, Playground, Swimming Pool, Shower/Dressing Rooms, Bus, Bus Loading Area, Parking Area, Highways, Auditorium, Lunchroom, Corridor, Stairs/Ramps, Lavatory, Classroom, Laboratory, Shops, Other (Specify).

18. **ACTIVITY:** (List activity during which injury occurred. Specify particular activity.)
Sports, Physical Education, Recreation, Classroom, Moving Equipment, Walking, Unauthorized, Other.

19. **EQUIPMENT:** (List equipment on which injury occurred.)______________
Was equipment being used? [ ]Yes [ ]No ______________
Was there any apparent malfunction? [ ]Yes [ ]No ______________
Did equipment appear to be used appropriately? [ ]Yes [ ]No ______________

20. **SURFACE:** (List surface on which injury occurred.) *Blacktop, Carpet, Concrete, Dirt, Gravel, Ice/Snow, Lawn/Grass, Mats, Stand, Synthetic (ie. tartin), Tile, Wood, Other (specify), Not Applicable.*

21. **DESCRIPTION:** (On the **BACK** of this form describe specifically how the accident happened.)

______________________ Title _________ ______________________
Signature of Person Making Report Principal's Signature

DISASTER EMERGENCIES

Over the last twenty years, there has been an average of 17 disasters per year that have necessitated a declaration of disaster by the President of the United States. In addition, there have also been many localized minor disasters that have resulted in numerous casualties. The schools of the nation have been involved in some of these, and any school may be on the brink of a disaster at any moment.

A disaster has been defined as a "great, sudden misfortune resulting in loss of life, serious injury, and property loss." In certain usage, the term refers to a sudden occurrence which kills 25 or more persons. Yet if it kills or injures but one person, it is still a misfortune.

Considering that most (perhaps as high as 90%) of all deaths due to major disasters could have been prevented through proper preparation, the value of disaster training becomes evident. No school health emergency program would be complete without attention to disasters. Wisdom dictates preparation for such emergencies as fires, floods, earthquakes, riots, etc. Experience indicates that the program should be organized to do the following:

- Prevent the occurrence of the disaster whenever possible.
- Minimize the number of casualties.
- Provide emergency rescue and first aid for the injured.
- Evacuate the injured to medical installations.
- Provide for emergency communication procedures.
- Provide for transportation, housing, and necessary care.
- Provide for the reconstruction of the lives of all involved.

If the school emergency program is part of the community civil defense program, the school should rehearse its procedures as part of the community rehearsal. Otherwise, on its own initiative, the school should go through simulated emergen-cies. Fire extinguisher and alarm systems are vital and should be maintained according to state and federal specifications. Even for minor disasters, the schools should have the things on the next page:

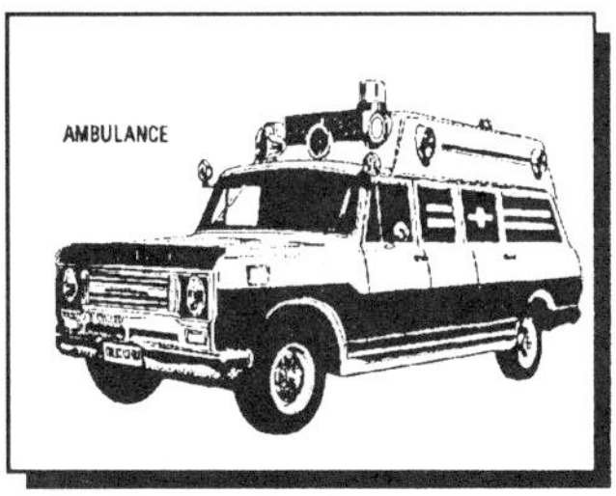

- Emergency rest rooms, one for boys and one for girls. Each should have at least two cots, adequate blankets, chairs, tables, wash basin, and other supplies.

- First aid supplies including splints, slings, etc.

- Emergency telephone numbers posted on all phones.

- Telephone numbers on file for the parents and physician of each student.

The hope for minimizing the effect of a disaster depends on the nature of its destructive force and its potential for predictability. Disaster agents vary in terms of their predictability. Probabilities can be calculated and plans made accordingly. For example, some areas of the country are more prone toward flooding; others, tornados; and others, earthquakes. The destructive forces may be ice, wind, rain, earth movement, flame, smoke, etc. Speed of onset, duration of impact, scope of impact, and intensity of impact are other variables. The damage may depend on the concentration of people in the area during a certain period of time.

A disaster may be divided into several phases and preparations made accordingly. These phases are as follows:

1. The pre-disaster phase is the normal everyday situation in the community. This is the time to make the preparations. What happens after this point depends very much on what happens during this phase.

2. The pre-impact phase begins with the earliest signs of possible danger. The duration of this phase varies greatly, but there may be time to put a warning system into operation.

3. The impact phase is the period when the disaster actually strikes.

4. The emergency phase is the period of response to the immediate demands presented by the disaster agent.

5. The recovery phase involves attempts to mitigate the long-term effects of the disaster agent and to return the situation to normal conditions.

Any school administrator who fails to be cognizant of the importance of school emergency health services is ignoring the very lives of those persons over whom he is directly responsible. He must be constantly aware of the possibility of medical emergencies.

POLICIES AND EMERGENCY PROCEDURES

Each school district should have a manual of policies and procedures for emergency situations including accidents and disasters. No school is immune from such emergencies. Basic emergency policies give direction to efforts designed to protect the students and school staff during an emergency. The written policies, if followed, also help protect the school personnel in case any legal action takes place following the emergency. If there are no written policies, the teacher's only recourse for action during an emergency is to do what appears to be common sense. The problem with common sense is that what appears to be common sense for one teacher may come in conflict with what appears to be common sense to the teacher in the next classroom. It is best to have a written plan that coordinates everyone's actions and provides management for the emergency.

The policies must be prepared in conjunction with other agencies in the community that may also be involved in the emergency. Such policies should be developed through cooperative efforts of teachers, physicians, nurses, and parents and should be clearly understood by all. The policies grow out of experience and are guided by the judgment of experts. Emergency policies should outline clearly the specific duties and activities for administrators, teachers, and other school personnel in conjunction with community resources. A committee may be assigned to write the policies, but ultimately they must be approved by the school administrator and the school board. These policies should concur with all the state laws and the regulations of education. Areas covered by school health policies include the following:

- A plan for training school personnel for emergencies.
- Adequate preventive measures.
- Effective health services to deal with emergencies.
- Procedures for communication with community resources.
- Responsibility and procedure for notifying parents.
- Procedure for taking children home or to a place of safety.
- A plan to instruct school personnel on giving first aid.
- The line of responsibility for various school personnel.

Safety and emergency care fits into all three areas of the school health program. Matters pertaining to safety generally fit into the environmental area. Safety education is a part of the health education class and is also a responsibility of all teachers, particularly those in physical education and the various laboratories. First aid and emergency care are a part of the health services area of the school health program. In order for proper care to be given to students requiring immediate medical attention, a school must be prepared for such a situation. The following is a general school procedure that can be followed:

1. Administer first aid to the injured and/or call for designated Emergency Medical Services (EMS).

2. Notify the principal and the school nurse who will contact the parents and make arrangements for additional care.

3. Contact the parent if the illness or injury is serious enough to require medical attention. Do not hesitate to secure medical care if parents cannot be reached, but make it clear that the school assumes no responsibility for the payment for services.

4. If a sick or injured child needs to go home, keep the child at school until a parent or relative can provide transportation home. If the child remains in school after an accident or emergency care, the student should be supervised and observed for any complications or indications of medical difficulties.

5. Prepare an accident report form and make as many copies as may be required locally, ie., the principal, the superintendent's office, the insurance company. The report should be completed as soon as possible following the emergency.

Follow local policies that may supersede or supplement these recommendations. If a written policy is not available, it is well to consider these steps:

- Every teacher should prepare a plan in writing, as well as possible, of what he or she would do in case of fire, explosion, riot, or natural disaster.

- Teachers should know where the first aid or emergency cabinets are in the school.

- In case of fire or fire drills, the teachers should always call the roll after the students are out of the building.

FIRST AID TRAINING

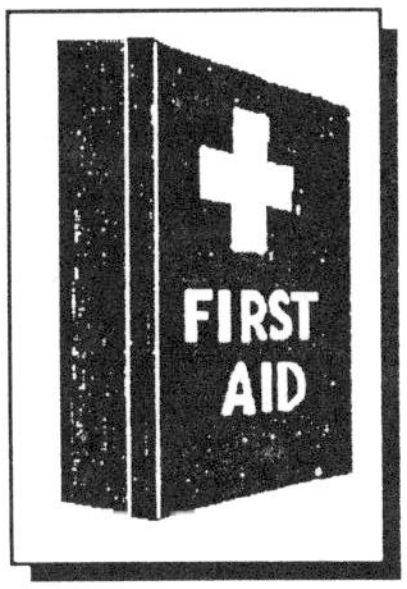

All too often, because they haven't had first aid training, when teachers are faced with emergency situations, they have to rely on common sense or hearsay. In extreme cases, teachers performing emergency care become so ill at ease themselves that they perform in an irrational manner and an injured student is injured further. Adequate first aid training would help avoid this problem. Knowledge and skills in performing first aid are tremendous sources of confidence when giving emergency care.

It is widely accepted that all school personnel should be trained in first aid. The Council of Chief State Officers and the Association of State and Territorial Health Officers strongly urge that teacher preparation institutions supply their students with adequate first aid training. Mayshark and Shaw in their book *Administration of School Health Programs* state that one responsibility of school administrators is to insure that all school employees receive some training in first aid and emergency care. The National Committee on School Health Policies of the National Education Association and American Medical Association suggest that everyone on a school staff be able to administer first aid. Training all school personnel in basic first aid principles is very important. Periodic inservice reviews and updating of emergency care practices are also important.

EMERGENCY SUPPLIES AND FACILITIES

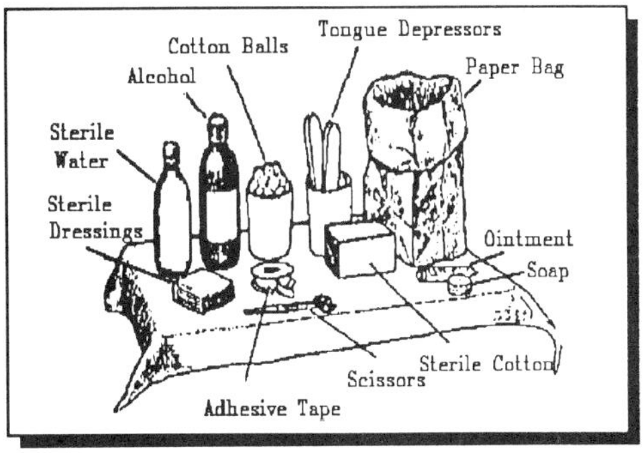

If a school is to have an effective emergency care program, it must have supplies and a location for handling emergency situations. In a recent survey, it was found that the degree of preparedness of supplies varied from nothing more than band-aids to well stocked. The survey further stated that the location of these supplies varied from the office to health rooms, clinics, and the nurse's room. One room should be selected and held in readiness for emergency situations. It may be best located near the physical education area due to the fact that many school accidents occur there.

In order for this room to fit the needs of the students, it should be well-stocked and inventoried. Let one competent person, well-trained in first aid, take control of that room and the supplies to be used for first aid measures. When the responsibility rests upon a single individual, there is no "passing the buck." A responsible person, with sufficient supplies, will greatly update a first aid program in any school. The phone numbers of the list of persons and services on the following page should be posted conspicuously near each school telephone:

- school physician
- substitute physician
- school nurse
- local health department
- local police station
- local fire station
- local ambulance service
- local hospital
- poison control center

A PLAN FOR ACTION

The ability to handle an emergency situation is increased when the situation has been considered beforehand. On the other hand, students may be adversely affected by poor planning. Consider the tragic example in Collinwood, Ohio where 176 lives were lost. Due to lack of proper evacuation planning, the students panicked and jammed against a locked exit door. Bodies were found piled 12 feet high against the door.

Each school should have prepared written plans regarding emergency care. Plans can't cover every contingency, but in an emergency, everyone is better off with one than without one. The difference may be comparable to "sand lot football" where they make up the plays as they go and argue about who is going to call the plays, and a well-trained team with a well-developed game plan. Allowances for variables and options are built into the plan. The plans for school emergencies should include instructions for contacting parents, arranging transportation, reporting first aid procedures, and evacuations. Each plan will differ according to local applications. It is imperative, however, that each school is prepared for emergencies, that the personnel review procedures often and, where possible, that procedures and practices be rehearsed in order to assure proficient handling of emergency situations.

RECORDS

An integral part of preparing for emergency care for students is the accumulation of records. These records understandably should contain the name of parents and how to get in touch with them in case of emergency. The nearest relative and neighbor should also be listed in the event the parents cannot be located. Some schools have signed permission slips on file for each student so that in an emergency situation medical care will not be delayed. Other schools believe the slips are unnecessary because in their role *in loco parentis* they already have the authority to authorize medical care.

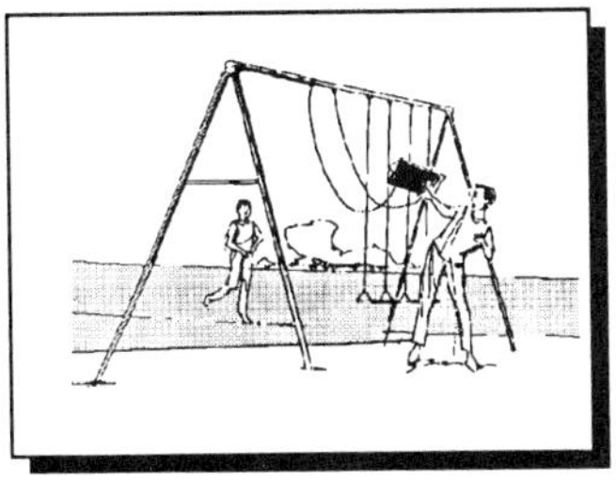

In addition to a health history of each student, the student's file should contain information on how to contact the student's parents or guardian and the names of the student's physician, dentist, and hospital. The student's history will aid in better emergency procedures and will protect a student from further injuries due to medical conditions not immediately visible to the first aid provider. To be of utmost usefulness, the record should be up to date, contain objective, not subjective data, and be used only by those with proper authority.

ORGANIZATION FOR SAFETY

Safety means freedom from accidents. Safety first means be safe before you proceed. That is virtually impossible if there is to be advancement and adventure in living.

With the American student spending such a great amount of time in school, it is important that the school environment be a safe place, free from accidents. With the increase of practical trades and in-school training going on in secondary education, safety becomes even more of a must. It seems only practical then, that every semester of school brings new students. It is a definite must that teachers repeat the rules of the class. This may seem repetitious to the teacher, but to the students, it will be new information that will protect them. It is when teachers fail to make clear their class rules for safety that they are held liable. This is extremely important in classes such as physical education, home economics, auto mechanics, arts and crafts, woodwork, chemistry and physics laboratories, and set construction projects for school plays, etc. where machinery is being used frequently.

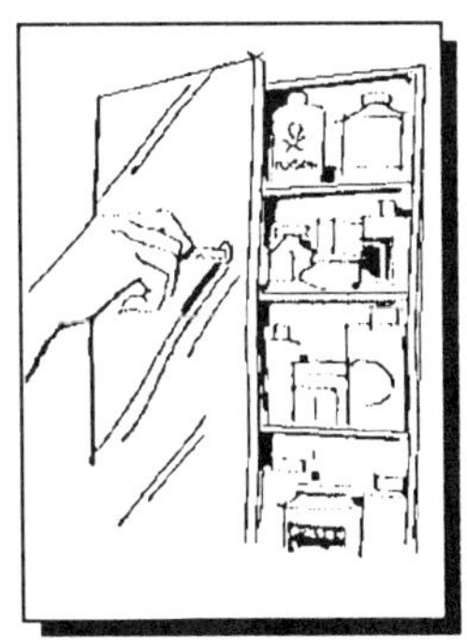

An excellent motto for classes of this sort is, "A place for everything and everything in its place." This should include students being in the proper place at the proper time. When this motto is enforced, it seems as if the first step in safety has been taken already.

Students often try to impress their peers by trying to show off, showing how close they can come to danger without actually getting hurt. This game might be thrilling or cute for the student, but more important, it is a hazard to him and those around him. This is one more reason why teacher supervision is so important. Accidents only take one second to occur!

SAFETY EDUCATION

There are a number of ways of teaching safety, and perhaps all have their place. It is generally preferable to teach safety in a positive manner rather than using "fear tactics." It is better to explain the "why" instead of just learning a list of "do's" and "don'ts." Rules are harder to remember than practical reasoning. The best time and place to teach safety is when and where it relates directly to its application in the regular class activities, when it is practical rather than theoretical. Physical education classes, shop classes, laboratories, and driver education programs are natural places to emphasize safety education.

Individual teachers can stress safety by including it in lectures where it could feasibly be brought up. The topic could then be discussed as long as students ask questions and seem interested. Lecturing may not be an effective way of teaching safety. Visual aids, demonstrations, guest experts, and role-playing activities are interesting ways of presenting safety topics. The goal is to get the students interested and involved.

The whole school can get involved in safety education campaigns. For example, the school could have a safety fair. As students become involved with the fair, their knowledge will grow in a fun way. Fairs are fun and will leave a positive tone on accident prevention. A number of activators that will get students thinking about safety include fire drills, earthquake drills, riot and bomb drills, the use of fire detection units, anti-drunk driving campaigns, safe driving programs, and first aid instruction.

Safety involves the steps taken prior to an event to keep the accident from happening. Education and motivation are the main points here. Most accidents are due to carelessness and ignorance of impending dangers. The responsibilities of those caring for children and youth must be stressed. The development of skills prior to engaging in hazardous sports is important. Steps must be taken to check equipment to see that it is functional and to control the situation to see that it is safe. Rules and regulations must be followed. Some safety points to consider are:

- Automobile safety. Encourage driver education programs, vehicle safety inspections, and street enforcement of traffic regulations. Don't overload vehicles, use safety restraints, and be courteous.

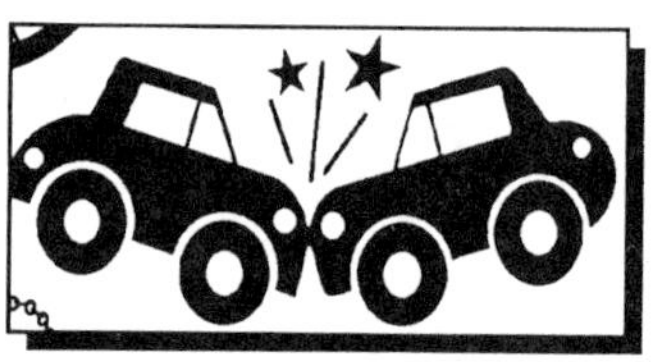

- Pedestrian and bicycle safety. Encourage the observance of safety regulators. Use clothing, lights, and reflectors that are highly visible.

- **Fire safety**. Avoid contact with open flame, hot surfaces, hot liquids, or chemicals. Use proper care with flammable substances and explosives. Avoid using improperly ventilated heaters. Avoid overexposure to the sun.

- **Water safety**. Provide proper supervision, particularly for small children. Provide swimming and water safety instruction. Place hazardous areas out of bounds--fence it off if possible. When swimming, have lifeguards and employ the buddy system. Do not dive into unknown areas. Make sure boats and equipment are safe. Follow the safety rules and provide instruction in effective artificial respiration.

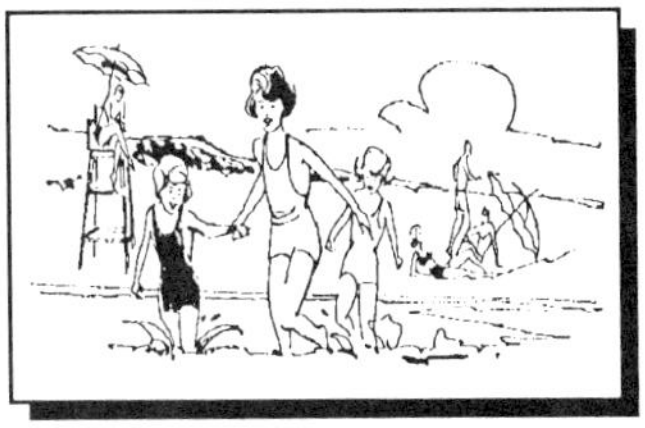

- **Poison safety**. Keep all potential poisons (medicines, paints, cleaning agents, insecticides, and petroleum products) out of the reach of children. Safely discard old unused medicines. Don't put hazardous substances in unmarked or improperly marked containers. Post the telephone number of the poison control center or hospital emergency room and keep a supply of syrup of ipecac available to use according to the directions of the emergency personnel.

- **Home and farm safety**. Prevent children from becoming trapped and suffocating in an unused refrigerator--take off the door. Keep plastic bags, etc. away from children. Don't let children play in areas where there might be a cave-in. Store and use all firearms, sharp tools, and knives properly. Dispose of broken glass and other dangerous rubble safely. See that machinery and farm animals are handled only by people who are properly trained and competent. Don't wear loose-fitting clothing that may get caught when working around machinery.

UNDERSTANDING RISK-TAKING BEHAVIOR

Some good programs related to risk-taking behavior have been developed recently. They help students understand the motivation for risk-taking behavior. There are risks involved in many activities, but the degree of risk depends on the skills and experience of the participants and environmental conditions. In risk-taking behaviors, there are both desirable and undesirable consequences. A person risks something to be gained against something to be lost. For example, a person may drives excessively fast to save some time, but he or she also increases the risk of suffering some delays due to an accident or being stopped for a speeding ticket. A person may engage in some "showing off" behavior to impress others, but if something goes wrong the person looks bad and is embarrassed.

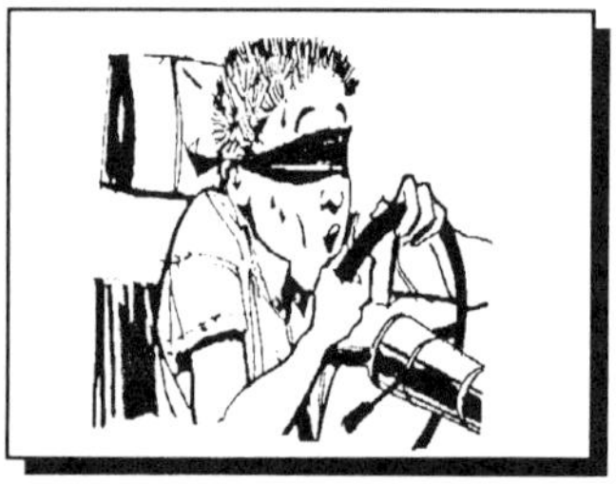

There are three elements that lead up to risk-taking behavior, 1) the hazards or inherent danger in the activity, 2) the perception of the danger, and 3) the decision to enter or refuse to enter the behavior. The key is the perception of the danger. Sometimes people are fully aware of the hazards when they decide to enter or not to enter the behavior. Sometimes they are only partially aware of the hazards, and sometimes people base their decision on ignorance. Many sports and recreational activities such as skydiving, sailplaning, skiing, motorcycling, and others are known for their risks. People have the right to choose to or not to participate in these activities, but before they make their choice they should be aware of the hazards involved and prepared to take steps to minimize the risks. Sometimes they enter risk-taking behavior without even thinking, sometimes they believe no hazards exist, and sometimes they believe they are invulnerable, indestructible, and invincible.

Safety education should help young people become prepared to evaluate the odds associated with the activities they consider. Safety should not keep people from having fun, but it should help keep them alive and healthy in order to have more fun. This may mean eliminating, reducing, or modifying some high-risk activities in order to increase the opportunity for enjoying other less risky activities.

SAFETY PROGRAMS

Safety programs are an important rebuttal to accidents. Every school should have some type of accident prevention program. Following are steps in organizing such a plan:

- Develop a policy of safety education
- Assign responsibility
- Promote faculty cooperation
- Determine nature and scope of program
- Develop program objectives
- Select course content and teaching methods
- Coordinate community safety efforts
- Evaluate
- Adjust program

The local board of health has the authority and responsibility by law to see that conditions within the school are safe and sanitary. If necessary, they have the authority to correct conditions and to bill the school for the expenses involved. Most cities or counties have a safety office. Sometimes it is in connection with the civil defense department. On a state and federal level, the Occupation Safety and Health Administration (OSHA) enforces certain safety codes. The National Safety Council provides information and encouragement along safety lines.

A number of student organizations can be established to help promote safety at school. Often students will respond better to programs initiated by fellow students than by school administration. The following are some examples:

School safety council. This is a council organized under effective faculty supervision to help in accident prevention and in social experience.

School safety patrol. This is a patrol that is designed to instruct, direct, and control the members of the student body and to assist teachers and parents in the instruction of school children in safe practices. They can direct student traffic, but not vehicles at crosswalks.

Fire patrol. This is a patrol inspection of buildings for fire hazards; the patrol should also periodically check emergency exits and fire escapes as well as be familiar with the use of fire-fighting equipment. The patrol should also direct regular fire drills.

Building and grounds patrol. This is a patrol to prevent disorders and accidents on the school premises, help crippled pupils, and greet and guide visitors.

CONCLUSION

The primary purpose of this chapter has been to alert prospective teachers to the need for safety measures in the classroom. When a school is free of accidents, it is no accident; it is the result of a good safety program. It may be difficult to give enough credit to good safety programs, because it is difficult to count the accidents that do not happen.

STUDY HELPS

1. Review the accident statistics to get a picture of the significance of accidents in this country generally and in the schools and among the school age population more specifically. Summarize your conclusions with a few comprehensive statements.

2. Explain why the common use of the word accident is often an obstacle to accident prevention efforts.

3. Wherein do the various definitions of the word accident agree and disagree?

4. Why does the definition of the word *accident* make a difference in safety and accident prevention programs?

5. What should be and should not be included in an accident report? Why?

6. In addition to the formal accident report, why is it important for a teacher to maintain personal notes about school accidents he or she has observed?

7. Define and give examples of the terms associated with accident analysis:

Factor	Cause	Final Factor	Multiple Factors
Phases	Pre-Event	Event	Post-Event

8. Why should schools have printed and approved policies and procedures for disasters and major emergencies?

9. What areas or types of problems should school emergency procedures attempt to cover with contingency plans?

10. What equipment, facilities, and supplies should be available within the school or immediately accessible to the school in case of an injury or disaster?

11. Why should schools require emergency preparedness training for all school personnel and what topics should be covered in such training?

12. Why do efforts to become organized for emergencies often result in a reduced need for such organization?

13. What are the main guiding principles relating to safety education in the secondary schools?

14. What are the three E's of safety and how are they implemented in the school setting?

Chapter 18

FIRST AID

This part of the unit is not last because it is least important. To the contrary, it is last because it is very important and should be remembered. It could become the most important lessons in the book. Prospective teachers frequently express a lack of confidence in their ability to handle a first aid emergency. Since the lack of confidence often stems from concern for the unknown, the information in this chapter may be of much help. Study it thoroughly.

FIRST AID AND EMERGENCY CARE

In order to carry out the health-related responsibilities of the teaching profession, it is essential that teachers have a knowledge of correct first aid procedures. Even in a setting as safe as the public schools, injuries and illnesses occasionally arise requiring the application of correct first aid. All teachers should be prepared so that when emergencies arise they will feel confident in dealing with the situation.

C.L. Anderson in his book, *School Health Practices*, gives the following justifications for attaining this knowledge:

> ***In an imperfect world of imperfect people, accidents will occur and emergencies will arise that require people skilled in first aid . . . Even in the best administered school with well-organized and well-functioning safety programs, serious accidents occur. All teachers should be prepared in first aid procedures so that when the emergency arises, they will be equal to the occasion and confident in their ability to deal with the situation.***

First aid has been defined as the immediate and temporary care given at the scene of an accident or sudden illness before the services of a physician can be obtained. For years, the American Red Cross was the premiere organization for teaching first aid, and they offer a variety of courses to the public free of charge. Today a number of organizations including the National Safety Council are teaching courses with such titles as First Aid, First Responder, and Emergency Care. Such courses vary in length from a few hours of basics to a few weeks of in-depth study. Although this lesson contains more than the basics, it does not provide the practical, hands-on experience. It is strongly advised that anyone wanting to learn first aid combine both the knowledge, such as provided here, and the skills which must be obtained as one practices under the watchful eye of a trained instructor.

SCHOOL FIRST AID POLICIES

Each local school district should make specific written policies for dealing with medical emergencies. Each teacher should be aware of and adhere to the policies in his or her district. Whatever first aid and emergency care knowledge a teacher has, including the information found here, it should be adjusted to comply with the policies of the local school district. The policies vary from district to district; for example, some districts require all teachers to have a current American Red Cross standard first aid certificate and to apply the knowledge and skills gained in that training as needed. On the other extreme, a few districts may still have a policy that teachers are to give *no* emergency medical care, but are to initiate procedures for securing the services of the local Emergency Medical Service (EMS) unit. The policies of most school districts fall somewhere between these two examples.

Local school policies should designate who is to give first aid under what circumstances. The policies may separate first aid into two major classifications:

I. Immediate Life Threatening Emergencies

II. Routine First Aid Procedures

Immediate life threatening emergencies are those situations which require immediate action if a life is to be saved, for there may not be enough time to wait for a designated first aid provider or the paramedics to arrive. Routine first aid are those situations where time is not that critical, and where the main thing to do is not let the situation get worse until trained emergency care providers arrive.

Some schools districts want *every teacher* to be a trained first aid provider. Other schools have at least one *designated first aid provider* on campus who is called to provide first aid. And the policy of some schools is to call the *emergency medical technicians* (EMTs) or paramedics immediately in all situations requiring first aid or emergency care. The designated first aid provider might be a health teacher or the physical education teacher, because they are most likely to have had first aid training. It could be a school nurse if the nurse is on campus. School policies should also designate procedures for calling for help. For example, should the teacher who witnesses an accident call for the ambulance directly or is the call routed through the principal's office? Some communities have the designated emergency *911* telephone number. A procedure for notifying an injured child's parents or guardian should also be a part of the school policy.

Commonly, the teacher will follow the sequence represented by the letters A B C P S S. This means they act swiftly in dealing with the four immediate life threatening conditions, treat for shock, stabilize the individual, and call for help.

A An obstructed Airway.

B No Breathing.

C Impaired Circulation due to severe bleeding.

P Poisoning.

S Shock Control.

S Stabilize the injured persons , don't move them.

Call for Help.

They act immediately in life threatening emergencies such as airway obstruction, stoppage of breathing, severe bleeding, and poisoning. For people who are trained to give CPR (cardiopulmonary resuscitation), the letter C also stands for no circulation due to heart failure. They also act to control shock and prevent further injuries--do not move the person, do not give medications, do not do anything that would increase the injury. They call for appropriate personnel to provide first aid and emergency care and notify school authorities and the injured child's parents.

Teachers should follow the school's emergency policies. Teachers may be found liable for negligence if they fail to give reasonable first aid care or if their care extends beyond recognized first aid.

GENERAL DIRECTIONS

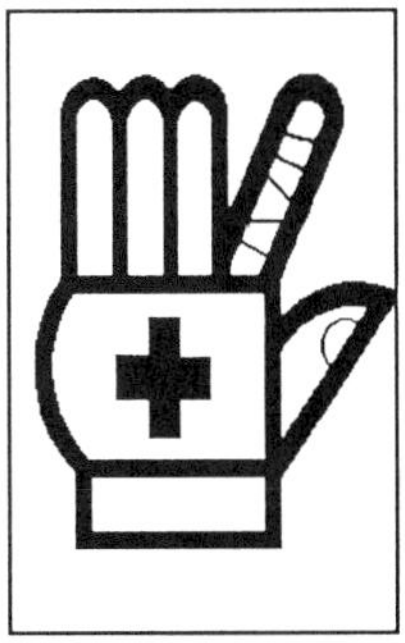

General directions are those things one should generally, but not always, do at a scene of an accident or sudden illness. One of the first general directions is to keep calm. Walk, not run. Speak, not shout. Calmness instills confidence. Talk in reassuring terms to the person who is injured or who has suddenly become ill and those around the scene. A general directive is, take command of the situation if you are the best prepared first aid provider present. Don't let some other well-meaning but incompetent person do the wrong thing; you take charge. Another general direction is to follow a plan based on priorities. An important general rule is, do not move the injured person until you are sure that moving will not make the situation worse. Also tell the injured person not to move.

ASSESSMENT

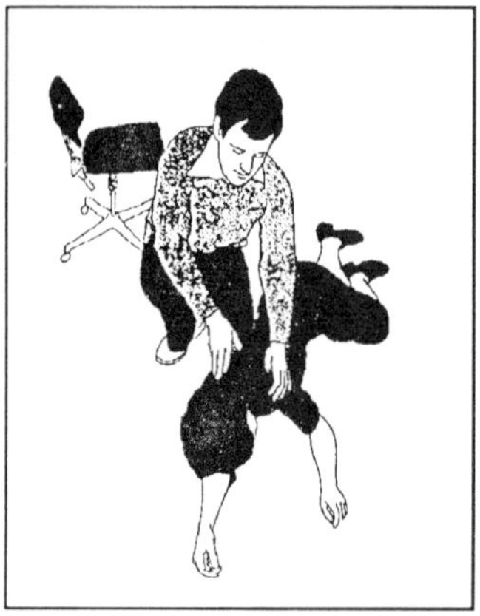

Before first aid is given, an assessment must take place. The purpose of the assessment is to determine priorities. An assessment may take a few seconds or a few minutes. Assessment is used when you first come on the scene and do not know many of the details about the problem. It starts with priority cases and will not be completed until the whole body has been checked, head to toe, and you are aware of all of the problems you can detect. The assessment involves most of the senses. It starts with what was said by those who called for help and what you hear from bystanders. It includes what you see as you approach the scene of the accident and what you see as you make the initial check of the injured person. During the assessment, you may feel parts of the body for indications of injury. Sometimes you may smell strange odors that may help indicate the nature of the problem or complications. Typically, the assessment is conducted in the position in which the person was found, usually lying down. If the person is up and moving about, ask them to lie down. Ask them to lie still until you have completed the assessment.

The first thing to check is breathing, and the easiest way to check breathing is to get the person to speak to you. So introduce yourself and ask a question. Say, "I'm Miss Smith, a teacher here at the school. I'm here to help you. What is your name? What seems to be your main problem?" If the person can speak, he or she is breathing. If the person does not speak, check for breathing (see BREATHING for details). If there is no breathing, you have found your first priority. Stop the assessment and deal with the breathing problem.

Next, check for serious bleeding. You are not worried at this point about minor bleeding, but a major hemorrhage. If a glance over the body reveals a serious bleeding problem, you have found another priority. Interrupt the assessment, and take care of the hemorrhage (see BLEEDING for details). Resume the assessment as soon as the hemorrhage is under control. As you continue the head-to-toe assessment, continue to look for bleeding. You may feel clothing that is wet from blood. If it is bleeding very freely, stop and control it; if it is not that serious, continue the survey and come back to deal with the wound when the assessment is completed.

Tell the person not to move until you have completed the assessment. Look and feel about the face, head, and neck for wounds, deformity, and discoloration. If the person is conscious, ask if he or she can feel any pain or numbness where you touch. Gently part the hair to look for scalp wounds. Do not move the head to look under it, look under the person only after you are assured there is no neck or spinal injury. Look at the eyes for unequal pupils or any other unusual signs. Look at and in the mouth for any injuries or foreign material. If you discover any evidence of poisoning (see POISONING for details), you have found another priority, stop and deal with it as circumstances indicate.

As the assessment continues, keep talking to the person and continue to ask if there is any pain or numbness as you touch their body. Feel the jaw, neck, shoulders, and arms. Press just hard enough so that if there was an injury the person would feel some pain. Also watch their eyes to see if they wince at your touch. As you get to their hands, ask them to squeeze your hand. If they can't, there may be spinal damage. Feel the ribs, abdominal area, hips, legs, and feet. As you get to the feet, ask the person to push his toes against your hand held at the sole of the foot. Again this is a check for spinal injuries. If you are sure there are no spinal injuries, you may roll the person onto his or her side so you can check for wounds to the back.

This completes the survey, and it is now time to take care of any injuries you have discovered. It is also time to take additional steps to control shock, (see SHOCK for details). The sequence of the assessment can be varied based on the circumstances. Its purpose is to detect any problems, particularly the priority problems. It is important to detect possible problems so that nothing is done to complicate them. Assessment is a part of first aid that is often overlooked, and this could be a basis of negligence in a liability case.

IMMEDIATE LIFE-THREATENING EMERGENCIES

The three crisis cases include emergencies involving stoppage of breathing (including heart stoppage), profuse bleeding, and poisoning. Immediate and urgent first aid is necessary in these situations; if the person does not receive immediate help, he or she could die. There is not time to wait for help to arrive. A teacher is not faced with these situations very often, but if and when they do occur, the teacher must act immediately, decisively, and more often than not, by himself. Being careful, remaining calm, and having confidence are important. In the majority of other injuries or illnesses, the primary responsibilities of the teacher are to obtain competent help, be sure further injury does not befall the person, and provide reassurance.

BREATHING

The body needs a continuous supply of oxygen to support life processes. If the brain does not receive oxygen for four to six minutes, irreversible brain damage and death will result. The air we normally breathe contains about 20 percent oxygen as we inhale. The air we exhale contains about 16 percent oxygen, so about 4 percent of the oxygen we breathe in goes from the air sacks in the lungs into the blood stream to be circulated to the body, including the brain. A number of things can interfere with this process.

Airway Obstruction

An airway obstruction is some type of blockage of the air passages into the lungs. The air passage may be blocked by either an anatomical obstruction or by a foreign object. There are two types of anatomical obstructions, the tongue or anaphylactic shock.

Anatomical obstruction. An anatomical obstruction is where parts of the person's own body blocks the airway. When the person is in a coma or heavily sedated by drugs and is lying on his or her back, the muscles that hold the jaw and tongue forward become so relaxed that the tongue drops back into the throat and blocks the airway. This problem can be solved simply by tilting up on the lower jaw or by turning the person on his or her side. The tongue attached to the lower jaw moves out of the air passage as the jaw is tilted. Turning a person on his or her side allows gravity to move the tongue out of the air passage. Either way may work; the person will gasp for air and soon return to normal breathing. Another type of anatomical obstruction occurs when people have a severe allergic reaction to a certain foreign substance, such as the venom from a honey bee sting. The reaction called *anaphylactic shock* causes the swelling of the linings of the air passages so that air can't get into the lungs. Death is sure if the person does not get some type of antihistamine to reduce the swelling. Except for securing immediate emergency care, there is little other first aid for this type of airway obstruction. Those with known allergic reactions should carry appropriate medication whenever they go on trips out of urban areas. In a city area, they can get to a hospital for treatment in time.

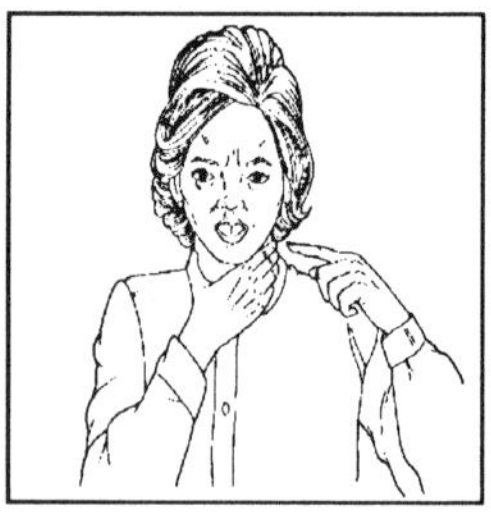

Foreign body obstruction. Another form of airway obstruction is foreign body obstruction. Among adults, this usually occurs when they are eating and try to swallow a hunk of food which gets caught in the throat. For children, the object could be any small object they could pick up and put into their mouth. With partial obstruction, the person can still cough and speak. This requires no first aid measure; they will soon recover on their own. With complete obstruction, they will be unable to speak or make any sounds.

They may give the universal sign of choking which is clasping one hand about the throat. The first aid provider should ask, "Can you speak?" If there is a negative response, the first aid provider should give first aid for choking.

First aid for choking. First aid for choking for a *conscious* adult is to give the Heimlich maneuver (abdominal thrust):

1. Stand, sit, or kneel behind the choking person with both arms around his or her waist.

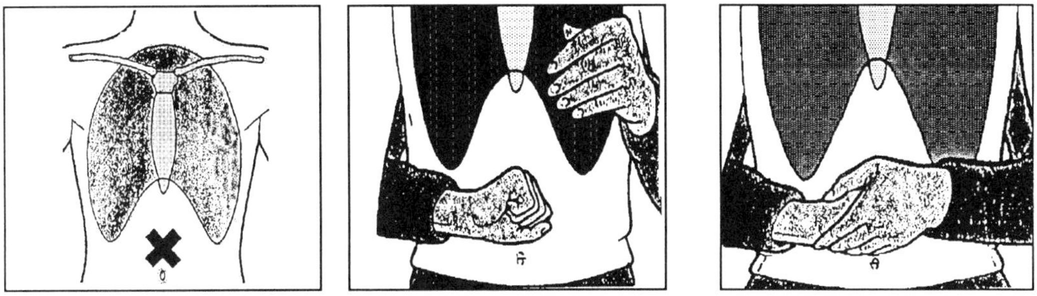

2. Make a fist with one hand and place the flat part of the thumb side of the fist against the abdomen. Find the thrust point halfway between the navel and the lower end of the sternum.

3. Grasp your fist with the other hand and press your fist into the choking person's abdomen with a quick, hard, upward thrust. This will compress the residual air in the lungs and will usually pop out the obstruction.

4. Repeat this abdominal thrust until the obstruction is expelled sufficient for breathing to resume.

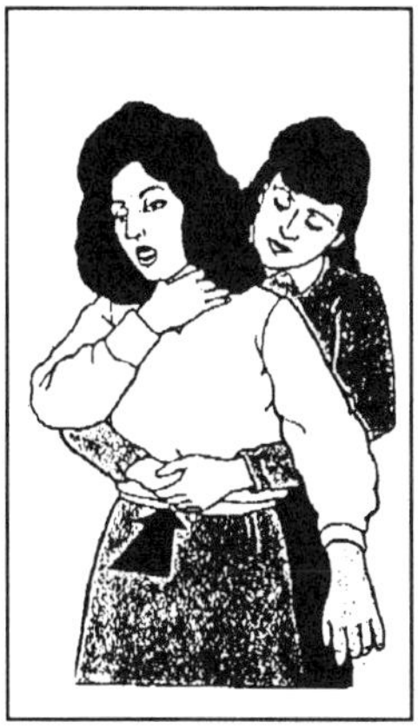

The Heimlich maneuver for an *unconscious* adult consists of the following:

1. Place the person on his or her back, kneel beside or straddle the person at the thighs facing the person.

2. Rest your fingers on the lower edge of the person's rib cage with the heel of your hand on the thrust point of the abdomen, halfway between the navel and the lower end of the sternum.

3. Place your other hand over the first hand and give a quick, hard, inward and upward thrust.

4. Repeat this abdominal thrust until the obstruction is expelled sufficient for breathing to resume.

Choking persons can perform the Heimlich maneuver on *themselves* by leaning over the back of a chair and directing a fall so that the back of the chair pushes into the abdomen at the thrust point. To perform the Heimlich maneuver on a *child*, place the child on his or her back as in the unconscious position and place the fingers on one hand on the thrust point of the abdomen and give a thrust. The pressure applied for an infant should be considerably less than that for an adult. For an *infant*, use only a couple fingers. For a person who is *pregnant or decidedly obese*, you will be unable to use the thrust point. Instead, if the person is conscious, clasp your hands around the lower part of the rib cage and squeeze suddenly or if unconscious place the flat of the hands over the lower part of the rib cage and push suddenly. Even if the Heimlich maneuver is completely successful in restoring breathing, the person should see a physician right away.

Pulmonary Resuscitation

As you approach a person who appears to be unconscious, the first thing you do is speak to them to see if they will respond. If there is no response, speak louder and touch or shake them. If there is still no response, check if they are breathing by placing your ear near their mouth and nose to listen for the sound of breathing. You may also feel their breath on your cheek and see their chest rise and fall with breathing. If there is no breathing, make sure there is an open airway by using the head tilt-chin lift method. Put one hand on their forehead and place the fingers of your other hand under their chin and lift, (if you suspect a neck injury gently lift the person's jaw without tilting the head). If their tongue was blocking their airway, they may gasp for air and start breathing. Check once more for breathing, and if there is still no breathing, start mouth-to-mouth resuscitation.

1. Check the mouth for any observable debris and remove any that may be found.

2. Pinch the nostrils with the fingers of the hand that is on the forehead and tilt the chin up with the fingers of the other hand.

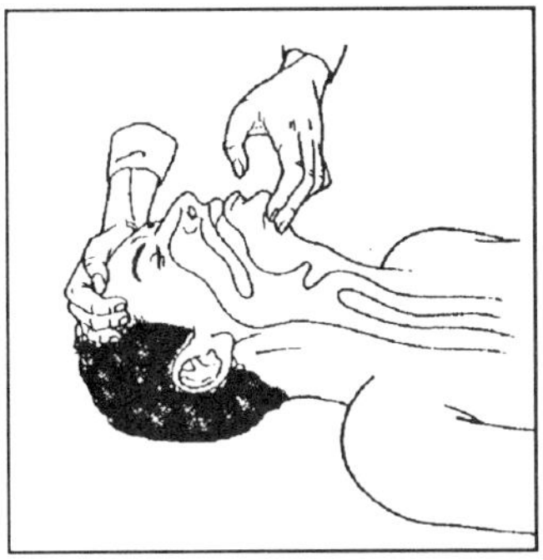

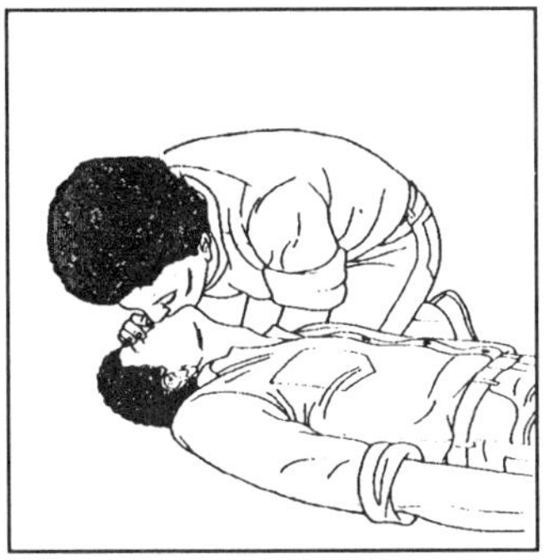

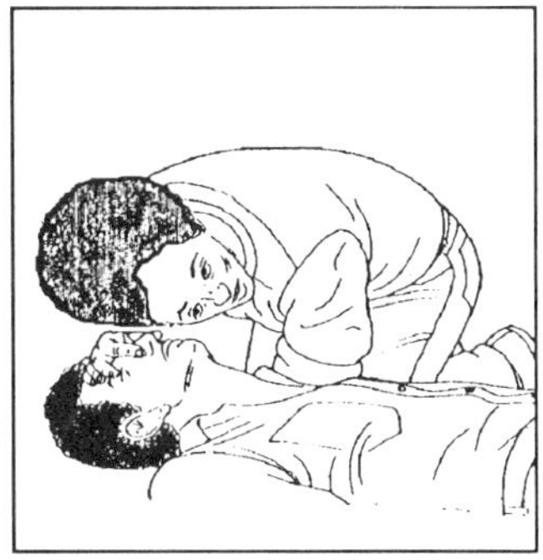

3. Take a deep breath and seal your mouth over the injured person's mouth; blow one deep breath.

   a. If you can't get air into the lungs, reposition the head and try again. If you still can't get air into the lungs there may be an airway obstruction problem. Use the Heimlich maneuver for an unconscious adult described above.

   b. If the lungs inflate, continue giving breaths at the rate of 12 to 15 breaths per minute (one breath every 5 seconds) for an adult. For a small child, give one breath every three seconds or 20 breaths per minute.

4. Between breaths, remove your mouth from the seal around the person's mouth and while you are taking a breath, turn your head to watch the chest movement as you listen to hear the exhaled air. In this position you will be able to tell if the person begins to breathe. You can also hear any sounds indicating that the person may vomit. If vomiting takes place, turn the person on his or her side so the vomitus can escape, clean away remaining material, and continue the resuscitation.

5. Continue rescue breathing until the person begins to breathe or until someone takes over for you.

Cardiopulmonary Resuscitation (CPR)

Pulmonary refers to the lungs, and *cardio* refers to the heart. Pulmonary resuscitation means artificial respiration or rescue breathing. If the heart is still going, pulmonary resuscitation is done by itself. But if the heart is not going, pulmonary resuscitation by itself will do no good. Both cardio and pulmonary resuscitation (CPR) are needed and that requires special training. After studying the above information you should be able to do the pulmonary part of CPR to save a life, even without practice. However the cardio part of CPR requires practice under a trained instructor. This lesson is not attempting to prepare you to do CPR. Nevertheless, CPR will be explained briefly so you will understand how it works. Hopefully, you will be encouraged to obtain CPR training from some other source.

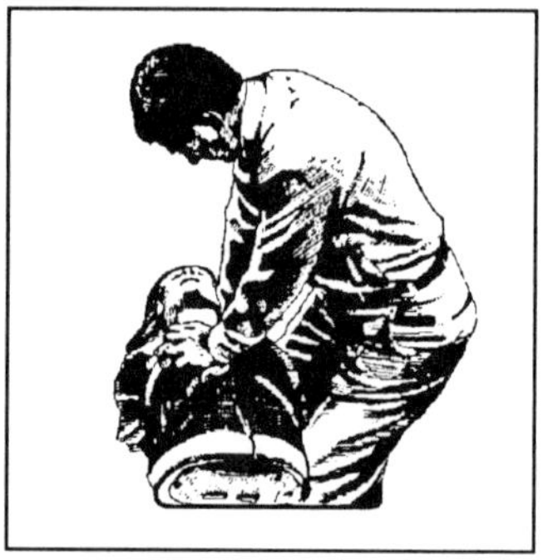

After giving the first one or two deep breaths in step three (3) above, a person trained in CPR would take up to 10 seconds to feel for a pulse in the groove on either side of the neck. If there is a pulse, they would continue giving pulmonary resuscitation as explained above. If there is no pulse, they would start doing chest compressions, squeezing the heart between the sternum bone and the vertebrae, to artificially pump the blood containing the oxygen to the brain. Cardio resus-citation, if done as effectively as possible, is still only 30 percent effective so it must be done perfectly to provide any chance of being effective. Feeling for the pulse is a critical part of CPR. If the heart has truly stopped, you can't do any harm--the person is dead and you can't make the situation worse. However, if the heart is beating weakly, but you don't feel it and you start to give compressions, you can make the situation worse. CPR training can mean the difference.

BLEEDING

The sight of blood often evokes an emotional response that may or may not be justified. A little loss of blood is not serious; a large loss of blood may be life threatening. The first aid provider's job is to assist the body's own methods for stopping bleeding. When chemicals in the blood and from the wound combine, clots form to stop the bleeding. If the first aid provider can slow down the flow of blood, the clots will gather at the wound. Direct pressure at the wound and elevation of the limb will help. A piece of clean cloth applied with pressure to the wound will provide a network of fibers that will collect the tiny clots and allow a larger clot to form that will help stop the bleeding. This combination of direct pressure, elevation, and a pressure bandage will control bleeding in most situations. In some severe bleeding situations, pressure at a pressure point may be needed. In rare situations, a tourniquet may be needed.

Mild Bleeding

In small wounds, bleeding will control itself. An adhesive compress (band aid) may be sufficient to cover the wound. Unless there is a problem with infection or unless the wound is large enough to require stitches, medical attention may not be necessary.

Severe Bleeding

If bleeding is moderate or severe, the injured person should lie down while the first aid provider does the following:

1. **Direct pressure and elevation.** Apply direct pressure over the wound with the cleanest cloth available. If the cloth becomes saturated, apply additional cloths. Do not remove any dressings. If the wound is on an extremity, elevate it. Elevation in conjunction with direct pressure may help in controlling bleeding of an extremity. Unless there is a possibility of a fracture to the limb, an arm or leg can be elevated higher than the heart.

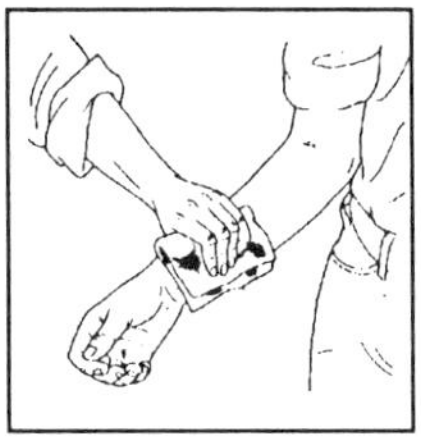

2. **Pressure point.** If pressure on the wound doesn't stop the profuse flow of blood, additional pressure at a pressure point may help slow down the flow of blood.

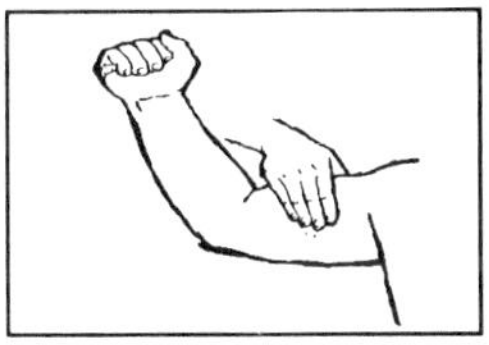

a) **Brachial artery.** Clasp your hand around the upper arm so that the flat part of the finger tips presses the artery against the inside of the arm against the arm bone. This technique stops most of the flow of blood to the arm so that clotting can occur. It should not be used longer than necessary, approx-imately 15 minutes.

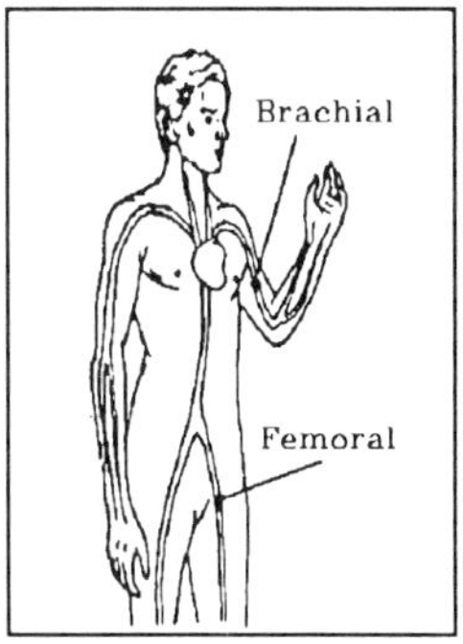

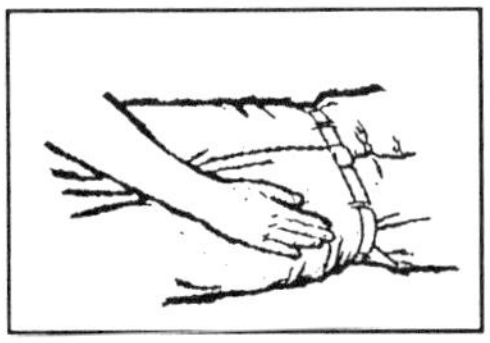

b) **Femoral artery.** Place the heel of one hand over the artery at the groin and place the other hand on top so your body weight will press the artery against the bone. Once bleeding is under control, apply more layers of dressing cloth over the wound and bandage firmly.

3. **Tourniquets.** A tourniquet is used only as a last resort to save a life at the risk of losing the limb. Because direct pressure and pressure points are effective, tourniquets are seldom needed, except perhaps when a first aid provider cannot be in two places at once. A tourniquet consists of a wide

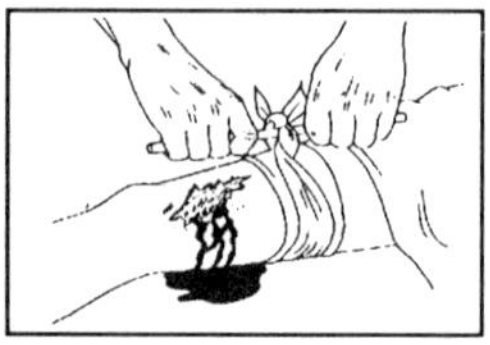

strip of cloth wrapped around the arm or leg above the wound and not over a joint. Tie two knots in the band and insert a short stick between the knots. Then twist the stick until the bleeding stops and then secure the stick. Note the time the tourniquet was put in place. Get the person to medical help immediately. Once applied, only a doctor should remove a tourniquet.

POISONING

Speed is important in dealing with any of the several types of poisoning. With oral poisoning, for example, treatment is best before the poisons leave the stomach or at least before they are absorbed through the intestinal lining. With inhaled poisons, such as carbon monoxide, it is important to get the person to fresh air as soon as possible. It is important to act swiftly in the event of a venomous snake bite. Contact poisons such as poison ivy should be washed off the body as soon as possible.

Poison control centers have been setup throughout the country to help individuals, hospital emergency rooms, and doctors deal quickly and properly with poisoning emergencies. The telephone number of the nearest poison control center is listed with the emergency numbers in the front of the phone book. They have nearly every type of poison or combination of substances that may be harmful on file so that the best treatment advice is available within seconds.

Oral Poisoning

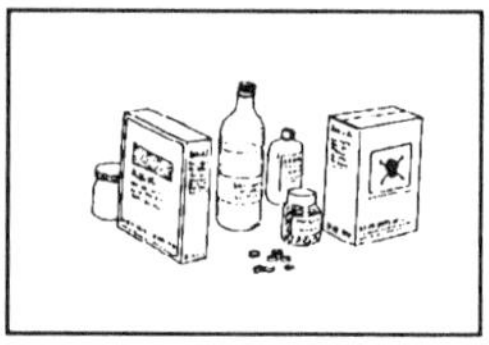

As the substances that cause oral poisons have become more numerous and complex, the recommended first aid procedures have become simpler. Poisons that may be swallowed are divided into two categories, depending on whether or not treatment includes inducing vomiting.

First aid for oral poisoning should include the following:

1. **Determine the nature of the poisoning**. This means try to identify the type of poison consumed, how much was taken, and how long it has been since it was taken. Also determine the age, sex, general health, and current condition of the person who consumed the poison. This should take just a few seconds.
2. **Call the Poison Control Center**. Dial the Poison Control Center in your area and give them the information about the nature of the poisoning found in No. 1 above. Then follow their directions. Stay on the line until they say they are

Poisons For Which You SHOULD Induce Vomiting	Poisons For Which You SHOULD NOT Induce Vomiting
Drugs and Medications	Acids and Alkalis:
Parts of Plants	Ammonia and Bleach
Spoiled Food	Drain and Oven Cleaners
Alcohol	Lye or Lime
Antifreeze	Metal Cleaners
Cosmetics	Rust Removers
Deodorant	
Laundry Detergent	Petroleum Products:
Mothballs	Furniture Polish
Perfume	Gasoline
Peroxide	Kerosene
Rat Poison	Paint Thinner
Suntan Lotion	Wood Preservatives

through talking to you.

3. **Dilute the poison**. In the meantime, while one first aid provider is on the phone to the Poison Control Center, a second first aid provider may attempt to dilute the poison. The amount of milk or water given to dilute the poison depends on which type of poison has been consumed.

    a. If the poison is of a type where you SHOULD induce vomiting, dilute with 4 or 5 glasses for an adult or 2 to 3 glasses for a child.

    b. If the poison was of a type where you SHOULD NOT induce vomiting, dilute with 1 or 2 glasses for an adult or 1/2 to 1 glass for a child.

If the poison is a noncorrosive type such as an overdose of medicine, the Poison Control Center will probably tell you to dilute profusely and to *induce vomiting* by giving the person an emetic such as syrup of ipecac. They will tell you how much to

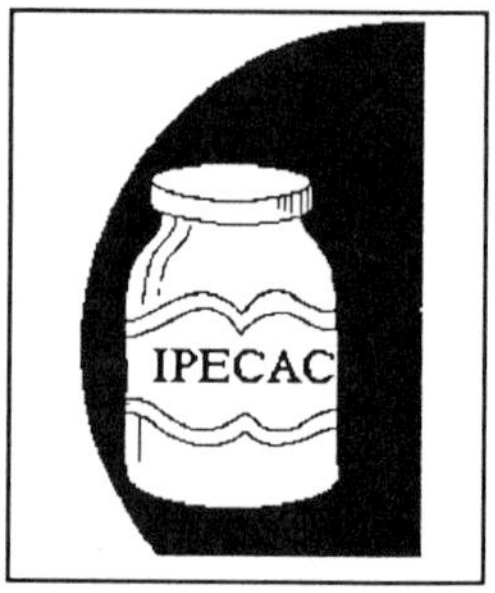

give and how to give it. You obviously have to have syrup of ipecac on hand in order to give it.

If the poison is a corrosive type substance such as a strong acid or alkali or petroleum product; or if the person is unconscious, is in convulsions, or complains of pain or a burning sensation in the mouth, the Poison Control Center will tell you *not to induce vomiting.* If a person who consumed strong corrosive substances were to vomit, it could threaten his or her life. For example, acids coming back up could seriously burn the trachea and, if aspirated, could burn the larynx, esophagus, and get into the lungs, causing death due to pneumonia.

The Poison Control Center will also direct you in regards to obtaining *medical help.* Note that it is a good idea to take the label of the poison container, the container, its contents, or the collected vomitus to the emergency room for identification. This will enable the physician to treat the person more effectively.

Drug overdoses can be life threatening. Treat this problem as an oral poison by calling the Poison Control Center and following their instructions. It is important to check for breathing, maintain an open airway, and check for normal body temperature. Give pulmonary resuscitation or CPR as needed.

Contact Poisons

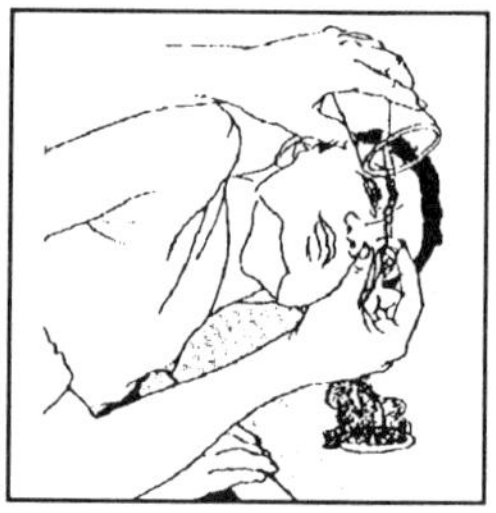

Chemicals in the eyes. Chemicals that may splash into the eyes should be washed away immediately. A chemistry laboratory or an industrial site using chemicals should have special eye washing devices. If such devices are not available, care should be taken so that chemicals washed from one eye do not flow into the other eye. Have the person lie on his back with his head turned to one side, then pour water from the bridge of the nose through the lower eye. Tilt the head to the other side and pour water through the other eye. Repeat this process continuously for at least 15 minutes. After that, bandage the eyes and transport the person to a medical emergency facility. The emergency facility should be notified about the problem in advance.

Chemicals on the body. Chemicals and poisons that get on the body should be washed off as soon as possible. A chemistry laboratory or an industrial site using chemicals should have a special shower available for such emergencies. In an outdoor setting, a person may contact poison ivy or poison oak. The exposed area of the body should be washed with soap and water.

Inhaled Poisons

Inhaled poisons are smoke, gases, and fumes. Warning signs include dizziness, headache, and weakness. Remove the affected person to fresh air and send for immediate medical care. Tell the emergency personnel to bring oxygen. Monitor the person's breathing and give pulmonary resuscitation or CPR if needed. Treat for shock. Elevating the head and chest slightly may ease breathing.

Bites And Stings

Bee sting. For some people, a bee sting can be a life-threatening emergency, and medical care may be needed immediately to combat anaphylactic shock. Preparation for field trips should include a check to see if anyone is allergic to bee stings. If so, his or her physician may recommend a medication for such an emergency. General first aid for honey bee stings includes removing the stinger, applying a cold compress, and calamine lotion for the relief of itching.

Snake bites. Venomous snake bites only occasionally result in death, but they frequently cause severe tissue damage and much suffering. A person who has been bitten by a snake should remain quiet with the bite lower than the heart. A constriction band tight enough to restrict blood flow, but not tight enough to stop circulation should be placed a few inches above the bite. The bite area should be washed with soap and water and covered with a dressing. The use of ice packs, incisions, and suction are generally not recommended first aid procedures. The person should be transported to medical facilities as soon as possible.

CONTROLLING SHOCK

Shock is defined as a condition in which the vital functions of the body are greatly suppressed. The characteristics of this condition are: a pale face, weak but rapid pulse, low blood pressure, irregular respiration through the mouth, a low temperature, moist and cold skin, eyes vacant and full, and dilated pupils.

A general rule of first aid is to always treat for shock. It may accompany any injury, and if not treated, will make the victim's condition worse. To avoid shock, the same measures are used as those to treat it. They are:

Position. Have victim lie down unless movement would increase injury. Elevate feet unless there is injury to head or chest. If unconscious or semiconscious, lay him on his side.

Temperature. Maintain body temperature but do not cause sweating. It may be as important to put some protection from the cold, such as blankets, under a person as it is over a person.

Comfort. Make the victim comfortable physically and psychologically. Loosen tight-fitting clothing. Talk to the person and give him or her encouragement.

Fluids. Give fluids by mouth if there is to be a delay in obtaining medical help, but do not give fluids if the person is unconscious, nauseated, has abdominal injuries, or if the person will likely undergo surgery.

First aid. First aid and care that will relieve pain and discomfort and control blood loss will help minimize shock.

STABILIZE

The main point in stabilization is to not let the situation get worse. A principle that has guided the practice of medicine over the years has been, "Do good if you can, but at least do not harm." In an emergency if a first aid provider can do the things mentioned above and treat for shock while waiting for help from professional medical personnel, he or she will be doing enough. It is important not to move a person who has been injured, especially if a bone fracture is possible. Other problems that don't require first aid should wait until medical personnel arrive.

FIRST AID FOR OTHER INJURIES

SKELETAL INJURIES

Skeletal injuries include fractures, sprains, and dislocations. Because of the chance of causing additional injury to a fracture and because it is often difficult to distinguish between a fracture and other skeletal injuries, the general rule is to treat all skeletal injuries as fractures. Added harm can easily take place if a person with a fracture is moved improperly. When giving first aid, it is important not to move a victim unnecessarily, particularly if there may be a back or spinal injury. A fracture can be made worse by movement.

Fractures

A fracture is a break in a bone. An open fracture is when there is a wound extending from the surface of the skin to the broken bone, and infection is an added risk of this type of fracture. Some of the indications of a fracture are the following:

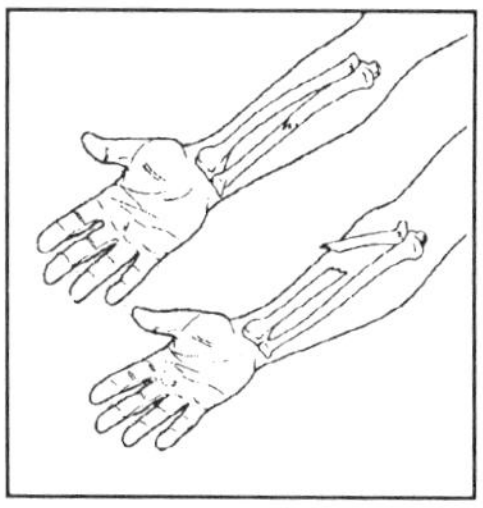

- Discoloration of skin
- Localized swelling
- Pain and tenderness
- Painful movement
- Bone deformity
- Numbness

Since sprains, strains, and dislocations can produce all of these same signs and symptoms except bone deformity, the abnormal shape of a bone shaft is a key indicator of a fracture. In the other cases, one just suspects a fracture and treats the injury as a fracture. Treatment for a fracture includes the following:

- Check for breathing and maintain it.
- Look for bleeding and control it.
- Never move the person before splinting unless life is threatened.
- Apply a splint at the site of the accident.
- Control shock, prevent infection, and treat other injuries.
- Call for Emergency Medical Services (EMS).

Very often in a school setting, the first aid providers should not attempt to apply a splint, they should wait and let the EMS apply the splint. The objective of the splint is to keep the broken bone ends and the adjacent joints from moving. An improvised splint should be padded to protect the skin under the splint. The splint should be tied above and below, but not over the fracture. The splint should be snug, but not tight enough to impair circulation; therefore, the ties should be checked frequently.

Sprains

A sprain is a stretching or tearing of the ligaments that hold the bone ends together. A sprain occurs at the joints such as the ankle, wrists, knees, and fingers. Since an x-ray is needed by the physician to rule out a fracture, in first aid it is best to treat a sprain as a possible fracture. Treatment for a sprain includes the following:

- Elevate the injured part.
- Apply cold packs at 25 minute intervals for 24 hours to minimize swelling. (Do *not* pack the injured part in ice.)
- Do *not* allow the person to try to walk on the injured part until the injury is checked by a physician.

Strains

A strain is a stretching or tearing of the muscles or tendons connecting a muscle to a bone. A burning pain is more apt to be felt along the bone and muscle rather than at a joint. Care for a strain includes the following:

- Rest the muscle involved and elevate the limb to minimize swelling.
- Apply cold packs to relieve pain for the first 24 hours then apply warm packs or heat to increase circulation and healing.

Dislocations

A dislocation occurs when a bone end is moved out of place. This may result from a blow or a fall. Shoulders and fingers are common sites for dislocations. Signs and symptoms of dislocations include swelling, deformity at a joint, discoloration, tenderness, and pain at movement. First aid for a dislocation includes the following:

- Do *not* move the injured joint.
- Use a sling or splint to immobilize the joint.
- Also use the sling to support and elevate the limb.
- Do *not* try to correct the deformity.
- Get medical care.

Individuals with possible spinal injuries should not be moved except by qualified and equipped emergency medical personnel unless there is imminent danger. Other skeletal injuries should be immobilized by trained first aid providers or emergency medical personnel. When in doubt concerning a skeletal injury, suspect the worst and treat it as a fracture. The victim's evaluation of his or her own injuries are important in determining the effect of the injury.

BURNS

Burns may be either thermal, chemical, or electrical. Chemical burns were treated previously in this lesson under contact poisons. Electrical burns sometimes present a special problem in attempting to extricate the burned person from a live electrical current. Think first of protecting yourself and make sure the current is turned off before touching the person. Electrical burns are treated the same as thermal burns except that the patient may also need intensive medical care for internal damage. Burns are described by degree with third degree being most serious. The descriptions and first aid treatment are as follows:

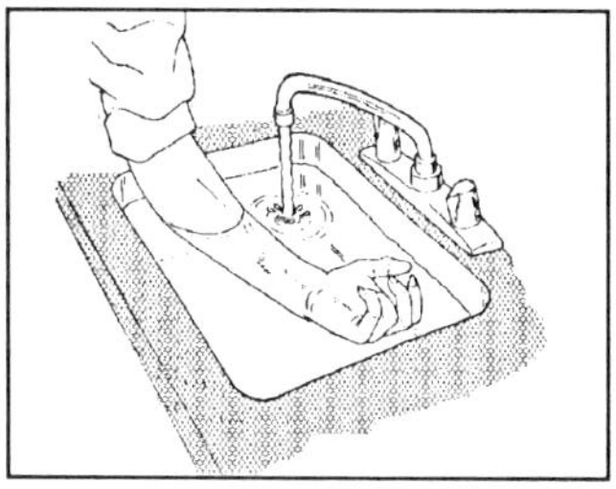

1st degree. The outside layer of skin becomes red like a sunburn. There may be mild swelling and pain. It can result from hot liquids, hot objects, chemicals, or the sun.

- Apply cold water applications or submerge the burned area in cold water for 10 minutes.

- Apply a dry dressing if it is necessary to protect an area from further irritations.

2nd degree. The skin appears red and blotchy. Blisters and swelling develop. Pain becomes more severe. What starts out looking like a first degree burn may end up as a second degree burn.

- Immerse the burned part in cold water (not ice water) for 10 minutes until the pain subsides.

- Do *not* break the blisters. Do *not* apply petroleum jelly or grease of any kind.

- Apply dry, sterile gauze or clean cloth as a protective bandage.

- If arms or legs are affected, keep them elevated.

- Seek medical care if the face or a large area of the body is burned.

3rd degree. There is deeper destruction and the burned area may appear either charred or white. Because nerve endings are destroyed, there may be little or no pain.

- Do *not* immerse an extensive burned area or apply ice water over it, because cold may intensify the shock reaction. However, a cold pack may be applied to the face or to the hands or feet.

- Do *not* remove adhered particles of charred clothing. Do *not* pull clothes over burned area. Do *not* apply any ointments or antiseptics to the burn. Do *not* touch the burn with anything except sterile or clean dressings.

- Cover burns with thick, dry, sterile dressings or a freshly ironed or laundered sheet or other household linen.

- Keep the person lying down. Keep burned arms or legs above the heart level.

- Watch for breathing problems and keep an open airway. Burns of the face are often associated with injury to the respiratory tract and may obstruct breathing as swelling increases. Prompt medical attention is imperative.

- Seek medical help immediately.

HEAT AND COLD EXPOSURE

The human body does an excellent job of keeping the body at the right temperature (98.6° F) in spite of changes in the temperature of the environment. However, the body has its limitations when it faces extremes.

Cold Exposure

If the core temperature of the body drops a mere four degrees, a person may go into *hypothermia,* which is the loss of the body's ability to make heat and a sure pathway to death, unless it is reversed through the application of heat from an outside source. Another problem is *frostbite.* When individual body cells become cold, they fail to function and the damage is similar to 1st, 2nd, or 3rd degree burns. The cells may actually freeze. First aid is to protect the body parts; do *not* rub the area or break the blisters. The person needs medical care.

Heat Exposure

People respond to high temperature and high humidity environments. In the same environment one person may go into heat exhaustion and another into heat stroke, and a third may experience heat cramps. Occasionally high school athletes experience heat exposure problems, such as at early football workouts. When more heat is produced than the body can get rid of through sweating, the body becomes overheated.

Heat exhaustion is manifest by excessive perspiration, headache, nausea, and weakness. The body temperature remains near normal. These symptoms can be relieved by resting in a cool place and avoiding strenuous activity and sunshine for a few days. Women are more likely than men to develop heat exhaustion.

Heat cramps may be associated with heat exhaustion or be independent of the other symptoms. Cramps are most apt to affect the muscles of the legs and abdomen. They can be helped by stretching them, massaging them, and applying heat.

Heat stroke is a life-threatening emergency. The symptoms include a very high body temperature, dry and hot skin, and a rapid pulse. The following immediate first aid steps must be taken to cool the body:

- Sponge the person with cool water or place the person in a tub of cool water, but avoid cooling the person too rapidly.
- Allow the person to rest in a cool, well-ventilated room. Monitor their temperature, and if it begins to rise, cool them down again.
- Call for or transport them to immediate medical care.

OPEN WOUNDS

Care for minor cuts and scratches includes cleansing the area with soap and water or a Phisohex solution and covering it with a band aid or sterile dressing, if necessary. For other wounds, cover with sterile gauze dressing and secure with a bandage. The student should have it checked by a physician. Dressings should not be changed at school unless written orders are obtained from the family physician.

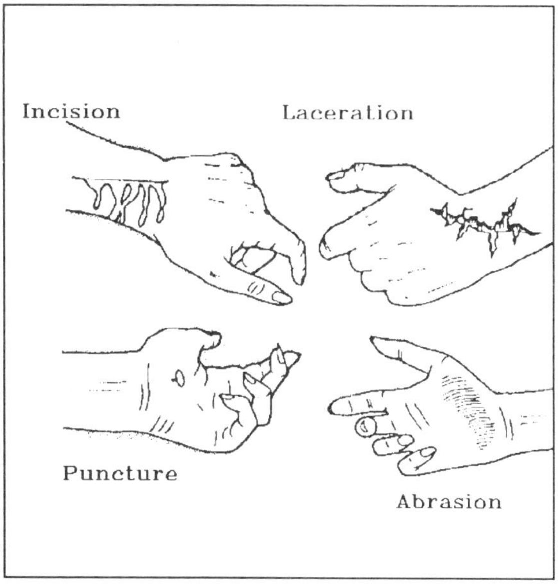

Abrasions

The outer layers of the protective skin are damaged. Abrased wounds usually result when the skin is scraped against a hard surface. Bleeding is limited. Danger of contamination and infection exist. First aid procedure is the following:

- Cleanse with soap and water and blot dry.
- Apply sterile dressing if necessary.

Incisions

An incised wound or cut frequently occurs when body tissue is cut on knives, rough edges of metal, broken glass, or other sharp objects. Bleeding may be rapid and heavy. First aid procedure is the following:

- Control bleeding.
- Apply sterile dressing and bandage.
- See doctor if wound is deep.

Lacerations

A lacerated wound displays jagged, irregular, or blunt breaking or tearing of the soft tissues, and is usually caused when great force is exerted against the body. Bleeding may be rapid and extensive. First aid procedure is the following:

- Control bleeding.
- Apply sterile dressing and bandage.
- See doctor if wound is deep.

Punctures

A puncture wound is produced by an object piercing skin layers, creating a small hole in the tissues. Puncture-producing objects include bullets and pointed objects such as pins, nails, and splinters. They usually cause little external bleeding, but may cause serious internal bleeding and infection. First aid procedure is listed on the following page.

- Clean the wound of any blood or fluids. It may not be necessary to cover the wound unless fluids continue to ooze.

- Watch for infection. If signs of infection such as swelling and red or white coloration around the wound and pus formation occur, contact a physician. If the wound was made by dirty object, it would be wise to go to a doctor at the first.

Impelled objects are a form of puncture wound. The object may be very small or very large. Any object penetrating the body should not be removed except by trained extrication crews under medical supervision.

Avulsion

An avulsed wound results when tissue is forcibly separated or torn from the victim's body. An amputation is a type of avulsion. There will be heavy, rapid bleeding. First aid procedure is the following:

- Control bleeding.
- Apply sterile dressing and bandage.
- An avulsed body part may be successfully reattached to a victim's body by a surgeon. Send the body part along with the victim to the hospital.

Blisters

Blisters caused by friction from shoes or boots appear on the heels, toes, and tops of feet. It is best to leave the blister unbroken. If the blister is not broken, protect it and avoid further pressure by putting a gauze pad with a hole for the blister over the blister with another gauze pad on top. If the blister is broken or needs to be broken, follow these steps:

- Wash the blister area clean.
- Sterilize needle.
- Puncture the blister from the edge with the needle.
- Gently press the fluid out with a clean cloth.
- Cover the blister with a dressing.
- Keep it clean.
- Get medical care at any signs of infection such as pus, redness, pain, or fever.

Do not attempt to remove the dead skin which formed the blister. Let it stay on as long as possible to provide protection to the tender underlying tissue and assist in the prevention of infection.

Nosebleed

Nosebleed is a frequent occurrence among students. Nosebleed can be caused by an injury to the soft tissues of the nose, a cold, high blood pressure, or strenuous physical activities. Sometimes it occurs spontaneously. With some people, the nasal membrane capillaries are close to the surface, and they are susceptible to nosebleeds, particularly in arid conditions. Nosebleeds are usually not serious and can be controlled quite simply.

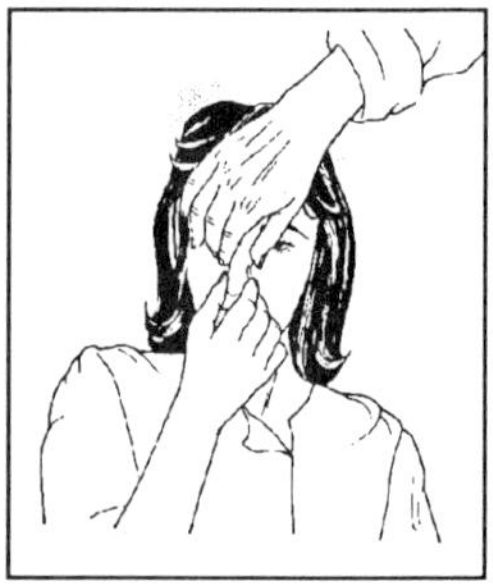

The recommended procedure for controlling nosebleed is to have the person sit down and squeeze the soft, flexible part on the tip of the nose firmly and lean forward for 10 to 15 minutes. If the bleeding continues, the person may need medical help. When the person leans forward, the blood accumulates in the front of the nose and this facilitates clotting. Encourage the person not to blow his or her nose for a few hours in order to not remove the clot. If a person leans back, the blood continues to run down the throat so clotting is less apt to happen, and nausea may occur.

Closed Wounds

Closed wounds can result in internal bleeding. A black eye or a bruise are examples of closed wounds that may not be serious. But a person can bleed to death without losing a drop of blood through the skin. Closed wounds with internal bleeding may result from falls or blows or from the impact of a automobile accident. Internal bleeding can also result from chronic conditions such as ulcers. Unexplained weakness and symptoms of shock may be due to internal bleeding. Vomiting or coughing up blood or blood in the urine or stool may indicate internal bleeding. First aid procedure is the following:

- If the person is unconscious, vomiting, or bleeding from the mouth place him or her on their side to avoid choking.
- Give nothing by mouth. Do *not* let the person eat or drink.
- Keep the person comfortable and warm.
- Get medical care immediately.

Head Injuries

Wounds to the head are potentially very serious and therefore require immediate medical attention. If there is a possible neck injury, do *not* move the person. Cover a scalp wound with a sterile dressing, but do *not* wash or clean it. Monitor for breathing and maintain an open airway. Information you can give the medical people about any changes in the person's status will be very helpful. Note the time of the injury and note changes in the following:

- Levels of consciousness such as alert, drowsy, or unconscious.
- Ability to remember information such as date or address.
- Speech patterns such as slurred speech.
- Size of pupils such as constricted, dilated, or unequal size.
- Ability to move or feel at various parts of the body.
- The characteristics of fluid coming from the nose, ears, or mouth.
- Tendency toward nausea or vomiting.

UNCONSCIOUSNESS

There are many causes of unconsciousness, such as physical shock, heat stroke, heat exhaustion, heart attack, convulsions, epilepsy, fainting, intoxication, diabetic coma and insulin shock, hemorrhaging, electric shock, and overdose of drugs. The first aid provider should determine what the cause is in order to give the proper first aid to the victim. Types of unconsciousness may be described as red, white, and blue.

Red. When the person is flushed, red-faced, with strong, slow pulse you should lay the person down with head slightly raised above level of rest of body. Apply cold wet cloth to head. If breathing stops, start artificial respiration.

White. When the person is pale, cold, clammy to touch, and has a weak pulse you should lay the person down with head slightly lower than rest of body. Keep the person warm. If breathing stops, start artificial respiration.

Blue. When the person has a bluish face, weak pulse, and irregular breathing, you should lay the person down and keep him warm. Start artificial respiration immediately if breathing stops.

Fainting

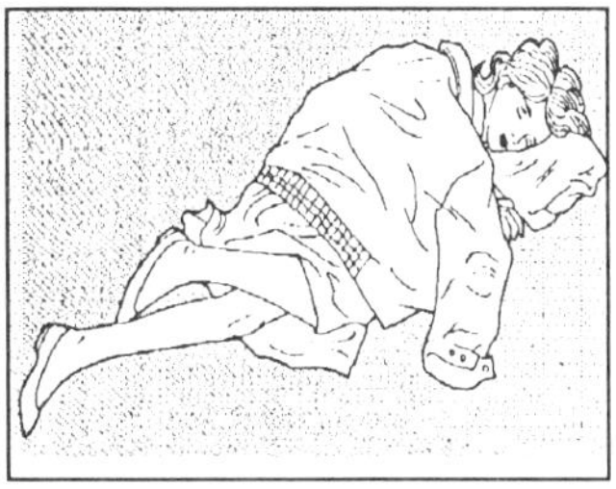

When the blood supply to the brain is interrupted momentarily, it may result in a loss of consciousness called fainting. Fainting can occur suddenly or be associated with warnings such as blurring of the vision, weakness, paleness, nausea, giddiness, and sweating. A person who feels these symptoms should lie down immediately if possible. If not, the person should sit or kneel and bend forward at the waist, putting the head down to get it lower than the heart. First aid for fainting includes the following:

- Act quickly, if you can, to prevent an injury during the fall.
- Keep the person lying down and loosen any tight clothing. A pillow for their head and a blanket may make them more comfortable. A moist washcloth for the face may also help.
- Get medical help if recovery is not rapid or if there is no known reason for their fainting.

Hyperventilation

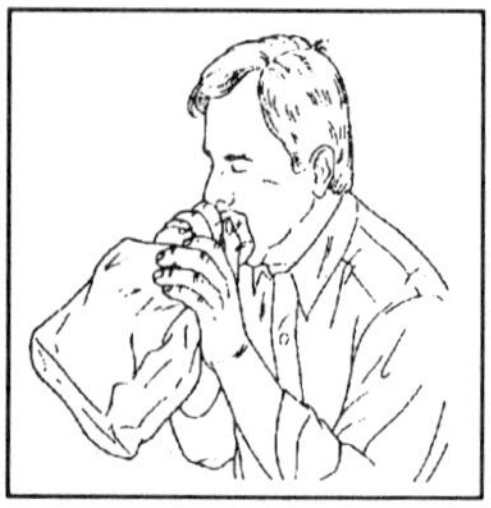

An uncontrollable episode of very fast breathing is hyperventilation. It is often associated with emotional stress. The rapid breathing may cause the person to get too much oxygen, and they may pass out. Symptoms include the feeling of not getting enough air, sharp and short pains in the chest, and a feeling of dizziness. For adults, it may be confused with a heart attack and medical care should be obtained immediately. For young healthy people, do the following:

- Be calm and encourage slower breathing.
- Have the person breath into a paper bag to reuse the same air.
- If the condition continues, get medical care.

Convulsions

Convulsions are associated with head injury, high fever, and epilepsy. First aid for epilepsy and diabetes is discussed more thoroughly in the lesson on chronic diseases. During the convulsion, the person's body may become stiff and move violently. First aid consists of protecting the person from injury and preventing choking.

- Clear away hard and sharp objects.
- Do *not* restrain the person. Do *not* put anything in their mouth.
- After the convulsions, if the person is unconscious, place the person on his or her side.
- Get medical care unless the seizures have become a reoccurring pattern for the person.

Heart Attack and Stroke

A heart attack is caused by a blockage in the coronary artery. Heart attacks are not likely to occur among high school students; the principal is a more likely candidate. Symptoms include a sudden constant pressure type pain in the chest. Frequently, the pain radiates to the left arm, shoulder, neck, and jaw. There is a shortness of breath, weakness, nausea, sweating, and a blueness of the lips and face. Call for an ambulance immediately. If the person has a history of heart problems, he or she may have medication (nitroglycerin tablets) you can help them take. Help the person find the most comfortable position, usually a reclining position. Loosen any tight-fitting clothing, cover the person lightly to maintain body temperature, and try to calm and reassure the person. If the person loses consciousness, check for breathing and pulse and use CPR if you are trained to use it.

A stroke is a blockage in the arteries going to the brain. Symptoms might include any or all of the following: weakness, paralysis on one side of the body, difficulty in breathing and swallowing, unequal pupils, confusion, dizziness, speech problems, and unconsciousness. Call for an ambulance immediately. Do *not* give fluids. Place the person on his or her side to prevent choking. Cover the person lightly to maintain body temperature. Monitor breathing and pulse and use CPR if it is needed and if you are trained to use it.

PSYCHOLOGICAL FIRST AID

There are many times when a teacher has an opportunity to render psychological first aid. Any type of physical injury or health emergency may require mental first aid. Remember, you are dealing with a whole person, not just his body. Students facing acute emotional stress resulting from bad news or disappointment may need help. Persons under the influence of drugs or experiencing a drug flashback may need psychological first aid. The basic principle of psychological first aid is to find ways of making effective human contact with the disturbed, worried, or frightened person. Give him reassurance that you will remain with him to protect him and help him. Give him verbal reassurance and physical reassurance by touching his hand, assuring him of your presence, kindness, and willingness to help.

So that a minimum amount of talking and a maximum amount of listening takes place, don't belittle the problem, criticize him, attempt to logically solve his problem for him, or try to talk him out of his fantasies. Be patient and show understanding, but don't give too much sympathy or pity. Give him reassurance that everything will be alright. Bolster his ego; show him that you care about him, but that you are not particularly anxious or overly concerned about his condition. Remain calm and confident, but remember your own limitations, and that it is only first aid until professional help is available.

FIRST AID SUPPLIES

Although school health rooms are usually stocked with first aid supplies, and assorted first aid kits are located in shops, labs, and physical education facilities, every teacher should have a small first aid kit in his or her classroom. It should contain band-aid type adhesive compresses, gauze squares, gauze roller bandages, adhesive tape, scissors, tweezers, a medicine dropper, a bottle of sterile water, a bar of soap, a clean cloth or two, and an adequate container. In areas where poisoning may occur, neutralizers, syrup of ipecac, and activated charcoal should be available.

You may notice that antiseptics are not listed. They should not be a part of a first aid kit in schools. Aspirin and other medications are not on the list. Antiseptics can do more harm than good in a first aid setting. Medications should not be administered in school unless specific orders are written by the family physician and parental consent is obtained for a special situation.

CONCLUSION

The aforementioned information should prepare you to handle emergency medical problems with calmness and confidence in a school setting or in other dimensions of life. You are prepared to meet your health-related responsibilities and thereby promote the well-being of your students. Take the time to review this lesson frequently. You might hope you will never need to use it, but in case you do, you will be prepared to take action.

FIRST AID CABINET INVENTORY

Suggested Supplies	Purpose
glass jars (2)	for applicators & blades
blades, wooden (500)	splints, depressors
wooden applicators (1000)	swabs, remove particles
toothpicks (750)	remove particles
tincture of green soap	wash injured parts
absorbent cotton roll	large pads for dressings
sterile gauze 3x3" squares (100)	dressings
sterile gauze 2x2" squares (100)	protect injuries
band-aids (100)	protect injuries
roller bandage 1" (12 rolls)	dressings
roller bandage 4" (12 rolls)	dressings
triangular bandage (4)	sling, area covering
safety pins (24)	for triangular bandage
adhesive tape/roll (1/2-2")	fasten splints & dressing
scissors (blunt or bandage)	cut dressings
tweezers	grasp small objects
eyedroppers (6)	apply oil
tourniquet (3) 1/2" rubber tube	check excessive bleeding
splints (metal or yucca) (10)	support
icebag (2)	relief of swelling
hot water bag with dover (2)	local relief of pain
mineral oil or petroleum jelly	relief of irritation
syrup of ipecac	induce vomiting - poison
paper cups (100)	receptacle

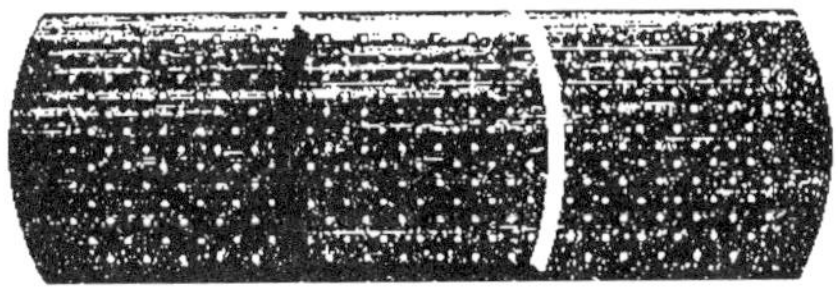

STUDY HELPS

1. What is the definition of first aid?

2. Why is it important to know and follow the policies of the school in which you teach regarding the giving of first aid?

3. Distinguish between: (1) Immediate Life-Threatening Emergencies and (2) Routine First Aid Procedures.

4. What should the letters A B C P S S remind you of in regard to setting priorities in first aid care?

5. What are general directions for first aid and what are some examples?

6. What is the purpose of assessment in first aid and how is an assessment conducted?

7. What are the steps of first aid for the following life-threatening emergencies?

    anatomical airway obstruction
    anaphylactic shock
    foreign body type airway obstruction
    stoppage of breathing
    severe bleeding
    oral poisoning
    chemicals in eyes
    chemical burns to the body
    inhaled poisons

8. What is the procedure in controlling shock when rendering first aid?

9. What does it mean to stabilize when rendering first aid?

10. What is the recommended first aid for the following problems?

fractures	sprains or strains	dislocations
1st degree burns	2nd degree burns	3rd degree burns
open wounds	puncture wounds	avulsion
nosebleed	closed wounds	
unconsciousness	hyperventilation	

INDEX

A

B

D

E

F

G

H

I

J

K

L

M

Q

R

S